American Medical Association
COMPLETE GUIDE TO PREVENTION AND WELLNESS

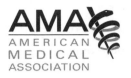

American Medical Association

COMPLETE GUIDE TO PREVENTION AND WELLNESS

What You Need to Know about Preventing
Illness, Staying Healthy, and Living Longer

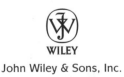

WILEY

John Wiley & Sons, Inc.

Published by John Wiley & Sons, Inc., Hoboken, New Jersey
Published simultaneously in Canada

Credits: CDC/Public Health Image Library: 146; National Cancer Institute: 127 (left); National Eye Institute, National Institutes of Health: 415 and 416; bar graph adapted from material in the 2006 Monitoring the Future Survey, National Institute on Drug Abuse: 468; Public Health Image Library: 127 (right); Food Pyramid courtesy of the US Department of Agriculture: 22; all other illustrations © American Medical Association.

For general information about our other products and services, please contact our Customer Care Department within the United States at (800) 762-2974, outside the United States at (317) 572-3993 or fax (317) 572-4002.

Wiley also publishes its books in a variety of electronic formats. Some content that appears in print may not be available in electronic books. For more information about Wiley products, visit our web site at www.wiley.com.

Library of Congress Cataloging-in-Publication Data:

American Medical Association complete guide to prevention and wellness : what you need to know about preventing illness, staying healthy, and living longer.
  p. cm.
 Includes bibliographical references and index.
 ISBN 978-0-470-25130-0 (cloth)
 1. Health. 2. Medicine, Preventive. 3. Medicine, Popular. I. American Medical Association.
II. Title: Complete guide to prevention and wellness.
 RA776.A435 2008
 613—dc22

                     2008032221

Printed in the United States of America

10 9 8 7 6 5 4 3 2 1

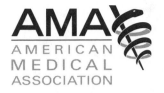

CONTENTS

Part Three PREVENTION AND WELLNESS THROUGHOUT LIFE

PART ONE

The Basics of Prevention and Wellness

NUTRITION, PREVENTION, AND WELLNESS

OF ALL THE STEPS YOU CAN TAKE to stay healthy and prevent disease, eating a nutritious diet is probably the most important. Healthy eating can help you maintain a proper weight and lower your risk for many of the most common chronic diseases such as heart disease and cancer. By contrast, poor nutrition, combined with physical inactivity and obesity, is a major health problem in the United States. This poor nutrition, or undernourishment, is not caused by lack of food. Food is widely available in this country, but the least expensive, easiest-to-find foods—fast food and high-fat, sugary, or salt-laden snack foods—tend to be the least nutritious.

Building a healthy diet

The food you eat is made up of three main nutrients: carbohydrates, protein, and fat. Carbohydrates are the body's main source of fuel and should make up 50 to 60 percent of your diet. Make sure the bulk of your carbohydrates come from whole grains. Healthy fat should make up no more than 30 percent of total daily calories, with protein providing the remainder. Use these elements like building blocks to construct a nutritious diet.

Carbohydrates

Simple and complex sugars, starches, and fiber from plant foods are the main components of carbohydrates. Carbs come in two types: simple and complex. Simple carbs are sugars, including the sugar found in fruit (fructose), the milk sugar lactose, and the white sugar in your sugar bowl (sucrose). Simple carbs taste sweet and are easy to digest. However, because they are so easily digestible, they can cause a sudden rise in blood sugar (glucose) levels—something a person with diabetes (or prediabetes) has to avoid.

Foods made from simple carbohydrates or starches, such as white bread, white rice, or white pasta, have been highly refined. This means that the fiber-rich outer bran and the nourishing inner germ of the grain have been removed, leaving only the vitamin-and-mineral-poor inside of the seed. This starchy leftover is digested quickly and speeds to the bloodstream, where it can sharply elevate blood sugar. For this reason, doctors tell people who already have elevated blood sugar levels to limit their intake of foods containing simple sugars.

Complex carbs, on the other hand, get absorbed into the bloodstream slowly. Because foods containing complex carbs—such as whole-grain breads, brown rice, cooked dried beans, and vegetables—take a longer time to digest, they don't reach the bloodstream all at once. Another benefit: these foods contain a lot more vitamins, minerals, and other nutrients than simple carbs.

FIBER

Fiber is a type of carbohydrate that is found in the cell walls of plants. Dietary fiber has been found to help reduce the risk for type 2 diabetes (see chapter 8)—one of the fastest-growing chronic diseases in the United States. Foods that contain a lot of fiber can help make the body's cells more sensitive to insulin, the hormone that enables the cells to use the sugar glucose, which they need to produce energy. (In people with type 2 diabetes, the body's cells are highly resistant to insulin, causing glucose to build up in the bloodstream.) In this way, high-fiber foods can help regulate blood sugar levels.

Fiber-rich foods can also help reduce the levels of artery-clogging LDL cholesterol (see page 199) in the blood, thus reducing the risk for heart disease, the nation's No. 1 killer among both women and men. Fiber-containing foods make you feel full, so they can help you keep your weight down. Fiber also helps keep the intestinal tract functioning well and reduces constipation. It also reduces the risk for diverticulosis (a condition in which small pouches develop in the walls of the large intestine; see page 342). The pouches can become inflamed, causing diverticulitis.

Fiber comes in two forms: soluble and insoluble. Soluble fiber can help control blood sugar levels and improve blood cholesterol. Insoluble fiber softens and bulks up stool to allow it to pass more easily through the intestines. Good sources of soluble fiber include cereal grains (such as barley, oatmeal, and oat bran), fruit (including citrus fruits, pears, prunes, apples, and bananas), legumes (including lima beans, kidney beans, and navy beans), peas (such as chickpeas and black-eyed peas), and vegetables (such as Brussels sprouts, broccoli, and carrots). Good sources of insoluble fiber include flaxseed (also an excellent source of heart-protecting omega-3 fatty acids; see page 8) and other seeds, whole grains (whole-grain bread, barley, brown rice, whole-grain breakfast cereals), carrots, cucumbers, zucchini, celery, tomatoes, and the edible skins of many fruits.

√ **Getting more fiber**

When adding fiber to your diet, start slowly and add fiber gradually, to avoid bloating and gas. Drink plenty of water when you start eating more fiber-rich foods or you could become constipated.

HOW MUCH FIBER DO YOU NEED?

How much fiber do you need every day to promote good health and prevent disease? A good rule of thumb is to eat about 28 grams of fiber for a 2,000-calorie diet. That sounds like a lot, but you can easily consume that much by following these tips:

- Choose breakfast cereals that have at least 5 grams of fiber per serving. Some cereals contain 10 grams or more of fiber. Cereals with wheat bran are especially beneficial for healthy digestion. For extra fiber and other nutrients, top your cereal with fruit.
- Eat whole fruit instead of—or in addition to—fruit juice. One orange contains three times the fiber of an 8-ounce glass of orange juice (and much less sugar).
- Add beans to your salads and soups, mix them into a casserole, or serve them as a side dish.
- Substitute whole-grain bread, pasta, and rice for the white variety.
- Serve more raw vegetables at lunch, dinner, and snack time.

Protein

The protein in food is made up of a chain of compounds called amino acids. The human body needs roughly 20 amino acids to make all of its proteins, which are the main components of muscles, organs, and glands. Every cell in the body and most body fluids contain proteins. The body needs even more protein to build and maintain the cells in muscles, tendons, and ligaments. Children and adolescents also need protein for growth and development.

Your body can manufacture only 10 of the 20 amino acids it needs. These 10 are called the nonessential amino acids because you don't need to get them from the food you eat. There are 10 other amino acids—the essential amino acids—that you can get only from your diet. If the protein in a food delivers all of the essential amino acids, it is called a complete protein. The protein contained in food that does not provide all the essential amino acids is known as an incomplete protein.

Foods derived from animals—including meat, poultry, fish, shellfish, eggs, and dairy products—supply complete proteins. Just make sure that when you eat animal-based foods you choose lean cuts of meat, poultry without the skin, and dairy products that are low in fat or fat-free, to help reduce your cholesterol level and your risk for heart disease.

Plant foods—including grains, fruits, and vegetables—do not provide all of the essential amino acids, and are called incomplete proteins. You can combine one incomplete plant protein with another at a meal to obtain all of the essential amino acids and form a complete protein. You can eat rice or corn with beans, for example, or peanut butter on whole-grain bread. You don't even have to combine plant proteins at the same meal—you could have rice at lunch and beans at dinner—to produce the right mix of essential amino acids.

Americans eat far more protein than they need. The quantity of protein that adults need to consume every day is pretty small—just 0.8 grams for every 2.2 pounds of body weight. If you are a 140-pound woman, you need only 51 grams of protein a day. A 200-pound man needs only 73 grams per day. You could accumulate 50 grams by eating one whole chicken breast, or by eating half a chicken breast, an 8-ounce glass of milk, and a cup of cooked beans. In general, protein should comprise from 12 to 20 percent of your daily intake of calories.

Eating too much protein can be unhealthy. For example, if you have gout (a form of arthritis), a diet high in animal protein may cause a flare-up. A high-protein diet can also place a heavy burden on the kidneys, which excrete in the urine excess waste from protein. As the kidneys clear the excess waste, they also eliminate large amounts of water, increasing the risk for dehydration, especially in a person who exercises vigorously. That's why people tend to lose weight fast at first on a high-protein diet—mainly from losing water. But along with the water loss, they're also losing muscle mass and calcium from their bones. Dehydration can also put a strain on the heart. So be cautious and talk to your doctor if you're considering going on a high-protein weight-loss diet.

Fats

Fat is an essential nutrient. It's the type of fat and the amount you consume that is important. Fat is a key source of energy and helps your body absorb vitamins A, D, E, and K. You also need fat for proper growth, development, and general good health. Fat imparts taste, consistency, and stability to food and helps you feel full. Both animal- and plant-derived foods contain fat.

The two main types of fat found in food are unsaturated and saturated. Unsaturated fat occurs in several forms. Some unsaturated fats can be good for you in moderation. Trans-unsaturated fats (trans fats) can be harmful. Saturated fats and trans fats raise total blood cholesterol and LDL cholesterol (the bad kind). Over time, abnormally high cholesterol can increase the risk for heart disease, heart attack, and stroke.

Dietary cholesterol—the kind present in animal foods such as egg yolks and lobster—also contributes to heart disease, but not as much as saturated fats and trans fats. For these reasons, the best course is to choose foods that are low in saturated fat, trans fats, and cholesterol.

In general, no more than 30 percent of your diet should come from fat—including daily intakes of less than 7 percent of calories from saturated fat, less than 200 milligrams of dietary cholesterol, and no trans fats. The recommendations allow up to 30 percent of daily calories from total fat. It's best to get most of your fat from unsaturated fats.

HEALTHY FATS

Healthy fats—including monounsaturated and polyunsaturated fats and plant sterols—are beneficial when consumed in moderation. These healthy fats can improve your blood cholesterol and reduce your risk for heart disease.

Monounsaturated fats

Monounsaturated fats, found mostly in olive, canola, and peanut oils, are the healthiest fats you can eat. They lower the level of total cholesterol in the blood, decrease harmful LDL cholesterol in the blood, and raise beneficial HDL cholesterol in the blood. Monounsaturated fats are usually liquid at room temperature.

NUTS ABOUT NUTS

Don't feel guilty the next time you reach for a handful of nuts at snack time. Although nuts are high in fat, the fatty acids they contain are mainly the monounsaturated or polyunsaturated kind, which are good for you. These fats have favorable effects on blood cholesterol, lower the risk for heart disease, and may increase longevity. Nuts are also good sources of protein, fiber, and many minerals. The different types of nuts provide different nutrients, so it's best to include a variety in your diet.

But keep in mind that nuts often come highly salted, and salt can increase blood pressure. Look for nuts that are unsalted or lightly salted. Nuts also contain a lot of calories—a handful a day is enough to get the health benefits. Store nuts in the fridge (or freezer) to keep them from becoming rancid.

Polyunsaturated fats

Polyunsaturated fats are found in corn, sunflower, safflower, flaxseed, and soybean oils, and in the oils of fatty fish such as salmon, mackerel, and tuna. Rich in omega-3 fatty acids and omega-6 fatty acids, polyunsaturated fats lower total cholesterol in the blood. However, in large amounts, they can also lower heart-healthy HDL cholesterol. Like monounsaturated fats, polyunsaturated fats are usually liquid at room temperature.

Omega-3 and omega-6 fatty acids

Omega-3 and omega-6 fatty acids are a type of polyunsaturated fat. They are called essential fatty acids because they are essential for health but cannot be made by the body. Instead, they must be obtained from food. Omega-3 fatty acids are found in fatty fish (such as salmon, mackerel, and sardines) and fish oils and in walnuts, flaxseed oil, and canola oil. The much more plentiful dietary sources of omega-6 fatty acids include cereals, whole-grain breads, most vegetable oils, eggs, poultry, and baked goods.

Caution with fish oil supplements

If you are considering taking fish oil supplements, talk to your doctor. Although they are generally considered safe, in some people who bruise easily, have a bleeding disorder, or take blood-thinning medication, they could cause more bleeding. Some studies have shown that consuming more than 3 grams of omega-3 fatty acids per day (equal to 3 daily servings of fish) may raise the risk for a kind of stroke caused by bleeding in the brain.

Fish oil supplements can also cause excessive gas and diarrhea when you first start taking them, but these effects quickly subside. Taking a time-release variety can help minimize these side effects. Also, remember that the FDA does not regulate dietary supplements, including fish oil, to make sure that they are safe and effective. In fact, most over-the-counter supplements of 1,000 milligrams of "fish oil" only contain 300 milligrams of the types of omega-3s that are best for you, so you would need to take a lot of these pills. And there are some concerns about mercury concentrations in fish oil supplements.

You need to balance your intake of omega-3 and omega-6 fatty acids—consuming too much of one and too little of the other may cause health problems. The typical American diet provides 10 to 30 times more omega-6 fatty acids than omega-3s. Health experts generally recommend that people consume fewer omega-6 fatty acids and more omega-3 fatty acids, bringing the balance to a ratio of four times more omega-3s than omega-6s.

What's the best way to get your omega-3s? As with all nutrients, it's always best to get them from food, but eating enough fish oil to realize the potential health benefits of omega-3s is not always easy. Health experts recommend consuming 3 servings of fatty fish (such as salmon, sardines, or mackerel) each week. Many doctors advise their patients to consume up to 3 grams of omega-3s every day—from food and, if needed, from supplements. Because many people find it difficult to get this amount from food only, they take fish oil supplements to reach 3 grams of omega-3s a day to balance their larger intake of omega-6s.

Plant sterols and stanols

Substances called plant sterols or stanols are fats found in nuts, seeds, and many other plant foods. When eaten regularly, plant sterols and stanols can slow the absorption of dietary cholesterol and substantially lower the level of total cholesterol and harmful LDL cholesterol in the blood. To make wider use of these heart-protecting properties, food scientists have teamed up with food manufacturers to add them to certain products such as margarines and salad dressings. Some studies have found that regularly eating foods containing plant sterols and stanols can reduce the risk for heart disease by about 25 percent. Ask your doctor about trying these products to help improve your cholesterol profile.

Fats in your diet

Certain fats that you eat, such as saturated fats, can have harmful effects on blood cholesterol and increase the risk for heart disease. There is evidence that they may also increase the risk for cancer. But some fats have beneficial effects on blood cholesterol and can reduce the risk for heart disease.

Types of Fat	Main Food Sources	Effects on Blood Cholesterol
GOOD FATS		
Monounsaturated fats	Most nuts, olive oil, canola oil, peanut oil, avocados	Lower total and bad LDL cholesterol, and raise good HDL cholesterol
Polyunsaturated fats	Sunflower oil, corn oil, safflower oil, flaxseed oil, soybean oil, cottonseed oil, fish	Lower total cholesterol but can lower good HDL cholesterol
Omega-3 fatty acids	Oily, cold-water fish, including salmon, tuna, lake trout, and herring, and flaxseed, wheat germ, canola oil	Lower total cholesterol, lower bad LDL cholesterol, and raise good HDL cholesterol
Plant sterols and stanols	Occur naturally in fruits, vegetables, nuts, cereals, and soybean oil; added to some tub margarines and salad dressings	Lower total cholesterol and bad LDL cholesterol
BAD FATS		
Saturated fats	Fatty red meat, dark poultry meat and skin, full-fat and 2% (reduced-fat) dairy products, butter, coconut oil, palm oil	Raise total and bad LDL cholesterol
Trans fats	Stick margarine, vegetable shortening, partially hydrogenated vegetable oils, some prepared and packaged baked goods and snacks including chips and crackers, french fries and other deep fried foods, some breakfast cereals	Raise total and bad LDL cholesterol, and may lower good HDL cholesterol
Dietary cholesterol	Egg yolks, shrimp and other shellfish, liver, full-fat dairy products	Raise total cholesterol, but not as much as saturated fats and trans fats do

UNHEALTHY FATS

Fats you need to watch out for include saturated fats, trans fats, and dietary cholesterol. These fats can have an unfavorable effect on cholesterol, raising total cholesterol and well as bad LDL cholesterol.

Saturated fats

Saturated fat is found mostly in foods that come from animals, including fatty cuts of meat, poultry with skin, whole and 2-percent (reduced-fat) milk, butter, cheese, and lard. But high amounts of saturated fat can also be found in some foods that come from plants, such as palm kernel oil, palm oil, coconut oil, and cocoa butter. Eating saturated fat increases the risk for heart disease and high blood pressure by raising the levels of total cholesterol and bad LDL cholesterol in the blood. You should restrict your intake of saturated fat to 10 percent or less of your total daily calories; many doctors recommend limiting saturated fat consumption to less than 7 percent.

In recent years, it was thought that a low-fat diet could protect against some common forms of cancer, such as breast cancer and colon cancer, but several studies have not found this to be the case for the general population. By contrast, there is some evidence that eating large amounts of animal fat and saturated fat may raise the risk for prostate cancer (see page 291) in men and endometrial cancer (see page 284) in women.

Trans fats

Unlike other fats, most trans fats are formed when food manufacturers turn liquid oils into solid fats like shortening and stick margarine. To do this, manufacturers add hydrogen to vegetable oil in a process called hydrogenation. Hydrogenation increases the shelf life and stabilizes the flavor of many popular foods. Trans fats are the reason french fries and doughnuts last so long and taste similar no matter which fast-food restaurant serves them. These damaging fats are also found in a variety of widely available foods including vegetable shortening, stick margarine, crackers and other snack foods, baked goods, pie crusts, and cookies. Any foods made with or fried in partially hydrogenated oils—deep fried chicken or fish, for example—also contain trans fats.

Eating foods that contain trans fats harms your heart in several ways. Trans fats elevate total blood cholesterol and bad LDL cholesterol. At the same time, trans fats may lower the level of good HDL cholesterol. This combination—high total cholesterol, high bad LDL, and low good HDL— is dangerous, producing an undesirable cholesterol profile that can lead to heart disease. Trans fats also increase the tendency of blood cells to cluster together into potentially artery-blocking clots. In addition, trans fats seem to trigger the immune system to increase inflammation in the body. Inflammation has been linked to an increased risk for heart disease.

What can you do to avoid trans fats? One way is to always read food nutrition labels (see page 34). Most nutrition experts say that the safest level of trans fat consumption is none. But keep in mind that food manufacturers may list an amount of trans fats of less than half (0.5) a gram as zero grams (0g) on the Nutrition Facts panel. As a result, you may see products that list "Trans Fat 0g" on the label but the ingredient list includes "shortening" or "partially hydrogenated vegetable oil." This means that the food contains small amounts (less than half a gram) of trans fats per serving. When eating out, ask the server if the oils used in food preparation are hydrogenated or partially hydrogenated, or if shortening is used for frying or baking. You can avoid trans fats easily by not ordering anything deep-fried.

TRANS FATS VS. SATURATED FATS

Trans fats' harmful effects on health have gotten lots of bad press, but it's important to keep things in perspective. Although gram for gram, trans fats are considered somewhat more harmful than saturated fats, too much of either can significantly raise the risk for heart disease, stroke, type 2 diabetes, and other health problems. And most important, Americans tend to eat about five times more saturated fats than trans fats, making saturated fats, in reality, a bigger health threat for most people.

Dietary cholesterol

Cholesterol is a fat that the body needs in small amounts. Distinguishing between the cholesterol that's in your blood (blood cholesterol) and the cholesterol that's in some of the food that you eat (dietary cholesterol) can be confusing. Blood cholesterol is a substance made by the liver to help the body manufacture hormones, vitamin D, and the bile acids that help the body digest fat and repair cells. Problems arise when the liver makes too much bad LDL cholesterol. LDL cholesterol is harmful because it lodges in the walls of arteries. HDL cholesterol is beneficial because it removes cholesterol from the arteries, delivering it to the liver, which eliminates it from the body.

Most of the cholesterol circulating in your body is produced in the liver; the rest is absorbed from the fats in food that you eat. You can control your cholesterol to some extent by limiting your intake of foods that are high in saturated and trans fats and cholesterol, which stimulate the liver to make more cholesterol. Trans fats and saturated fats have the most harmful effects on blood cholesterol levels, by raising the level of bad LDL cholesterol and lowering the level of good HDL cholesterol. However, your blood cholesterol profile is largely influenced by genetic factors you inherited.

Dietary cholesterol refers to the cholesterol that is present only in some foods of animal origin—not plant-based foods. Common food sources of cholesterol include egg yolks, shrimp, lobster, red meat, full-fat dairy products, and organ meats (liver, kidney, and brains). Dietary cholesterol does not raise blood cholesterol as much as saturated fats and trans fats do, but the recommendation is to limit your intake of dietary cholesterol to less than 300 milligrams a day. People who have high blood cholesterol or heart disease are advised to restrict their intake to less than 200 milligrams a day. The yolk of one large egg contains about 214 milligrams of dietary cholesterol. Doctors generally recommend that healthy people consume no more than four egg yolks each week. People with heart disease should have one or fewer egg yolks each week. (Egg whites have no cholesterol.)

USING FATS WISELY

You can help lower your blood cholesterol by replacing saturated fats with unsaturated fats. But also keep in mind that limiting the total amount of fat and oil helps keep your calorie intake moderate, which, in turn, helps you control your weight. When buying fats or oils, keep these tips in mind:

- Choose liquid vegetable oils that are high in unsaturated fats—including canola, corn, olive, peanut, safflower, sesame, soybean, and sunflower oils.

- Buy only margarine made with unsaturated liquid vegetable oils as the first ingredient. Choose soft tub margarines that contain no partially hydrogenated oils.

- Limit butter, and never use lard, fatback, or solid shortenings. Lard and fatback are high in saturated fat and cholesterol, and stick margarine and solid shortenings (usually) contain trans fats. (Some familiar brands of shortening are now made with no trans fats.)

- Buy light or nonfat mayonnaise and salad dressing instead of the regular kind that is high in fat.

- Look for margarines and salad dressings that contain plant sterols or stanols (see page 9), which, when consumed regularly, can significantly improve blood cholesterol.

Vitamins

Although nutritional deficiencies are not common in the United States, they can occur in people with eating disorders, alcoholism, gastrointestinal disorders that interfere with proper food absorption, or prolonged diarrhea. They can also occur in women during pregnancy or when they are breast-feeding, in menstruating women who have heavy periods (iron-deficiency anemia), in people who are following a calorie-restricted diet, and in the elderly (especially those who remain indoors during most of the day and don't get vitamin D from the sun). For this reason, most doctors agree that taking a daily multivitamin supplement is an acceptable form of health "insurance," but they advise against taking megadoses of single supplements, which can lead to serious health problems.

Vitamins are classified into two categories: fat soluble (A, D, E, and K) and water soluble (B complex and C). Fat-soluble vitamins are found in fats and oils in foods and are stored in body fat. Water-soluble vitamins dissolve in water and mix easily in the blood. Your body stores only small amounts of water-soluble vitamins and excretes them in urine. For this reason, you need to consume them regularly to maintain an adequate supply. Some vitamins are antioxidants—chemicals that prevent damaging changes in cells that can produce chronic inflammation, which may play a role in many common diseases including heart disease, some cancers, and Alzheimer's disease, and many of the effects of aging.

Vitamin D: More important than you thought

Researchers are finding that vitamin D not only can make bones and teeth stronger, but also has an effect on the immune system, the ability of the pancreas to make insulin, and the functioning of the heart. Insufficient vitamin D is now thought to play a role in the development of heart disease, some autoimmune disorders such as rheumatoid arthritis, colon cancer, and even influenza. It now appears that getting a certain amount of sun every day is essential for good health, although excessive sun exposure is harmful because it can lead to skin cancer and some other problems such as cataracts (see page 408) and age-related macular degeneration (see page 413) .

Vitamin D is a fat-soluble vitamin that your body makes after exposure to ultraviolet (UV) rays from the sun. The UV rays from sunlight trigger the skin to make vitamin D. Sunlight is your major source of vitamin D. A much smaller amount is contained in certain foods, especially cod liver oil and vitamin-D-fortified milk and orange juice. Your body needs vitamin D to adequately absorb calcium. Without enough vitamin D, your body has to take calcium from its stores in your skeleton, which weakens existing bone and prevents the formation of strong, new bone.

Spending as little as 10 or 15 minutes in the sun several times a week is enough to get your recommended dose of vitamin D. Sunscreen that has a sun protection factor (SPF) of 8 or more blocks the UV rays that your skin needs to form vitamin D, so put on your sunscreen after you get about 10 minutes of sun exposure. Always use sunscreen if you will be out in the sun longer than 10 or 15 minutes.

If you live in a northern climate, you're probably not getting enough vitamin D from the sun during the winter months. Many elderly people who are confined to their homes, nursing home residents, and dark-skinned people may also be deficient. In this case, you may need to take a vitamin D supplement. But talk to your doctor first.

Antioxidants

Antioxidants are substances in food that protect against free radicals, which are potentially damaging molecules made during the normal chemical and physical processes that take place in cells. During these processes, called oxidation, energy is produced. Oxidation is an essential activity of all life systems, but in excess it can damage cells and contribute to the development of disorders ranging from arthritis to heart disease to Alzheimer's disease. Free radicals and oxidation can also be caused by environmental and lifestyle factors. For example, smoking and exposure to radiation can increase free radical production in the body and cause cell damage that can lead to cancer.

Antioxidants—such as vitamins A, C, and E, and beta carotene—may be the antidote to excessive oxidation by free radicals, protecting cells against

Vitamins at a glance

Vitamin	Function	Good food sources	Symptoms of deficiency
FAT-SOLUBLE VITAMINS			
Vitamin A	Antioxidant; required for growth and development and healthy immune function, vision, and skin	Fortified milk, carrots, sweet potatoes, winter squash, eggs, cheese, cod, halibut, fish oils	Visual disturbances, respiratory infections, dryness of the skin, faulty bone formation
Vitamin D	Increases calcium absorption; builds strong bones and teeth.	Sunlight, cod liver oil, salmon, mackerel, fortified milk, fortified orange juice, fortified breakfast cereal	Decreased bone mass
Vitamin E	Antioxidant; helps form blood cells, muscle, and lung and nerve tissue; boosts the immune system	Nuts, soy beans, green leafy vegetables, wheat germ oil, whole wheat, whole-grain cereals	Numbness, tingling, or burning pain in the hands and feet from nerve damage; dry skin and hair; poor wound healing; bruising; anemia; muscle weakness
Vitamin K	Helps blood clot.	Green leafy vegetables, plant oils, dairy products	Impaired blood clotting
Beta carotene	Antioxidant; used by the body to make vitamin A	Orange and deep yellow vegetables and fruits (carrots, sweet potatoes, winter squash, cantaloupe, pumpkins, mangoes)	Long-term inadequate intake can cause the same symptoms as vitamin A deficiency (above)
WATER-SOLUBLE VITAMINS			
Vitamin B1 (thiamine)	Helps convert food into energy	Fortified breakfast cereals and breads, pork, organ meats, legumes, seeds, nuts, brewer's yeast	Muscle weakness, heart failure
Vitamin B2 (riboflavin)	Plays a role in energy production; helps maintain healthy eyes, skin, and nerve function	Milk, eggs, cheese, organ meats, green leafy vegetables, fortified breakfast cereals and breads	Sore throat; inflamed skin; red, tearing, itchy eyes; anemia
Vitamin B3 (niacin)	Needed for fat metabolism, proper digestion, and a healthy nervous system	Meat, beans, fortified breakfast cereals and breads	Mouth ulcers; pellagra (which causes diarrhea, a scaly rash, and disorientation)

Vitamin	Function	Good food sources	Symptoms of deficiency
Vitamin B5 (pantothenic acid)	Essential for numerous chemical reactions needed to sustain life	Eggs, liver, fish, poultry, whole-grain breads, legumes	Deficiency is rare; causes daytime sleepiness, fatigue, headache, tingling in the hands and feet, leg muscle weakness, increased susceptibility to infections
Vitamin B6 (pyridoxine)	Helps convert carbohydrates into glucose (sugar), to produce energy; essential for the metabolism of fats and protein; promotes health of the nervous system, skin, hair, eyes, mouth, and liver	Wheat germ, liver, peanuts, brewer's yeast, legumes, potatoes, bananas	Deficiency is rare; causes itchy skin rash, irritability, depression, confusion, nerve damage
Vitamin B9 (folate, folic acid)	Needed for new cell formation, normal red blood cell production, and DNA production	Fortified breakfast cereals and breads, organ meats, green vegetables, eggs	Diarrhea, appetite loss, weight loss, weakness, inflamed tongue, headache, heart palpitations, irritability
Vitamin B12 (cyanocobalamin)	Needed for normal blood formation and a healthy nervous system; helps produce DNA	Eggs, liver, organ meats, milk, chicken, cheese, fortified breakfast cereals	Deficiency is most common in older people; produces neurological problems such as numbness, tingling, difficulty with balance, memory loss, dementia
Biotin	Needed for metabolism of fats and carbohydrates	Egg yolk, fish, nuts, bananas, grapefruit, strawberries, organ meats,	Deficiency is rare; produces hair loss, skin rashes, weight loss, nausea, numbness in the hands and feet, muscle pain
Vitamin C	Antioxidant; needed to maintain healthy connective tissue, collagen, bones, and teeth	Citrus fruits, tomatoes, cauliflower, broccoli, spinach, potatoes	Scurvy, a disease that produces muscle pain, weakness, irritability, anemia, bleeding, gum disease, loosening of teeth

free-radical damage. The minerals selenium, magnesium, copper, and zinc also have antioxidant properties. Studies are currently under way to find out whether antioxidants, by limiting the production of free radicals, might help prevent or delay the development of some of the most common chronic diseases such as heart disease and cancer. Researchers are also looking at whether antioxidants can help slow the aging process.

Antioxidants consumed in foods seem to have a much more powerful effect than those provided in supplements. Studies that look at the therapeutic value of high doses of vitamins, which usually test them in isolation, have not found them to be effective at preventing illness. This may be because very high doses of specific nutrients can interfere with normal body processes, such as the balance of chemical reactions in the body.

Phytochemicals

Phytochemicals are naturally occurring substances in plant foods that can help keep you healthy. Fruits, vegetables, and legumes (dried beans and peas) contain hundreds of phytochemicals, which work together with vitamins and minerals to protect against cancer, heart disease, and other disorders. The vitamins, minerals, fiber, and phytochemicals in plant foods combine to produce a health-protecting and disease-fighting effect that you can't get from vitamin supplements. Eating a variety of fruits, vegetables, and legumes gives you all of these nutrients together.

Minerals

Minerals are called inorganic chemical compounds because they are made from neither plants nor animals. They work in the body to regulate hormones and support the activities of enzymes (proteins that promote and accelerate the rate of chemical reactions). Minerals are grouped into two categories: major and trace. The body needs the major minerals—calcium, magnesium, and phosphorus—in relatively large amounts, while the trace minerals are required in only minute amounts. Consuming a balanced and varied diet is the best way to obtain minerals and to maintain a proper mineral balance.

Major Minerals

Mineral	Function	Good Food Sources	Symptoms of Deficiency
Calcium	Maintains normal heart, muscle, and nerve function; keeps teeth and bones healthy	Dairy products, oysters, salmon, collard greens, spinach, kale, broccoli, oranges	Arm and leg muscle spasms, heart palpitations, bone softening or brittle bones, poor growth, reduced bone mass, tooth decay, depression
Chromium	Regulates blood sugar by boosting effects of insulin	Whole grain cereals, brewer's yeast, liver, beer, poultry	Poor blood sugar control; numbness, tingling, or burning sensations in the hands and feet from nerve damage
Copper	Essential for healthy functioning of the heart and for making hemoglobin and collagen; helps in energy production and iron absorption	Organ meats, oysters, whole grains, nuts, shellfish, dark-green, leafy vegetables	Anemia, low white blood cell count, skeletal defects
Fluoride	Inhibits tooth decay and stimulates new bone formation	Fluoridated water, grains, vegetables, seafood, seaweed, cheese, tea, coffee	Increased risk for tooth decay and decreased bone mass
Iodine	Essential for production of thyroid hormone, which is crucial for normal growth and development	Seafood, iodized salt, eggs, dairy products, drinking water	Moderate deficiency produces goiter; severe deficiency produces abnormally low levels of thyroid hormone in adults and growth retardation in infants
Iron	Essential for red blood cell development and transport of oxygen in the bloodstream	Meat, fish, beans, spinach, molasses, kelp, broccoli, seeds, brewer's yeast	Anemia, paleness, weakness, fatigue, shortness of breath, heart palpitations, deformed nails, headaches

(continued)

Mineral	Function	Good Food Sources	Symptoms of Deficiency
Magnesium	Promotes muscle and nerve function; maintains teeth and bones	Brown rice, nuts, green leafy vegetables, grains, seeds, beans, peas, wheat germ, whole grains, bananas, oranges, strawberries	Heart failure and other heart disorders, high blood pressure, low potassium levels, nervousness, kidney damage and stones, irritability, muscle spasms
Manganese	Needed for proper muscle, nerve, and enzyme function; helps produce cholesterol and fatty acids in the liver	Seeds, unrefined grains, tea, beans and other legumes, vegetables	Not known
Molybdenum	Needed for the activity of certain enzymes	Milk, beans, peas, breakfast cereals, and bread	Symptoms are rare, but include rapid heart rate, headache, nausea, vomiting, disorientation, and coma
Phosphorous	Helps form genetic material; builds strong bones and teeth; maintains acid-base balance; needed for energy production	Protein-rich foods, such as meats, fish, and dairy products; dried beans and peas, nuts, breakfast cereals	Bone fractures, irritability, weakness, blood cell disorders, stomach and intestine disorders, poor kidney function
Potassium	Maintains body's fluid balance; transmits nerve signals; regulates blood pressure; prevents irregular heartbeat	Bananas, oranges and orange juice, apricots, starchy vegetables, nuts, seeds, yogurt, fruit	Muscle weakness, confusion and seizures; disturbed heart rhythm
Selenium	Antioxidant; essential for healthy functioning of the heart muscle	Seafood and organ meats, plants (depending on the selenium content in soil)	Symptoms are rare, but include muscle weakness, pain, and tenderness
Zinc	Involved in wound healing, the normal fluid balance of the skin, taste, and smell; works with more than 70 different enzymes	Meat, liver, eggs, seeds, whole grains, peanuts, cheese (Vegetarians should consume foods high in zinc or use zinc supplements to offset their lack of animal protein.)	Severe weight loss, apathy, depression, growth retardation, delayed sexual maturity, hair loss, anemia, night blindness, impaired wound healing

To supplement or not to supplement?

That's a good question. If you are pregnant, are nursing a baby, or have a chronic medical condition such as diabetes, hypertension, or heart disease, talk to your doctor or pharmacist before purchasing or taking any dietary supplements. While vitamin and mineral supplements are widely used and generally considered safe for children, you may want to check with your doctor or pharmacist before giving any dietary supplements to your child. If you plan to use a dietary supplement in place of a medication or in combination with any medication, talk to your doctor first. Many supplements contain ingredients that have strong biological effects and can interact with some medications. In addition, the safety of supplements is not regulated by the FDA.

Some supplements can have unwanted effects during surgery, so it's important to fully inform your doctor about any vitamins, minerals, herbals, or other supplements you're taking, especially before elective surgery. You may be asked to stop taking these supplements at least two to three weeks before the procedure to avoid potentially dangerous supplement-drug interactions—such as changes in heart rate or blood pressure, or increased bleeding—that could adversely affect the outcome of your surgery.

Taking a combination of supplements or using them together with medications (either prescription or over-the-counter) could produce adverse effects, some of which can be serious. For example, the prescription drug warfarin, ginkgo biloba (an herbal supplement), aspirin (an over-the-counter drug), and vitamin E (a vitamin supplement) can all thin the blood. Taking any of these products together can increase the risk for internal bleeding.

While your body needs essential nutrients to stay healthy and avoid disease, taking megadoses of some nutrients can be harmful and may not be protective. Doctors think that the explanation for this may be that the combinations of multiple nutrients found in foods have more power to protect the body from free radical damage than do single nutrients taken alone in supplements. Bottom line: Try to get most of your nutrition from a healthy, well-balanced diet and, if you want to take a supplement, a single multivitamin without megadoses of nutrients is best.

MyPyramid

The U.S. Department of Agriculture introduced a new and improved food guide pyramid in 2005, called MyPyramid, which is designed to help people choose foods that match their specific calorie needs. It also includes an important new element: regular exercise. The updated pyramid depicts a stick figure climbing stairs to encourage physical activity. To learn more about MyPyramid, visit www.mypyramid.gov.

MyPyramid

To make sure you consume a varied and balanced diet, try to eat foods from each group every day. The Web site helps you make smart choices from every food group, find your balance between food and physical activity, get the most nutrition from your calories, and stay within your daily calorie needs. The message is: Eat less, eat smart, and move more every day.

MyPyramid Guidelines at a Glance

Grains	Vegetables	Fruits	Milk	Meat and Beans
Eat about 5 to 8 ounces of cereals, breads, crackers, rice, or pasta every day. Make at least half of your grains whole grains.	Eat about 2½ to 3 cups of vegetables each day, especially green leafy veggies, orange veggies, and dried beans and peas.	Eat about 2 cups each day. Choose fresh, frozen, canned, or dried versions. Whole fruit gives you more nutrients and fewer calories than juice.	Eat about 3 cups each day. Choose low-fat or fat-free products. If you don't or can't consume milk, choose lactose-free products or calcium-fortified foods and beverages.	Eat about 5½ to 6½ ounces each day. Choose low-fat or lean meats and poultry. Bake, broil, or grill them. Choose more fish, beans, peas, nuts, and seeds.
1 ounce is about 1 slice of bread, 1 cup of breakfast cereal, or ½ cup of cooked rice, cereal, or pasta.	1 cup is a cup of raw or cooked vegetables or vegetable juice, 2 cups of raw leafy greens, or 1 cup of cooked dried beans or peas.	1 cup is a cup of fruit or 100% fruit juice, ½ cup of dried fruit, or 1 small apple, 1 large orange, 1 large banana, 32 seedless grapes, or 8 large strawberries.	1 cup is a cup of milk or yogurt, 1½ ounces of natural cheese, or 2 ounces of processed cheese.	An ounce is 1 ounce of meat, poultry, or fish; ½ cup of cooked dried beans or peas; one egg; 1 tablespoon of peanut butter; ½ ounce of nuts or seeds; or 2 ounces of tofu.

These amounts are based on a 2,000-calorie daily diet and are for people who get less than 30 minutes of moderate physical activity each day, beyond normal daily activities. If you are more physically active, you may be able to eat more while staying within your calorie needs.

Find your balance between food and physical activity:

- Stay within your daily calorie needs.
- Be physically active for at least 30 minutes most days of the week.
- To prevent weight gain, you may need to engage in about 60 minutes of physical activity each day.
- To sustain a weight loss, you'll need at least 60 to 90 minutes a day of physical activity.

Know the limits on fats, sugars, and salt:

- Get most of your fat intake from fish, nuts, and vegetables.
- Limit solid fats like butter, stick margarine, shortening, and lard, and foods that contain them.
- Check the Nutrition Facts Label to keep saturated fats, trans fats, and sodium low.
- Choose food and beverages low in added sugars. Added sugars contribute calories with few, if any, nutrients.

Dietary Guidelines for Americans

The Dietary Guidelines for Americans are the cornerstone of governmental nutrition policy and nutrition education. Designed to recommend good eating habits for people over age two, the Dietary Guidelines promote health and reduce risk for the major chronic diseases. The guidelines give recommendations for physical activity as well as healthy eating.

Get enough nutrients for your calorie needs

Key recommendations

- Consume a variety of nutrient-dense foods and beverages from the basic food groups while choosing foods that limit the intake of saturated and trans fats, cholesterol, added sugars, salt, and alcohol.
- Get the recommended intakes within your energy needs by adopting a balanced eating pattern, such as that suggested by MyPyramid or the DASH eating plan (see page 27).

Manage your weight

Key recommendations

- To maintain your body weight in a healthy range, balance the calories you take in from foods and beverages with the calories you expend.
- To prevent gradual weight gain over time, make small reductions in calorie intake and increase physical activity.

FIGURING DAILY CALORIE NEEDS

The information you see on food labels is based on a 2,000-calorie-a-day diet. This one-size-fits-all approach can be misleading, because people can have widely different calorie needs based on many factors, including their level of activity, age, and gender. This chart will give you an idea of how many calories you can consume each day to maintain energy balance (calories in = calories out) based on your gender, age, and activity level. (The numbers are estimated and rounded to the nearest 200 calories and were determined using an equation from the 2002 Institute of Medicine Dietary Reference Intakes report.)

To lose 1 pound per week, your body needs to burn 3,500 more calories in a week than you consume. You can do this by burning 500 more calories each day (by becoming more active) or by eating 500 fewer calories each day, or by burning 250 more calories and consuming 250 fewer calories. You can lose weight faster by both eating less and being more active.

Gender	Age (years)	Daily Calorie Intake Based on Activity Level		
		Inactive	Moderately Active	Active
Girls and boys	2 to 3	1,000	1,000–1,400	1,000–1,400
Females	4 to 8	1,200	1,200	1,400–1,800
	9 to 13	1,600	1,600	1,800–2,200
	14 to 18	1,800	1,800	2,400
	19 to 30	2,000	2,000	2,400
	31 to 50	1,800	1,800	2,200
	51+	1,600	1,600	2,000–2,200
Males	4 to 8	1,400	1,400–1,600	1,600–2,000
	9 to 13	1,800	1,800–2,200	2,000–2,600
	14 to 18	2,200	2,400–2,800	2,800–3,200
	19 to 30	2,400	2,600–2,800	3,000
	31 to 50	2,200	2,400–2,600	2,800–3,000
	51+	2,000	2,200–2,400	2,400–2,800

Be physically active

Key recommendations

- Engage in regular physical activity and shun sedentary activities to promote health, psychological well-being, and a healthy body weight.

- To reduce the risk for chronic disease in adulthood, engage in at least 30 minutes of moderate-intensity physical activity—above your usual activity—on most days of the week.

- For most people, engaging in physical activity of a more vigorous intensity or longer duration secures even greater health benefits.

- To help manage body weight and prevent gradual weight gain in adulthood, get 60 minutes of moderate- to vigorous-intensity activity on most days of the week. Don't eat too much more just because you are exercising more.

- To sustain weight loss in adulthood, get at least 60 to 90 minutes of daily moderate-intensity physical activity. Some people may need to consult with their doctors before participating in this level of activity.

- Include aerobic exercise for heart health, stretching exercises for flexibility, and resistance exercises for muscle strength and endurance.

Eat your food groups

Key recommendations

- Consume plenty of fruits and vegetables. Two cups of fruit and 2½ cups of vegetables per day are recommended for a 2,000-calorie daily diet.

- Choose a variety of fruits and vegetables each day. Select from dark green leafy vegetables, orange vegetables, beans and other legumes, starchy vegetables, and other types of vegetables several times a week.

- Eat 3 or more ounces of whole-grain foods per day, with the rest of the recommended grains coming from enriched products. At least half the grains should be whole grains.

- Consume 3 cups per day of fat-free or low-fat milk, yogurt, or low-fat cheeses.

Know your fats

Key recommendations

- Consume less than 10 percent of your daily calories from saturated fats and less than 300 milligrams per day of cholesterol from food. Keep trans fat consumption as low as possible because there is no safe limit for trans fat consumption.

- Keep your total fat intake between 20 and 35 percent of total calories, with most fats coming from polyunsaturated and monounsaturated fat sources, such as fish, nuts, and vegetable oils.

- When selecting and preparing meat, poultry, and dairy products, make sure that they are lean, low-fat, or, preferably, fat-free.

- Limit your intake of fats and oils that are high in saturated and trans fats by choosing products low in such fats and oils.

Eat the good carbs

Key recommendations

- Choose fiber-rich fruits, vegetables, and whole grains often.

- Choose and prepare foods and beverages with little added sugars or calorie-containing sweeteners, in amounts suggested by MyPyramid (see page 22) and the DASH eating plan (see next page).

- Reduce the incidence of tooth decay by practicing good oral hygiene and by cutting down on sugar- and starch-containing foods and beverages.

Know about sodium and potassium

Key recommendations

- Consume less than 1 teaspoon (2,300 milligrams) of salt per day.

- Choose foods with little salt and avoid adding salt while cooking or at the table. At the same time, consume potassium-rich foods (see page 20), such as fruits and vegetables.

- People with high blood pressure, African Americans, and middle-aged and older adults should try to consume no more than 1,500 milligrams of sodium per day (less than a teaspoon), and meet the potassium recommendation (4,700 milligrams per day) by eating potassium-rich foods.

Be moderate with alcohol

Key recommendations

- Those who choose to drink alcoholic beverages should do so sensibly and in moderation—no more than one drink per day for women and no more than two drinks per day for men.

- Alcoholic beverages should not be consumed by some people, including those who have alcohol dependence, women of childbearing age who may become pregnant, women who are pregnant or breastfeeding, children and adolescents, people taking medications that can interact with alcohol, and those with certain medical conditions.

- Alcoholic beverages should be avoided by people performing activities that require attention, skill, or coordination, such as driving or operating machinery.

Handle food safely

Key recommendations

To avoid food-borne illness from microorganisms such as bacteria:

- Wash your hands, all food contact surfaces, and fruits and vegetables thoroughly. Meat and poultry should not be washed or rinsed (to minimize the spread of bacteria to other surfaces).

- Separate raw, cooked, and ready-to-eat foods when shopping, preparing, or storing foods.

- Cook foods to a safe temperature to kill microorganisms.

- Refrigerate perishable food promptly and defrost foods properly.

- Avoid raw (unpasteurized) milk or any products made from unpasteurized milk, raw or partially cooked eggs or foods containing raw eggs, raw or undercooked meat and poultry, unpasteurized juices, and raw sprouts.

The DASH eating plan

What you choose to eat affects your chances of developing many of the most common chronic diseases, including heart disease, type 2 diabetes, cancer, and high blood pressure. Following an eating plan called the Dietary

Approaches to Stop Hypertension (DASH) and eating less salt (sodium) has been shown to help lower blood pressure. (Visit the Web site at dashdiet.org.) Developed by scientists at the National Heart, Lung, and Blood Institute, the DASH diet is recognized as an overall health-promoting diet that may also lower the risk for heart disease, cancer, and other disorders because it's low in total fat, saturated fat, trans fats, and cholesterol, as well as salt. In addition, the diet calls for an abundance of vegetables, fruits, fiber, and whole grains, along with lean protein sources and low-fat dairy products.

The menus and recipes in the DASH eating plan allow 1,500 to 2,300 milligrams of sodium per day. The 1,500 milligram level reduces blood pressure the most and is the amount recommended by the Institute of Medicine as the level most people should try to achieve. In general, the lower your salt intake, the lower your blood pressure is likely to be.

The DASH eating plan follows heart-healthy guidelines to limit harmful fats and cholesterol. It focuses on increasing your intake of foods that are rich in nutrients—primarily minerals (such as potassium, calcium, and magnesium), protein, and fiber—that are expected to lower blood pressure. The diet has other health benefits as well: it protects your heart, can help you lose weight or maintain a healthy weight, and meets your nutritional needs in a balanced way. The chart below gives an example of the DASH eating plan based on a diet with 2,000 calories a day. Use it to help plan your meals.

The DASH eating plan at a glance

Food Group	Daily Servings	Serving Sizes	Examples and Notes	Significance of Each Food Group to the DASH Eating Pattern
Grains	6–8	1 slice bread; 1 oz dry cereal, ½ cup cooked rice, pasta, or cereal	Whole-wheat bread and rolls, whole-wheat pasta, English muffin, pita bread, tortillas, bagel, cereals, grits, oatmeal, brown rice, unsalted pretzels and popcorn	Major sources of energy and fiber, as long as you choose higher-fiber options
Vegetables	4–5	1 cup raw leafy vegetable, ½ cup cut-up raw or cooked vegetable, ½ cup vegetable juice	Broccoli, carrots, collards, green beans, green peas, kale, lima beans, potatoes, spinach, squash, sweet potatoes, tomatoes	Rich sources of potassium, magnesium, and fiber

Food Group	Daily Servings	Serving Sizes	Examples and Notes	Significance of Each Food Group to the DASH Eating Pattern
Fruits	4–5	1 medium fruit; ¼ cup dried fruit; ½ cup fresh, frozen, or canned fruit; ½ cup fruit juice	Apples, apricots, bananas, dates, grapes, oranges, grapefruit, grapefruit juice, mangoes, melons, peaches, pineapples, raisins, berries, tangerines	Important sources of potassium, magnesium, and fiber
Fat-free or low-fat milk and milk products	2–3	1 cup milk or yogurt, 1½ oz cheese	Fat-free (skim) or low-fat (1%) milk or buttermilk; fat-free, low-fat, or reduced-fat cheese; fat-free or low-fat regular or frozen yogurt	Major sources of calcium and protein
Lean meats, poultry, and fish	6 or less	1 oz cooked meats, poultry, or fish; 1 egg	Select only lean; trim away visible fats; broil, roast, or poach; remove skin from poultry	Rich sources of protein and magnesium
Nuts, seeds, and legumes	4–5 per week	⅓ cup or 1½ oz nuts, 2 Tbsp peanut butter, 2 Tbsp or ½ oz seeds, ½ cup cooked legumes (dry beans and peas)	Almonds, hazelnuts, peanuts, walnuts, pecans, cashews, mixed nuts, sunflower seeds, peanut butter (without partially hydrogenated oils), kidney beans, black beans, red beans, chick peas, lentils, split peas	Rich sources of energy, magnesium, protein, and fiber
Fats and oils	2–3	1 tsp soft margarine, 1 tsp vegetable oil, 1 Tbsp mayonnaise, 2 Tbsp salad dressing	Soft margarines (without partially hydrogenated oils), vegetable oils (such as canola, corn, olive, or safflower), low-fat mayonnaise, light salad dressing	The DASH study has 27 percent of calories as fat, including fat in or added to foods
Sweets and added sugars	5 or less per week	1 Tbsp sugar, 1 Tbsp jelly or jam, ½ cup sorbet or gelatin, 1 cup lemonade	Fruit-flavored gelatin, fruit punch, hard candy, jelly, maple syrup, sorbet and ices, sugar	Sweets should be low in fat

THREE MINERALS IMPORTANT FOR CONTROLLING BLOOD PRESSURE

If you have high blood pressure, increasing your consumption of foods containing the minerals potassium, calcium, and magnesium can help improve your blood pressure. Potassium balances sodium in the body, helping to control blood pressure and reduce the risk for stroke. Calcium has been shown to lower blood pressure. To achieve this beneficial effect, you need to consume 1,000 to 1,500 milligrams of calcium each day. Magnesium helps lower blood pressure.

Calcium-rich foods include dairy products (even those that are low-fat and fat-free) and green leafy vegetables. Potassium-rich foods include many fruits, vegetables, dairy foods, and fish. The best sources of magnesium are whole grains, green leafy vegetables, nuts, seeds, and legumes.

You can easily boost your intake of these key minerals by eating from 5 to 13 servings of fruit and vegetables each day and consuming 3 servings of fat-free milk or yogurt daily.

Vegetarian diets

There are three main types of vegetarians—ovolactovegetarians, who shun meat, poultry, and fish but consume eggs and dairy foods; lactovegetarians, who consume dairy products but not eggs; and vegans, who consume only plant foods. Some vegans even refuse to use products that come from animals, such as honey, leather, fur, silk, and wool.

Generally, a vegetarian diet can be very healthy. Vegetarians tend to have a lower risk of developing heart disease, high blood pressure, and certain types of cancer. They're also less likely to be overweight. But vegetarians can develop iron deficiency anemia or malnutrition if they aren't careful about what they eat. Vegans also have a high risk of developing vitamin B_{12} deficiency because most food sources of vitamin B_{12} come from animals. Fortified breakfast cereals are one of the few sources of vitamin B_{12} from plant foods, so they can be an important dietary source of vitamin B_{12} for vegans. Most strict vegetarians and vegans who do not consume foods that come from plants and are fortified with vitamin B_{12} should consider taking a dietary supplement that contains vitamin B_{12}.

Vitamin B_{12} deficiency symptoms can be slow to appear because it can take years to deplete the normal body stores of vitamin B_{12}. Breast-fed infants of women who follow strict vegetarian diets have very limited reserves of vitamin B_{12} and can develop a vitamin B_{12} deficiency within months. If undetected and untreated, vitamin B_{12} deficiency in infants can cause permanent brain damage. That's why it's so important for moms who follow a strict vegetarian diet to talk to their doctor about vitamin B_{12} supplements for their infants and children.

If you are not a vegetarian, it's still a good idea to try to serve your family one or two vegetarian meals a week. Eat vegetarian at breakfast or lunch only and then have meat, poultry, or fish at dinner. Here are some ways to turn family meals into vegetarian feasts:

- Go Mexican. Serve bean burritos or enchiladas, guacamole tacos, or black bean chili for dinner or lunch.
- Have eggs for dinner. Scramble them, fry them (in oil spray), put them into a casserole or omelet, or add a hard-boiled egg to a salad.
- Create a chef salad supper with a variety of vegetable ingredients, such as leaf lettuce, spinach, beets, bell peppers, cucumbers, peas, red onions, zucchini, and crunchy jicama. Top it with beans, reduced-fat cheese, or tofu for protein.
- Make an Asian stir fry with lots of veggies and add nuts or tofu on top. Serve over brown rice or soba (buckwheat) noodles.
- Dish up pasta with marinara or pesto sauce, or in an olive oil and vegetable broth. Or make vegetarian lasagna with spinach and low-fat ricotta filling. Serve a green salad on the side.
- Stuff winter squash with bread and nut stuffing and serve with a green vegetable such as Brussels sprouts, cabbage, asparagus, or kale.
- Make a vegetable or bean soup. Experiment with vegetables you've never tried.

Healthy cooking and shopping

Providing healthy meals does not need to be time-consuming or expensive. Healthy meal planning incorporates fresh foods instead of processed ones. It also incorporates abundant fruits and vegetables, whole grains, and lean sources of protein, and uses healthful cooking methods—less frying and more baking, broiling, steaming, roasting, stewing, or boiling. Follow these easy cooking tips for reducing the amount of fat in your meals:

- For crispy fish, roll it in cornmeal and bake it.
- For crispy chicken, remove the skin; dip it in skim milk mixed with herbs and spices; roll it in bread crumbs, cornflakes, or potato flakes; and bake it.
- Take off poultry skin before or after cooking it.
- Use a nonstick pan with vegetable cooking oil spray or a small amount of liquid olive or vegetable oil instead of lard, butter, shortening, or stick margarine (any fat that is solid at room temperature is likely to have saturated or trans fats and is not healthy).
- Trim visible fat before you cook meats.
- Chill meat and poultry broth until the fat becomes solid, and skim off the fat before using the broth.
- Add herbs and spices to your recipes to enhance flavor and make up for the lower amounts of fat, sugar, and salt.

MAKING SMART BEVERAGE CHOICES

Choose water or diet or low-calorie beverages instead of sugar-sweetened drinks.

For a quick, easy, and inexpensive thirst-quencher, carry a water bottle and refill it throughout the day.

- Don't stock the fridge with sugary beverages. Instead, keep a pitcher or bottles of cold water in the fridge.
- Serve water with meals.
- Make water more interesting by adding slices of lemon, lime, cucumber, or watermelon, or drink sparkling water.
- Add a splash of 100 percent fruit juice to plain sparkling water for a refreshing, low-calorie drink.
- When you do opt for a sugar-sweetened beverage, go for the small size. Some companies are now selling 8-ounce cans and bottles of soda, which contain about 100 calories.
- Be a role model for your friends and family by choosing healthy, low-calorie beverages.

- Substitute low-fat or fat-free cheese, milk, mayonnaise, and cream cheese for the full-fat kinds.

- Use two egg whites instead of one whole egg to lower the amount of cholesterol in recipes (egg whites, unlike the yolk, are cholesterol-free).

- Prepare macaroni and cheese with nonfat milk and low-fat cheese.

When grocery shopping, make a list of the foods you intend to buy to limit impulse buying of high-fat and high-sugar foods. Buy fresh, whole foods instead of packaged or processed rice mixes, soups, and snacks. Frozen or canned vegetables can be okay if they do not have added sugar or salt. Remember the following guidelines when you're at the supermarket:

- Buy more vegetables, fruits, and whole grains. Frozen vegetables can be a cheaper and sometimes healthier alternative to "fresh" supermarket vegetables (which are not always as fresh as home-grown vegetables).

- Select fat-free milk (instead of 2 percent or whole milk) and low-fat cheeses and other dairy products.

- Choose fish, lean cuts of poultry such as chicken breasts or drumsticks (instead of the wings or thighs), and lean cuts of meat such as round, sirloin, and loin.

- Read nutrition labels on food packages.

- Stock your pantry with healthy foods you can turn into quick, easy meals.

- Instead of sugary soft drinks, purchase healthy drinks such as 100 percent fruit juices with *no* added sugar, low-sodium vegetable juices, and sparkling water.

Portions and servings

What's the difference between a portion and a serving? A "portion" is how much food you choose to eat at one time, whether in a restaurant, from a package, or in your kitchen. A "serving" is the amount of food listed on a food package's Nutrition Facts panel. Sometimes the portion size and serving size match, but many times they do not. Keep in mind that the serving size on the Nutrition Facts panel is not a recommendation for the amount of food you should eat. It's just a quick way of telling you the number of calories and types of nutrients in a certain amount of food.

HOW TO READ FOOD LABELS

The Nutrition Facts panel is the part of a food package label that lists serving size, the number of servings in the package, the number of calories in a serving, and the percent of daily values (which are the same as the recommended daily allowances) of many important nutrients—fat, carbohydrate, protein, cholesterol, fiber, sugar, sodium, vitamins A and C, and the minerals iron and calcium (no daily values have been set for protein, sugar, or trans fat). For more information to help you read food labels, go to the FDA Web site (http://www.cfsan.fda.gov/label.html).

Nutrition Facts

Serving Size 1/2 cup (114 g) — ①
Servings Per Container 4

Amount Per Serving — ②

Calories 90	Calories from Fat 30

% Daily Value*

Total Fat 3 g	5%
Saturated Fat 0 g	0%
Cholesterol 0 mg	0%
Sodium 300 mg	13%
Total Carbohydrate 13 g	4%
Dietary Fiber 3 g	12%
Sugars 3 g	
Protein 3 g	

③ ④

Vitamin A 80%	•	Vitamin C 60%
Calcium 4%	•	Iron 4%

⑤

* Percent Daily Values are based on a 2,000 calorie diet. Your daily values may be higher or lower depending on your calorie needs.

	Calories	2,000	2,500
Total Fat	Less than	65 g	80 g
Saturated Fat	Less than	20 g	25 g
Cholesterol	Less than	300 mg	300 mg
Sodium	Less than	2,400 mg	2,400 mg
Total Carbohydrate		300 g	375 g
Dietary Fiber		25 g	30 g

⑥

Calories per gram:
Fat 9 • Carbohydrate 4 • Protein 4 — ⑦

⑧ *Many factors affect cancer risk. Eating a diet low in fat and high in fiber may lower risk of this disease.*

⑨ ☐ GOOD SOURCE OF FIBER
☐ LOW FAT

What food labels can tell you

1 To make it easy to compare different brands of the same food, all serving sizes of the food are required to be the same.

2 This line shows the total calories in 1 serving and how many calories from fat are contained in the serving.

3 This section displays the amounts of different nutrients in 1 serving so you can easily compare the nutrient content of similar products and add up the total amounts of a given nutrient that you eat in a day.

4 The percent of daily values is indicated for each nutrient. Percents of daily values are based on a diet of 2,000 calories per day, but that may be too high for many people (see page 24).

5 This area shows the percent of daily values for vitamins A and C, iron, and calcium.

6 This section helps you calculate your daily allowance of various fats, sodium, carbohydrates, and fiber for both a 2,000- and a 2,500-calorie-per-day diet.

7 The number of calories in 1 gram of fat, carbohydrate, and protein are shown here.

8 The federal government has approved the use of certain health claims on packaged foods. Examples include:

- A diet low in fat and rich in fruits and vegetables may reduce your risk for some cancers.
- A diet rich in fruits, vegetables, and grains may reduce the risk for heart disease.
- A low intake of calcium is one risk factor for osteoporosis.

9 Terms such as "low," "high," and "free" on food labels must meet strict definitions. For example, a food described as low-fat must have no more than 3 grams of fat per serving; a low-sodium food must have no more than 140 grams of sodium per serving; and a low-calorie food must have no more than 40 calories per serving.

Each of the 5 to 13 servings of fruits and vegetables you need to eat in a day is pretty small. For example, 1 serving translates into 1 medium-sized piece of fruit, ½ cup of cut-up fresh or canned vegetables or fruit, and 1 cup of raw leafy vegetables or salad. It may help to compare recommended food serving sizes to everyday objects. For example, ¼ cup of raisins is about the size of a large egg. See other serving size comparisons below. (Remember that these size comparisons are approximations.)

Serving size	Looks like
3 ounces of meat or poultry	A deck of cards
1 cup of cereal	A fist
½ cup of cooked rice, pasta, or potato	Half a baseball
1 baked potato	A fist
1 medium fruit	A baseball
½ cup of fresh fruit	Half a baseball
1½ ounces of low-fat or fat-free cheese	Four stacked dice
½ cup of ice cream	Half a baseball
2 tablespoons of peanut butter	A Ping-Pong ball

Since the 1970s, restaurant serving sizes have grown dramatically—and so has the average waist size of Americans. People are eating enormous amounts of food in one sitting, making it harder and harder for them to maintain a healthy weight and contributing to the soaring rates of obesity in this country. These ever-larger portions served outside the home are also affecting how much we eat at home.

Making an effort to cut back on portion size is a great way to help keep your calorie intake in check. But it's not easy. Fast-food restaurants are enticing customers to order larger portions with special deals. Getting a larger amount of food for a little extra money may seem like a good value, but you end up with more food and a lot more calories than you need. Here are some other ways to fight portion distortion when you eat out:

- **Share your meal.** Order a half-portion, or order an appetizer as a main meal. Examples of healthy appetizers include bean dip with pita, soup, bruschetta (toasted bread topped with a tomato and olive oil sauce), shrimp cocktail, and tomato or corn salsa over a baked potato.
- **Choose menu items with a low-fat preparation.** Look for or ask for foods that have been prepared with little or no added fat. Look for the terms "baked," "broiled," "roasted," "grilled," "steamed," "poached," or

"simmered." Choose or request skinless cuts of poultry and lean cuts of meat. Avoid deep-fried foods.

- **Take half of your meal home.** Ask for half of your meal to be boxed up so you won't be tempted to eat more than you need.

- **Eat slowly and enjoy your food.** It takes a while for the brain to register when you are full. Take your time by sitting down at a table to eat—without the TV on. Don't eat on the run or while you're doing something else at the same time, such as driving.

- **Stop eating when you begin to feel full.** Focus on enjoying the setting and your friends or family for the rest of the meal.

- **Avoid large-size sugary soft drinks.** They contain a boatload of calories. Instead, try drinking water with a slice of lemon, iced tea, or low-sodium tomato juice.

- **Choose a restaurant that serves healthy foods.** Look for restaurants that serve nutritious meals such as salads, grilled or steamed entrées, or soup.

- **Go easy with salad toppings.** When eating a healthy salad, don't ruin it by covering it with high-fat cheese, meat, or hard-boiled eggs or by drenching it in high-fat dressing.

Be on the lookout for sodium

Sodium, or table salt, is an essential nutrient. Your body needs it to balance the water and minerals and to maintain the normal functioning of the nerves and muscles. But most people in this country eat much more salt than their body needs. The excess salt makes your body retain water, which increases the volume of blood and can elevate blood pressure, especially if you're overweight or sensitive to the effects of salt.

More than one out of four people with normal blood pressure and more than half of people with hypertension in this country are salt sensitive. Some people have an increased susceptibility to being salt sensitive, including older people, African Americans, and those who have a family member who is salt sensitive or who has high blood pressure. No simple test exists for salt sensitivity, so doctors generally recommend that everyone limit their daily salt consumption to no more than 2,300 milligrams, or about 1 teaspoon of table salt, a day. This 1-teaspoon daily total includes all of the salt and sodium you consume throughout the day—from packaged foods as well as what you use in cooking and at the table. If you have high blood pressure, the benefits are even greater if you reduce your salt intake to less than 1,500 milligrams a day, as recommended in the DASH eating plan (see page 27). Lower-sodium diets can keep blood pressure from rising and help blood pressure medications work more effectively. In general, the lower your sodium intake, the lower your blood pressure is likely to be.

The hard part in keeping sodium intake down is that only 10 percent of dietary sodium comes from the salt people add to their food at the table. This underscores the importance of reading food labels (see page 34). To really see a reduction in your salt intake, always carefully check the salt or sodium content in the prepared, preserved, and processed foods you buy. Choose those that indicate that they are low-sodium, reduced-sodium, sodium-free, or with no salt added. A good rule of thumb is to look for less than 140 milligrams of sodium per serving.

Watch out for foods that are especially high in sodium such as luncheon meats, prepared cheeses, canned vegetables and soups, the flavor packets in rice and pasta mixes, sausages, smoked meats and fish, potato chips and other snacks, some baked products, and condiments such as mustard, ketchup, and soy sauce. Club soda can also be high in sodium. A number of food additives—including monosodium glutamate (MSG), sodium nitrate, sodium benzoate,

> **✓ Use food labels to make healthy choices**
>
> Read food labels carefully, especially noting the type of fat in the food, the total fat grams per serving (look for fewer than 3 grams), the amount of sodium (look for fewer than 140 milligrams), and the fiber content (look for more than 3 grams). Stay away from processed and commercially packaged convenience foods because they are often high in sodium and fat.

baking powder, and baking soda—add sodium to foods. Look for them on the ingredient list on packages. When you buy bottled seasonings, such as chili powder, garlic powder, and onion powder, check the label to make sure they don't contain added salt.

Food safety

Food-borne illnesses are prevalent and the germs that cause them are constantly changing. The most common food-borne infections are those caused by the bacteria Campylobacter, Salmonella, and Escherichia coli (E. coli) 0157:H7, and by a group of viruses called Norwalk and Norwalk-like viruses. Below, you'll find a list of the most common food-borne illnesses and learn how you can protect yourself against them.

- **Campylobacteriosis** This infection is the most frequently identified bacterial cause of diarrheal illness in the world. Undercooked chicken (or other food that has been contaminated by juices dripping from raw chicken) and unpasteurized milk are common sources of this infection.

- **Salmonellosis** The next most common food-borne infection is caused by Salmonella bacteria, which are widespread in the intestines of birds, reptiles, and mammals. The infection can spread to humans in a variety of different foods, including raw or undercooked eggs or egg products, raw milk or raw milk products, contaminated water, meat and meat products, and poultry. Raw fruits and vegetables contaminated during slicing have been implicated in several food-borne outbreaks.

- **E. coli 0157:H7 infection** This bacterium is found in cattle and other farm animals. Humans get sick when they consume food or water that has been contaminated with microscopic amounts of cow feces.

- **Norwalk and Norwalk-like virus infection** This group of viruses is a very common cause of food-borne illness, although it is rarely diagnosed because the laboratory test is not widely available. Unlike many food-borne pathogens found in animals, Norwalk-like viruses spread primarily from one infected person to another. Infected kitchen workers can contaminate a salad or sandwich as they prepare it, if they have the virus on their hands. Infected fishermen sometimes contaminate oysters as they harvest them.

The foods most likely to be contaminated with a bacterium or virus are raw foods of animal origin, including raw meat and poultry, raw eggs, unpasteurized milk, and raw shellfish. Foods that mix the products of many individual animals, such as bulk raw milk, pooled raw eggs, or ground beef, are especially risky because an organism in any one of the animals can contaminate the batch.

Eating raw fruits and vegetables can also be chancy. Washing produce can lower the risk of contamination but won't eliminate it. Some outbreaks of food poisoning have been traced to fresh produce that was processed under unsanitary conditions, primarily from contaminated water used for washing and chilling the produce after harvest. Unpasteurized apple cider and other fruit juice can also become contaminated from organisms in the fruit used to make it.

The following precautions can help you reduce your risk of acquiring a food-borne illness:

- **Cook meat, poultry, and eggs thoroughly.** Use a thermometer to measure the internal temperature of meat and make sure you have cooked it enough to kill any bacteria. For example, you should cook ground beef to an internal temperature of 160°F. Eggs should be cooked until the yolk is firm. No more eggs over easy!

- **Don't contaminate one food with another.** To avoid cross-contaminating foods, always wash your hands, utensils, and cutting boards in warm soapy water after they have been in contact with raw meat or poultry and before they touch another food. Put cooked meat on a clean platter, not back on the surface that held the raw meat.

- **Refrigerate leftovers right away at 34°F to 40°F.** Bacteria can grow quickly at room temperature, so refrigerate leftover foods if you or your family won't be eating them within two hours. You don't have to wait for cooked food to cool before placing it in the fridge, but large volumes of food will cool more quickly if you divide them into several shallow containers for refrigeration.

- **Wash all produce.** Rinse fresh fruits and vegetables in running tap water to remove visible dirt and grime and then place them in a bath of water to which you have added a splash of white vinegar. You'll be surprised to see how much debris comes off in the water. Remove and discard the outermost leaves of a head of lettuce or cabbage. Be careful not to contaminate cut-up fruits or vegetables while slicing them on the cutting board, and avoid leaving cut produce out at room temperature for too many hours.

- **Wash your hands.** Don't become a source of a food-borne illness yourself. Wash your hands with soap and water before preparing food and wash them again after handling raw meat, poultry, eggs, or fish. Wash them again if you sneeze into your hands or blow your nose. Avoid preparing food for others if you have diarrhea. Changing a baby's diaper while preparing food is a bad idea that can easily spread bacteria.

- **Report food-borne illnesses to your local health department.** Your local public health department is an important part of the food safety system. Calls from concerned citizens are often the way outbreaks are first detected. If a public health official contacts you to find out more about an illness you had, always cooperate. In public health investigations, it can be as important to talk to healthy people as to those who are sick.

TOP 10 WAYS TO IMPROVE YOUR DIET

Eating less and eating smarter by including more nutritious foods—and avoiding less nutritious ones—are the single most effective ways to stay healthy, avoid illness, and, possibly, live longer. The chart below shows 10 easy steps you can take to improve your diet.

1. Limit portion sizes to reduce calories.
2. Eat more fruits, veggies, and fiber.
3. Eat fast food rarely—and never supersize it.
4. Limit saturated fat and try to avoid all trans fats.
5. Cut down on your intake of sugar and simple starches (such as white bread and white rice).
6. Eat less salt.
7. Consume more calcium and vitamin D.
8. Become a sometime vegetarian.
9. Boost your intake of omega-3 fatty acids by increasing your intake of fatty fish to at least three times a week.
10. Substitute olive oil for most other oil in cooking, on salads, and as a dip for bread.

2

LIVE YOUNGER LONGER WITH EXERCISE

THERE'S AN OLD SAYING that exercise won't necessarily help you live longer, but it will help you live younger longer. Now doctors know that, in some cases, exercise can indeed extend life and help you live younger longer. Research has shown that increased levels of fitness can boost longevity and reduce mortality rates from all causes of death. In studies of people who were very inactive or who fell into the "low fitness" category, death rates were lowest for those who subsequently increased their activity. This indicates that even a modest increase in physical activity can provide enormous health benefits.

Any form of physical activity can improve health, including activities you perform during your everyday life that wouldn't necessarily be called exercise—walking the dog, climbing stairs, gardening, dancing, or pulling the kids around the block in a wagon. Adding a regular exercise program to the mix would benefit your health even more. At the very least, physical activity increases what doctors call your functional reserve. That's a fancy way of saying how much strength and energy you have to lead an active life. Put simply, leading an active life enables you to keep on being active, putting off (or avoiding altogether) the time when you have to depend on other people to perform your daily tasks.

Instead of talking about the very least that exercise can do, let's look at the most a physically active life can give you. Take heart disease: regular exercise can help improve your blood cholesterol levels and reduce your risk for heart disease. And arthritis: exercise relieves joint pain and stiffness, builds strong muscles to support the joints, and increases joint flexibility. This chapter will explain many more important ways that regular exercise can maintain wellness and prevent disease. It will also show you how to sustain a regular exercise plan—one that you can follow for the rest of your life.

How exercise keeps you healthy

If exercise could be packed into a pill, it would be the most commonly prescribed medication in the world. Physical activity provides health benefits for every part of the body. Studies have found that people who participate in physical activity on a regular basis can reduce their risk for a number of the most common chronic diseases—including heart disease, stroke, type 2 diabetes, high blood pressure, and colon cancer—by 30 to 50 percent. Active people also have lower rates of premature death compared with people who are the least active. In terms of the health benefits of exercise, the advice is simple: If you are doing none, do some; if you are doing some, do more. Regular physical activity improves your health in the following ways:

- Reduces your risk of developing heart disease—and the risk of dying from it.
- Cuts your risk for stroke.
- Slashes your risk of having a second heart attack if you have already had one.
- Lowers total blood cholesterol and raises HDL, the "good" cholesterol.
- Lessens your risk of developing high blood pressure.
- Helps reduce blood pressure in people who have high blood pressure.
- Lowers your risk for type 2 diabetes.
- Reduces the risk for colon cancer.
- Helps you achieve and maintain a healthy body weight.

- Reduces feelings of depression and anxiety.
- Promotes psychological well-being.
- Reduces stress.
- Helps build and maintain healthy bones, muscles, and joints.
- Reduces the risk of falling in older people.
- Improves your sleep.
- Enhances flexibility and balance.
- Relieves arthritis pain.
- Results in fewer hospitalizations, doctor visits, and medications.

Exercising to prevent heart attack and stroke

Over the past three decades, the United States has seen a steady decline in the death toll from heart disease and stroke. Despite this decline, heart disease remains the leading cause of death, and stroke the third leading cause of death, in both women and men in this country. Lifestyle improvements and better control of the risk factors for heart disease and stroke have been major factors in this decline to date. Many of the risk factors for heart disease—such as smoking, high blood pressure, unfavorable blood cholesterol levels, obesity, type 2 diabetes, and physical inactivity—can be reversed or controlled by adopting a healthy lifestyle. In fact, the United States has seen positive changes in the national trends for smoking, high blood pressure, and abnormal blood cholesterol, but obesity and physical inactivity are getting worse as physical activity at work and home continues to decline sharply. These recent trends of more obesity and less physical activity appear to be reversing the decades-long trend of reductions in heart disease and stroke rates.

Exercise can help prevent heart disease and stroke in a number of important ways. Physical activity can help lower your chances of having a heart attack by:

- Boosting your levels of HDL, the good cholesterol.
- Helping you lose excess fat or maintain a healthy weight.
- Lowering your blood pressure.
- Improving the ability of your cells to respond to insulin, reducing your risk for type 2 diabetes.

- Reducing the risk for blood clots.
- Increasing your heart's ability to pump more blood with less effort.
- Improving your circulation by increasing blood flow to the heart.
- Increasing your overall fitness level.
- Moderating stress, a possible risk factor for heart disease.

If you already have heart disease, you can still benefit greatly from an exercise program—especially if you combine it with a heart-healthy diet and stress-reduction activities. Physical activity is also important in the treatment of people who have high blood pressure, chest pain, a prior heart attack, nerve disease, and even heart failure (see page 230). Cardiac rehabilitation programs that combine physical activity with a reduction in other risk factors have shown that it is possible to actually reverse some forms of heart disease.

Exercising to prevent cancer

There's strong evidence that physical activity helps lessen the risk of cancers of the colon and the breast. Several studies have also reported links between exercise and a reduced risk of prostate, lung, and endometrial (lining of the uterus) cancers. Here's how exercise seems to fight the different forms of cancer:

COLON CANCER

Physical activity may help to prevent the development of colon cancer. Activity helps maintain regular bowel movements, which lessens the time the colon is exposed to potentially cancer-causing substances in stool. Exercise also seems to have a positive impact on the immune system and on inflammation in the body, two factors that may affect colon cancer risk.

BREAST CANCER

Physically active women seem to have a lower risk of developing breast cancer compared with women who are inactive. Physical activity causes changes in hormone levels, body mass, and immune function that may help prevent tumor development.

PROSTATE CANCER

Inactive men have higher rates of prostate cancer than men who are very physically active. While men who are active have a reduced risk for prostate cancer, doctors don't yet know the exact biological mechanisms that explain this connection.

LUNG CANCER

A few studies have found higher rates of lung cancer among people who are physically inactive compared with those who are active, even after accounting for smoking. The relationship between exercise and lung cancer risk is less clear for women than it is for men. Investigators think that improvements in lung function and air exchange in active people may explain how physical activity helps lower the risk for lung cancer.

ENDOMETRIAL CANCER

Women who are inactive have higher rates of endometrial cancer compared with physically active women. Increases in body weight and corresponding changes in levels of sex hormones such as estrogen, brought about by a lack of exercise, appear to be the primary explanations for the link between inactivity and endometrial cancer.

Exercising to prevent type 2 diabetes

Type 2 diabetes affects more than 20 million people in the United States, accounting for 95 percent of all diabetes cases. (Type 1 diabetes is much less common.) Type 2 diabetes is a major risk factor for heart disease and stroke. Most common in adults over age 40, type 2 diabetes affects 8 percent of the U.S. population age 20 and older. It is strongly linked to obesity (more than 80 percent of people with type 2 diabetes are overweight), inactivity, and a family history of type 2 diabetes. Hispanics and African Americans have an exceptionally high risk for the disease. The prevalence of type 2 diabetes has tripled in the last 30 years, and much of the increase is due to the dramatic upsurge in inactivity and obesity.

If you exercise regularly, you can prevent or delay the development of type 2 diabetes in a number of ways. Regular exercise helps your cells use the sugar circulating in your bloodstream (glucose) more efficiently by making the cells more sensitive to the hormone insulin. Insulin enables cells to take in and use glucose for energy. If you both exercise and lose weight, you will improve your cells' sensitivity even more. But that's not the whole story. Physical activity also helps to reduce your risk for type 2 diabetes by reducing body fat, especially in the abdominal area.

Exercising to prevent osteoporosis

Osteoporosis is characterized by a low level of calcium and minerals in the bones. This condition sets the stage for bone fragility, resulting in an increased risk for fractures, especially after a fall. Both men and women can develop osteoporosis, but the disorder is much more common in women, primarily after menopause.

Bone is living tissue that responds to exercise by becoming stronger. People who exercise regularly generally achieve greater bone mass (bone density and strength) than those who don't. Bone mass peaks during your 30s. After that time, most people begin to lose bone. In women, this bone loss accelerates after menopause. If you are over the age of 20, you can help prevent bone loss with regular exercise. Even if you already have osteoporosis, you can minimize any further bone loss with weight-bearing exercise.

Weight-bearing exercise is good for your bones because it puts an extra workload on the bones, making them stronger. Examples of weight-bearing exercises include walking, hiking, jogging, climbing stairs, playing tennis, dancing, and lifting weights. Examples of exercises that are not weight-bearing are swimming and bicycling. While swimming and bicycling help build and maintain strong muscles and have excellent benefits for your heart, they are not the best ways to strengthen and maintain your bones.

Strength training (see page 52) two to three times per week is an excellent way to keep your bones strong. Make the exercise more taxing by slowly adding more weight or doing more repetitions over time. Work on all of the muscles in your arms, chest, shoulders, legs, abdomen, and back to make the bones attached to those muscles stronger.

Exercising to prevent Alzheimer's disease

You've probably read or heard about studies showing that mental exercises—like doing crossword puzzles or learning a new skill or language—may prevent the mind-shattering effects of Alzheimer's disease. Physical exercise might also have a protective effect. Regular physical activity is linked to a lower risk for dementia (loss of intellectual function that interferes with the activities of daily life) and Alzheimer's disease.

Encouraging studies have been conducted in nursing home residents who already have Alzheimer's. After a year of exercise, their mental condition showed a slower-than-usual decline. Physical activity also lessened the frequency of unwanted common Alzheimer's behaviors such as wandering, pulling at clothing, making repetitive noises, and swearing. Exercise also enhanced residents' communication and social participation.

Doctors are unsure how the underlying mechanism works, but studies have found that animals who exercise regularly have fewer amyloid plaques (the abnormal collections of dead and dying nerve cells and protein fragments that characterize the brains of Alzheimer's patients at autopsy) than animals who are inactive.

An epidemic of inactivity

In spite of the health advantages that exercise provides, inactivity is widespread in the United States and increasing. More than 60 percent of American adults fail to get the recommended amount of regular physical activity—and 25 percent of all adults are completely inactive. Inactivity generally increases with age, is more common among women than men, and is more prevalent among people with a low income and less education than those with a high income or education.

Only one in four American adults performs vigorous, leisure-time physical activity lasting 10 minutes or more at least three times a week. An additional one third of adults are not active enough to receive any health benefits. Of young people ages 12 to 21, only one out of four engages in light to moderate activity, such as walking or bicycling nearly every day. About half regularly engage in vigorous exercise, but 25 percent report no vigorous physical activity. Half of all high school students don't have to take physical education classes.

To add to this trend, few occupations provide opportunities for physical exertion. A hundred years ago, men and women labored physically to earn their living, often from sunup to sundown, but such extreme physical work has declined markedly from that time. Calorie requirements (the amount of calories you need to balance your daily exertion and maintain a stable weight) started to fall during the Industrial Revolution. By the end of World War II, more and more labor-saving devices rolled off factory assembly lines to meet the demands of a more prosperous population that could afford to buy the machines.

Today the labor-saving devices that have freed us from labor-intensive work—such as our telephone, our TV, and our computer—have brought unintended health consequences. Most of the time, when we work, we sit. And when it's time to relax, we sit again—in front of the TV, at the movies, or at a restaurant. The resulting lack of exercise triggers the very processes that cause the most common chronic diseases: overweight and obesity, heart disease, high blood pressure, type 2 diabetes, and osteoporosis.

A sedentary lifestyle, combined with the profusion and easy availability of inexpensive, calorie-dense food, is directly responsible for the rapidly rising rates of obesity in this country. Many people eat more calories than they expend in physical activity. Doctors refer to this disparity as an energy imbalance. Evolution equipped the human body to efficiently survive famines and to thrive when adequate food supplies became available. But evolution never prepared us for a time like this—when we generally expend low levels of energy in our daily life and food is abundant, convenient, and often tempting. It's hard to turn down a second helping at a meal or a luscious dessert. In response, our efficient body stores all those extra calories as fat for a future time when food is scarce and our body needs to burn the stored fat for energy. But that time never comes, and the excess calories continue to accumulate, and we get fatter and fatter.

The three types of exercise

Exercise falls into three categories—aerobic, strength training, and flexibility—and each type provides different health benefits. Aerobic exercise strengthens your heart, while strength training builds muscle and bone. Flexibility exercises increase the range of motion of your joints. An ideal exercise regimen includes all three to ensure total fitness.

Aerobic exercise

Aerobic exercise is any type of activity that uses the large muscles of the arms and legs in a continuous and rhythmic fashion. Aerobic fitness is also called cardiovascular fitness because it improves the ability of the heart, blood vessels, and lungs to supply oxygen and fuel to the body during continuous physical activity.

Aerobic activities make your cardiovascular system stronger, lowering your risk of heart disease and high blood pressure. Regular aerobic exercise also increases your endurance, enabling you to go farther and sustain the activity longer. The following activities give you the heart-strengthening, cancer-checking benefits of aerobic exercise, and most also help build strong bones:

- Walking
- Running
- Jogging
- Bike riding
- Cross-country skiing
- Water aerobics
- Swimming
- Dancing
- Stair climbing
- Elliptical training
- Rowing
- In-line skating
- Skipping rope

✓ Drink plenty of water

Vigorous exercise can deplete your body's supply of fluids because of the water loss from breathing and perspiration, especially in hot or humid weather. Drink water before you exercise, during your workout, and for about two hours afterward. Drinking water is the best way to quench your thirst. Sports drinks can replace the electrolytes lost during vigorous exercise, but most sports drinks contain lots of sugar. If you do only moderate exercise, such as walking, stick with water. Otherwise, you might just drink back all of the calories you burned during your exercise.

Do aerobic activities at a moderate pace at first, so you can keep going longer and won't get discouraged. A good rule of thumb is that you should try to achieve a level of exercise that is at least brisk enough for you to break a light sweat, but not so vigorous that you are breathless; you should still be able to carry on a conversation. Try to exercise enough to reach your target heart rate (see page 64) and then keep it there for at least 20 minutes after a warm-up period. Build up your exercise time gradually. Once you get in shape, your session could last from 30 to 60 minutes depending on the type of exercise you are doing and how briskly you do it. For example, jogging requires more energy than a brisk walk, so jogging will take less time than walking to achieve the same conditioning effect. But try to work up to a total of 60 full minutes of exercise each day. The bottom line: If you are doing nothing, do something; if you are doing something, do more.

After exercising within your target heart rate zone, slow down gradually. For example, swim more slowly or change to a more leisurely stroke. You can also cool down by changing to a less vigorous exercise, such as from running to walking. This slowed pace allows your body to readjust gradually. Stopping abruptly could cause dizziness and other problems. When you exercise, the rhythmic motion of the muscles "milks" the veins, improving blood return to the heart. If you stop abruptly, blood can pool in your extremities (where the arteries and veins are widened to supply more blood to the muscles), reducing blood return to the heart and possibly leading to lowered blood pressure, which can cause dizziness.

HOW YOUR BODY ADJUSTS TO AEROBIC ACTIVITY

During aerobic exercise, your body goes through many changes to adjust to the increased need for oxygen and energy. Here are some of the adjustments your body has to make to sustain aerobic activity:

- Faster, deeper breathing to allow you to take in more oxygen
- An increased heart rate to propel blood faster from your lungs to your muscles and back
- Widening of the small blood vessels (capillaries) to enable oxygen to get to the muscles and waste products to be removed faster. As you increase your exercise, more capillaries form in your muscles to streamline oxygen transport and waste removal.
- A higher body temperature, to enable your body to discharge heat as you exhale and release heat, water, and minerals as you perspire
- The release of brain chemicals called endorphins that trigger positive moods and soothe pain

AEROBIC ACTIVITY WARDS OFF HEALTH PROBLEMS

Performing aerobic exercise regularly can help you avoid or manage some serious medical conditions. It can also make you feel better, both physically and emotionally. But keep in mind that the benefits of aerobic exercise do not stay with you if you don't keep it up. The longer you have

Exercise may improve Parkinson's disease

Regular exercise when you're young may help protect your brain against the kind of cell damage that causes Parkinson's disease. Exercise seems to trigger certain brain cells to discharge chemicals called neurotrophic factors, which help brain cells fight damage from Parkinson's. Regular physical activity may also slow the progression of the disease in people who already have it by somehow repairing or counteracting the damage.

been exercising, the more slowly you will lose your conditioning if you stop exercising for a period of time.

Heart disease

Aerobic exercise improves blood cholesterol levels, reducing the risk for heart disease. It also makes your heart a more efficient pump and helps you avoid weight gain. If you've already had a heart attack, aerobic activity can reduce your risk of having a second one.

High blood pressure

Aerobic exercise can help reduce blood pressure. Regular aerobic exercise such as brisk walking, done over several months, can lower blood pressure by about 10 points—enough to normalize blood pressure in some people.

Unfavorable cholesterol levels

Exercise can improve your cholesterol profile by lowering your total cholesterol level, raising good HDL cholesterol, and lowering bad LDL cholesterol in the blood. It also improves your body's ability to clear triglycerides (potentially harmful blood fats) from the blood more quickly.

Stroke

More favorable blood pressure and cholesterol levels translate into less buildup of plaque in the walls of the arteries. The less the buildup of fatty deposits in the blood vessels that lead to the brain, the lower the risk for stroke.

Type 2 diabetes

By enabling you to keep down your weight, aerobic exercise cuts your chances of becoming overweight or obese, key causes of type 2 diabetes. Exercise also reduces your risk for type 2 diabetes by making your cells more sensitive to the effects of insulin.

Infections

Aerobic exercise seems to improve the immune system's ability to fight infection. People who engage in regular physical activity are less vulnerable to the viruses that cause colds, the flu, and other common infections.

Depression

Aerobic exercise performed on a regular basis can lessen the symptoms of depression, anxiety, and other mood disorders.

Osteoporosis

Walking, jogging, and other weight-bearing aerobic exercises help prevent the bone thinning that leads to osteoporosis. Reducing your risk of osteoporosis lowers your risk for fractures—the main cause of loss of independence in older people.

Strength training

Exercises that build muscle go by a variety of names, including strength training, resistance training, weight training, or weight lifting. Strengthening exercises are safe and effective ways of building muscle mass for people of all ages, including those who are not in perfect health. In fact, people with health conditions—including heart disease or arthritis—often benefit the most from an exercise program that includes lifting weights a few times each week. Strength training, as a supplement to regular aerobic exercise, can also have a positive impact on your mental and emotional health.

THE HEALTH BENEFITS OF STRENGTH TRAINING

You will gain a wealth of benefits when you do strengthening exercises regularly, especially as you grow older. It is also a powerful way to cope with and reduce the symptoms of many chronic conditions, including arthritis, diabetes, osteoporosis, obesity, and depression.

Strengthening exercises, when done correctly, augment your flexibility and balance, which lowers your chances of falling. Strength training also increases bone density and reduces the risk for fractures, important considerations for older people, especially women after menopause, who can lose 1 to 2 percent of their bone mass every year in the first years after menopause.

Strength training can be helpful for weight control, because people who have more muscle mass have a higher metabolic rate. If your body has more muscle, it burns calories more quickly. Muscle consumes calories when you are active, while stored fat uses very few calories. An increased metabolic rate is helpful for both weight loss and long-term weight control.

Strength training is also beneficial for people with type 2 diabetes. Just 16 weeks of strength training can bring dramatic improvements in blood sugar control—improvements comparable to taking diabetes medication. People with diabetes who do strength training gain muscle and strength, lose body fat, and are less likely to experience depression than those who avoid strengthening exercise.

Strength training is vital for heart health because heart disease risk is lower when your body is leaner. People who already have heart disease gain not only strength and flexibility but also aerobic capacity when they perform strength training three times a week as part of their cardiac rehabilitation program. Many doctors recommend strength training as a way to reduce the risk for heart disease and as a therapy for patients in cardiac rehabilitation programs.

And don't believe anyone who tells you that you can't boost your muscle size and strength as you age. In fact, scientists have found that nursing home residents in their late 80s and early 90s are able to triple their strength and increase the size of their muscles by 10 percent in just eight weeks with strength training. The take-home message: A good deal of the muscle loss seen with aging can be prevented and even reversed. The research showed little difference between building old muscle and building young muscle. You may need to work your older muscles more slowly and carefully, but the outcome is the same—more strength, which translates into more independence as you get older.

GETTING STARTED WITH WEIGHTS

When you're just starting out on strengthening exercises, use a low-weight dumbbell or machine weight to determine what load you can handle comfortably and safely. You can also use tubing and elastic bands for strength training, or work against your body to build muscle mass by doing push-ups, leg lifts, and pull-ups. The following guidelines will help you gauge your exercise intensity so you can see whether you are using the correct amount of weight and doing the right number of repetitions. Complete each repetition by counting to two when raising the weights and counting to four when bringing them down.

- Were you able to complete 2 sets of 10 repetitions without too much strain?

  No: Reduce the weight to an amount that you can lift 10 times; rest for one or two minutes, then repeat for a second set.

  Yes: Continue to the next question.

- After completing 10 repetitions, do you need to rest because the weight is too heavy to complete more repetitions?

  Yes: You are working at the proper intensity and should not increase the weight.

  No: Continue to the next two questions to find out how to safely increase the intensity of your workout.

- Could you have done a few more repetitions without a break?

  Yes: If you can do only a few more repetitions (not the entire next set of 10) without a break, then at your next workout, do the first set of repetitions using your current weight and the second set using the next weight up. For example, if you're currently using 1-pound dumbbells, use 2- or 3-pound dumbbells for your second set.

- Could you have done all 20 repetitions at one time, without a break?

  Yes: At your next session, use heavier dumbbells for both sets of repetitions.

After the first week or so of strength training, start doing each exercise with weights that you can lift at least 10 times with only a little difficulty. If a given exercise seems too difficult—if you can't do at least 8 repetitions—then the weight you're using is too heavy and you need to scale back.

After two weeks of doing your strength-training routine, evaluate the difficulty of each exercise with your current level of weights. By the end of the second week, the exercises may feel too easy. For instance, you may be able to easily lift a 5-pound dumbbell more than 12 times. You can now step up your weights to 6- or 7-pound dumbbells and see how the exercise feels at the new weight level.

It's important to adhere to your strength-training regimen as much as you can. You may find yourself making a few false starts before you succeed at making the program a regular part of your life. There may be times when interruptions, such as vacation, illness, or family or work demands, conspire to prevent you from doing your strength-training exercises for a week or two—or even longer. Try not to feel guilty or disappointed in yourself. Just resume your routine as quickly as you can. You may not be able to pick up exactly where you left off—you may need to decrease your weights a bit—but stay with it, and you will regain the lost ground.

It is very important to breathe properly during weight-lifting. Never hold your breath and bear down. This can have adverse effects on your heart and blood vessels. Also, hernias (bulges of soft tissue through weak areas in muscle walls) can result from straining. Try to breathe out as you lift or press against resistance, and breathe in as you lower the weight or return to your starting point.

STRENGTHENING EXERCISES

The popularity of programs such as Pilates has focused attention on the body's core, the muscles in the abdomen, back, and pelvis. These muscles make up the body's center of gravity when you stand, lift, and walk. The midsection is an area that often comes to mind when we think of "letting yourself go." But strengthening your core is worth the extra effort: it can improve your posture, provide support for your spine, and make you stronger and leaner. Core strengthening is a strength-training exercise that can also help you avoid that midsection spread.

In addition to taking up Pilates classes, you can strengthen your core muscles by performing exercises at home, perhaps with a fitness ball. Choose a fitness ball that's the correct size for your height. Balls come in different diameters; ask an expert which size is best for you. Most people start out with a 55- or 65-centimeter ball. Softer balls seem to make the exercises a little easier, so pick a relatively soft ball to start. The key to exercise ball workouts is keeping your balance while on the ball.

On the next two pages are some basic strengthening exercises. These exercises build muscle by forcing the muscles to work against the weight of your body. It's a good idea to alternate strength-building exercises with aerobic exercise. Try to do the following exercises three or four times a week. Try to do each one 5 times and then gradually build up to 10 to 15 repetitions as you get stronger.

Strengthening Exercises

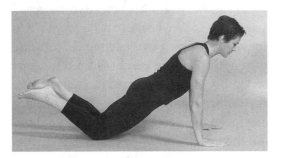 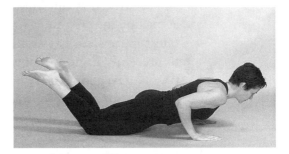

Modified push-up

Get on your hands and knees on the floor and shift your weight forward, with your hands aligned under your shoulders and your feet raised off the floor (left). Bending your elbows, lower your body from the knees up until your chest almost touches the floor, keeping your hands in the same position on the floor and using your abdominal muscles to keep your back straight (right). Still keeping your back straight, push up until your arms are almost straight (but not locked) at the elbows. Repeat as many times as you can without straining. (For an extra challenge, try holding each position for a few seconds.)

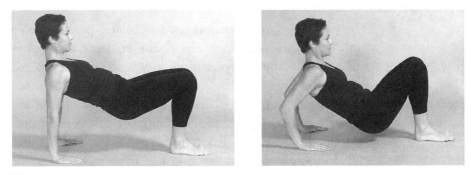

Triceps press

Sit on the floor with your knees bent at a 45-degree angle, your feet flat on the floor, hip-distance apart, and your hands on the floor behind you, fingertips pointing forward. Lift your hips off the floor (left). Bending at the elbows, lower your bottom until it almost touches the floor (right), hold for a count of five, and straighten the arms, returning to your starting hips-up position.

Abdominal curl

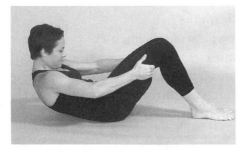

Lie on your back with your knees bent and your arms holding the backs of your thighs. Press the small of your back into the floor as you lift your head and upper body until most of your upper back is off the floor. Hold for a count of two. Lower your body to the floor, keeping the small of your back pressed to the floor (to work your abdominal muscles and avoid straining your back). As your strength increases, increase the number of repetitions. A more difficult way to do sit-ups is with your arms over your chest, hands on the shoulders, or with your hands placed lightly behind your neck.

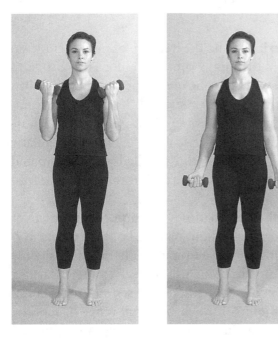

Biceps curl

Standing with your back straight, your knees bent slightly, and your feet slightly apart, hold two hand weights (start with 1- or 2-pound weights) up to your shoulders, with your elbows bent up at your sides (left). Slowly bring the weights down to your thighs, palms facing forward (right). Slowly raise the weights back up to your shoulders, keeping your elbows at your sides. When you can repeat the exercise 12 times, increase the weights by 1 pound.

Pump-up

Standing with your back straight, knees bent slightly and feet slightly apart, hold two hand weights (with ends close to or touching each other) at chest level, elbows bent out to the sides parallel to the floor and shoulders down (left). Lower the weights slowly to thigh level, keeping the ends of the weights close together (right). Slowly raise the weights back up to your chest. When you can repeat the exercise 12 times, increase the weights by 1 pound.

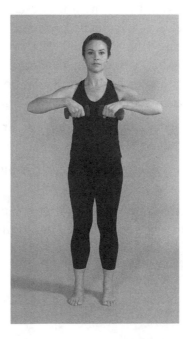

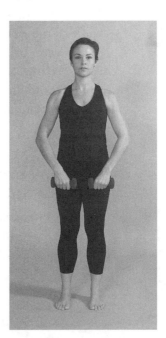

Flexibility exercises

Stretching exercises give you flexibility and the freedom of movement to do the things you need to do—and the things you like to do. They also keep your joints healthy. Stretching exercises alone may improve your flexibility, but they will not improve your endurance or strength. You have to do aerobic exercise to boost your endurance and strength training to build muscle mass for greater strength. Stretch before and after you do your regularly scheduled strength and aerobic exercises—this is called warming up and cooling down. For best results, stretch at least three times a week, for at least 20 minutes each session.

Do each stretching exercise three to five times a session. Slowly reach for the correct position, as far as possible without pain. Relax, then repeat, trying to stretch farther. Stretching should never hurt. It may feel slightly uncomfortable, but not painful. You need to push yourself to stretch farther, but not so far that it hurts. Do your stretching exercises on both sides of your body and try to put your joints through their full range of motion. Never bounce during a stretch, because you could easily hurt yourself. Breathe deeply and slowly in through your nose and out through your mouth. Deep, slow breathing will help you de-stress.

Taking yoga or Pilates classes or stretching along with a video are excellent ways to extend and tone your muscles and limber up your joints. Doing simple stretches of your arms, back, and legs in the morning is also a good way to increase your flexibility. The key muscles to stretch are the hamstrings in the backs of the thighs and the muscles in the lower back and shoulders. Follow these recommendations for getting the most benefit out of your stretching and reducing the risk for injury:

- If you feel pain, ease up on your stretch. Pain is a sign that you have extended too far.
- Stretch slowly and smoothly to avoid muscle injury. Don't bounce or jerk.
- Stretch as far as you comfortably can and hold your stretch for 30 seconds to give your muscles and joints the full benefits of the stretch.

Flexibility Exercises

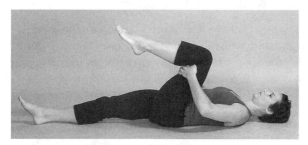

Lower back and buttocks stretch

Lie on your back on the floor with one leg stretched out straight and the other leg bent up. Pressing your lower back gently to the floor, reach behind the thigh of the bent leg and pull it slowly toward your chest. Maintain the position for at least 30 seconds and release. Repeat with the other leg.

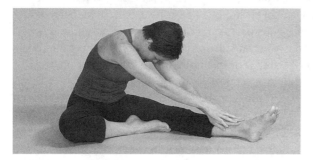

Hamstring stretch

Sit with one leg extended in front of you and the other leg bent. Reach forward with both hands along your extended leg as far as it feels comfortable. Bend from your hips, keeping your back straight. Maintain the position for at least 30 seconds. Repeat with the other leg.

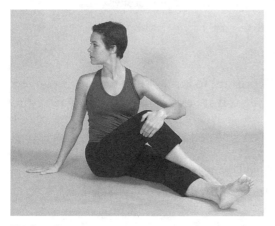

Back twist

Sit up with your legs out in front of you on the floor. Cross one leg over the other with your knee bent and foot flat on the floor. Keeping your back straight and buttocks on the floor, take hold of the bent knee with the opposite hand and gently turn to bent-knee side, rotating your hips and looking over your shoulder. Maintain the stretch for at least 30 seconds. Repeat on the other side.

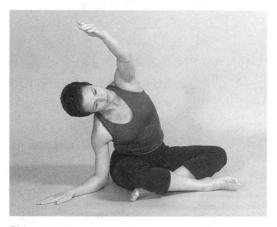

Side stretch

Sit cross-legged on the floor. Inhale and raise one arm to the ceiling and, exhaling, bend from the waist to the opposite side, sliding the other hand along the floor and keeping your buttocks on the floor. Maintain the stretch for at least 30 seconds. Inhale as you return to the center, dropping your raised arm and lifting the other arm and repeating the bend to the other side.

THE BENEFITS OF CROSS-TRAINING

Cross-training is a technique that enables you to fight boredom while gaining extra benefits from your fitness program. Cross-training is performing two or more different types of exercise—either in one workout or alternately in consecutive sessions. If you walk or jog, for example, you could also lift weights twice a week or take a yoga class. You can engage in more than one type of aerobic exercise—bike riding and walking, or swimming and stair climbing, for example—to vary your workouts even more. Bringing variety into your exercise sessions can help keep you motivated.

No single type of physical activity can provide all the health benefits gained from exercise. For example, aerobic exercise enhances heart health because of the sustained use of large-muscle groups. But aerobic activity doesn't necessarily help develop muscle mass, especially in the upper body. On the other hand, weight training builds muscle mass, but doesn't necessarily improve joint flexibility. Only a combination of the different types of exercise can give you the optimal, all-around fitness your body needs.

Cross-training helps make your entire body stronger, not just your legs or arms. Cross-training also lowers your risk for injury by spreading out the impact of activity over various parts of your body. If you do get injured, you can still exercise while avoiding the injured area. For example, if you injure your ankle or knee, you may still be able to swim.

You can do a different type of exercise each day or have fun with more than one on the same day. If you decide to do different types of exercise on the same day, try changing the order in which you do them from day to day to ward off monotony.

WHEN TO STOP EXERCISING

Exercise is good for you but it's important to know when to stop. If you feel any of the following symptoms while you are exercising, stop right away and see your doctor:

- Chest pain or pressure
- Irregular, rapid, or fluttery heartbeat
- Severe or unexpected shortness of breath
- Dizziness or faintness
- Sudden onset of change in vision, weakness in one arm or one leg, speech difficulty, or confusion

If you have any of the following conditions, you should temporarily suspend your exercise program, or at least cut back until you feel better, and then resume your exercise gradually:

- Significant infections, such as pneumonia

- Fever, which can cause dehydration and a rapid heartbeat
- Foot or ankle sores that won't heal
- Joint swelling
- Recent eye surgery

How long, how often, and how hard?

Once you decide to take the exercise challenge, consider three factors that make up the backbone of any good exercise program: frequency, duration, and intensity. The bottom line is: If you're doing nothing, do something. If you're already exercising, do more—exercise for longer periods and at greater intensity.

If you have been inactive or if you are overweight, start out slowly. The best approach is to start with light or moderate activity—such as walking,

---

A DOZEN EASY WAYS TO STAY FIT

Exercise can add a spring to your step—and maybe even years to your life. Take the following actions to make regular exercise a part of your life so you can stay fit and enjoy yourself while doing it.

Follow the 10,000 Steps Program (see page 74).

Start lifting weights.

Take a yoga class.

Walk for 30 minutes every day.

Swim daily at the local community center.

Play actively with your kids.

Take the stairs instead of the elevator, especially if you are only going up or down a couple of floors.

Work out to an exercise DVD.

Walk through the local mall in the winter.

Strengthen your core with Pilates exercises.

Sign up for an aerobics class at the community center or gym.

Work with a personal trainer to establish a weight-training routine.

biking, swimming, or following an exercise DVD—that uses the large muscle groups in the legs. Gradually increase the duration of the activity first. Once you are exercising more than 30 minutes a day, keep increasing the duration of your activity, but also gradually increase the intensity of the activity. Mixing in some light weights adds value once your heart and lungs are fit. The key is to get moving—and be more physically active than you already are.

Frequency

Exercising regularly is one of the most important aspects of any exercise program. Frequency refers to the number of times each week that you perform a given activity. Ideally, you need to do something aerobic (see page 49) every day. If you don't exercise daily, you won't get all of the benefits of regular physical activity and you won't get stronger or build your endurance or improve your fitness. Of course, if you're just starting to exercise after being sedentary for a long time, start with just slow walking, three times a week. Try to spread your exercise sessions throughout the day to maximize the benefits, especially if you don't have time for one long workout.

Once you have been exercising three times a week for a few weeks, try to include another exercise day in the week, and then another. Gradually work up to daily exercise. Of course, there will be days when you're not feeling up to exercising or the weather is bad, but your overall goal should be to get at least half an hour of exercise every day.

Whenever you miss more than a week of exercising, you may need to restart at a level lower than where you were when you stopped. If you miss a few sessions because of a minor illness such as a cold, wait until you feel better before you start exercising again. After a minor injury, wait until the pain goes away to start up again. Resume your exercising at one half to two thirds your normal level, depending on the number of days you missed and how you feel while you're exercising.

Whatever your reasons for missing the exercise sessions, don't worry about the missed days. Just get back into your routine and think about the progress you'll be making toward your overall fitness goal. When it comes to strength training (see page 52), one to two days a week is enough for the muscles in your trunk, but the muscles in your arms and legs require three to five sessions per week for optimal results. Allow a day between weight-training sessions to let your muscles rest.

TIPS FOR A SAFE AND EFFECTIVE EXERCISE PROGRAM

The following tips can help you get the most out of your exercise program.

Check with your doctor. If you have a chronic health problem such as obesity, diabetes, heart disease, or high blood pressure, ask your doctor to recommend the types of physical activities that are right for you.

Start slowly. Fit more physical activity into your daily routine and gradually work up to the 60-minute daily goal to improve your health and manage your weight.

Set goals. Set short- and long-term goals and celebrate each success.

Track your progress. Keep an activity log to monitor your progress. Write down when you worked out, what activity you did, for how long you did it, and how you felt during the workout.

Think variety. Choose a variety of physical activities to help you meet your goals, avoid boredom, and keep your body and mind challenged.

Be comfortable. Wear comfortable shoes and clothes—ones that are right for the activity and the conditions.

Listen to your body. Stop exercising and call your doctor if you experience any pain (especially chest discomfort or pain), dizziness, severe headache, or other unusual symptoms while you work out. If the symptoms do not go away, get medical help right away. If you are feeling fatigued or sick, take time off from your routine to rest. You can ease back into your exercise program when you start feeling better.

Eat a healthy diet. Choose a variety of nutritious foods every day. Your health and weight depend not only on your exercise regimen, but also on the fuel you put into your body.

Get support. Ask your family and friends to support you or join you in your activity. Form walking groups with coworkers, play with your children outside, or take a dance class with your partner or friends.

Duration

How long should you exercise? That depends on your age, your fitness level, and the intensity of your exercise. If you are inactive now, you should begin slowly with a 10- to 15-minute walk or other short session, three times a week. As you become more fit, you can do longer sessions or more frequent short sessions. But for most people, the current recommendation still stands: accumulate at least an hour of exercise on most, if not all, days of the week.

But you don't have to accomplish this goal in one long session. You can have multiple 10- or 15-minute workout sessions throughout the day. Make the most of those 15 minutes whenever you can. Try climbing 10 flights of stairs at work, walking for 10 or 20 minutes at lunch, and swimming for half an hour after work. There are a variety of ways to accumulate your 60 minutes in short bursts of exercise every day—walk the dog a couple of times a day, pull the kids around the block a few times in a wagon or sled, lift weights for 10 or 15 minutes, or work out with an exercise video for a few minutes.

Intensity: The target heart rate

When you first start exercising, it's important to exercise at a comfortable pace. For example, when jogging or walking briskly you should be able to keep up a conversation comfortably. If you don't feel back to normal within 10 minutes of stopping exercise, you're pushing yourself too much. Labored breathing or prolonged weakness during or after exercising means that you are exercising too hard, so you need to cut back.

How intense should your workout be? The best way to find out is to use your heart rate. Your maximum heart rate is the fastest your heart can beat. There are several formulas for calculating maximum heart rate, but the simplest is to subtract your age in years from 220. If you are 30 years old, for example, your maximum heart rate is 190 beats per minute; if you are 60 years old, your maximum heart rate is 160 beats per minute. Exercise above 75 percent of your maximum heart rate may be too strenuous unless you are in excellent physical condition. Exercise below 50 percent gives your heart and lungs little conditioning. Therefore, the best activity level is 50 to 75 percent of your maximum rate. This 50 to 75 percent range is called your target heart rate zone. The desired level of intensity for an exercise should be between 55 and 75 percent of your maximum heart rate (up to 90 percent if you are a highly trained athlete).

When you begin your exercise program, aim for the lower part of your target zone (50 percent) during the first few months. As you get into better shape, gradually build up to the higher level of your target zone (75 percent). After six months or more of regular exercise, you can exercise at up to 85 percent of your maximum heart rate if you want. But you don't have to exercise that hard to stay in good condition.

To find your target zone, look for the age category closest to your own age in the table below and read the line across from it. For example, if you are 30, your target zone is 95 to 142 beats per minute. If you are 43, the closest age to yours on the chart is 45. Your target zone is 88 to 131 beats per minute.

Target heart rate

Age	Target Heart Rate Zone 50–75%	Average Maximum Heart Rate 100%
20 years	100–150 beats per min	200 beats per min
25 years	98–146 beats per min	195 beats per min
30 years	95–142 beats per min	190 beats per min
35 years	93–138 beats per min	185 beats per min
40 years	90–135 beats per min	180 beats per min
45 years	88–131 beats per min	175 beats per min
50 years	85–127 beats per min	170 beats per min
55 years	83–123 beats per min	165 beats per min
60 years	80–120 beats per min	160 beats per min
65 years	78–116 beats per min	155 beats per min
70 years	75–113 beats per min	150 beats per min

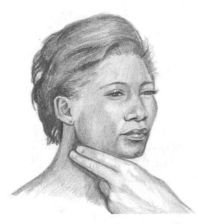

To see if you are staying within your target heart rate zone, take your pulse right after you stop exercising. Here's how to do it:

- When you stop exercising, quickly place the tips of your first two fingers lightly over one of the blood vessels on your neck located to the left or right of your Adam's apple.

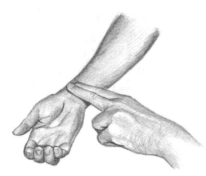

- Another readily accessible pulse spot is on the inside of your wrist, just below the base of your thumb.

- Count your pulse for 10 seconds and multiply the number by six to get the number of beats per minute.

- If your pulse falls within your target zone, you're doing fine. If it is below your target zone, exercise a little harder next time. And if you're above your target zone, exercise a little less strenuously. Don't try to exercise at your maximum heart rate—you'd be working too hard.

- Once you're exercising within your target zone, check your pulse at least once each week during the first three months and once in a while after that.

Some people find that exercising within their target zone seems too strenuous. If you start out lower, that's okay, too. You will find that with time you'll become more comfortable exercising and can increase into your target zone at your own rate. Once you reach a moderate level of fitness, it might be difficult to reach your target heart rate by simply walking, unless you walk at a rate of at least 1 mile in 15 minutes.

Here's another quick way to gauge the level of your exercise intensity: the talk test. The talk test method of measuring exercise intensity is simple. A person who is active at a light intensity level should be able to sing while doing the activity. One who is active at a moderate intensity level should be able to carry on a conversation comfortably while engaging in the activity. If a person becomes winded or too out of breath to carry on a conversation, the activity is considered vigorous.

In general, moderate-intensity physical activity refers to any activity that burns 3½ to 7 calories per minute. These levels equal the effort a healthy person might make while walking briskly, mowing the lawn, dancing, swimming for recreation, or bicycling. Vigorous intensity can be applied to any activity that burns more than 7 calories per minute. Examples of such activities include jogging, doing heavy yard work, performing high-impact aerobic dancing, swimming continuous laps, or bicycling uphill.

Another good strategy is to increase your general activity level in everyday life. Take the stairs instead of the elevator or walk to the grocery store from the farthest parking space you can find instead of searching for the closest spot.

COMPARING THE INTENSITY OF VARIOUS ACTIVITIES

You can perform a moderate amount of physical activity in a number of ways. Be sure to choose activities you enjoy and that fit into your daily life. The amount of activity you perform is determined by the activity's duration, intensity, and frequency, so you can do the same amount of activity in longer sessions of moderately intense activities (such as brisk walking) as you can do in shorter sessions of more strenuous activities (such as running). The list below shows examples of moderate amounts of activity, from those at the top of the list that are minimally vigorous to those toward the bottom of the list that are very vigorous and require less time to get the same effects.

- Washing and waxing a car for 45 to 60 minutes
- Washing windows or floors for 45 to 60 minutes
- Playing volleyball for 45 minutes
- Playing touch football for 30 to 45 minutes
- Gardening for 30 to 45 minutes
- Wheeling self in wheelchair for 30 to 40 minutes

- Walking 1¾ miles in 35 minutes (20 minutes/mile)
- Shooting baskets for 30 minutes
- Bicycling 5 miles in 30 minutes
- Dancing fast (social) for 30 minutes
- Pushing a stroller 1½ miles in 30 minutes
- Raking leaves for 30 minutes
- Walking 2 miles in 30 minutes (15 minutes/mile)
- Doing water aerobics for 30 minutes
- Swimming laps for 20 minutes
- Playing wheelchair basketball for 20 minutes
- Playing basketball (a game) for 15 to 20 minutes
- Bicycling 4 miles in 15 minutes
- Jumping rope for 15 minutes
- Running 1½ miles in 15 minutes (10 minutes/mile)
- Shoveling snow for 15 minutes
- Stair climbing for 15 minutes

Getting started

Before you start an exercise program, check with your doctor to make sure you're healthy enough to exercise, and to find out at what level you should begin. Most doctors agree that walking is the safest and easiest way to start being more active. Walk to more places more often—to the post office or the grocery store, from the farthest parking space at the mall, and up as many stairs as you can find.

Remember that exercise doesn't have to be strenuous to benefit your health. Even moderate exercise, such as walking, can significantly affect your health in many positive ways. Later, when you build up your strength and endurance, you can try more vigorous activities, such as jogging, stair climbing, or rowing.

Each exercise session should include a 5-minute warm-up. Begin exercising slowly to give your body a chance to limber up and get ready for more vigorous exercise. Start at a medium pace and gradually increase it by the end of the 5-minute warm-up period.

If you plan to do highly vigorous activities such as jumping rope, jogging, or stationary bike cycling, warm up for 5 to 10 minutes by jumping rope or jogging slowly, warming up to your target heart rate zone (see page 64). It's a good idea to stretch before your warm-up and after your exercise session. You can find many stretching exercises in running books or online. Below are three stretches you can use before your warm-up and after your cool-down period. Each of these exercises helps stretch different parts of your body. Stretch slowly and steadily, and don't bounce when you stretch.

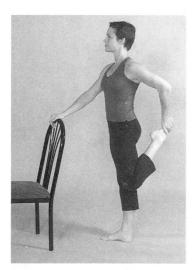

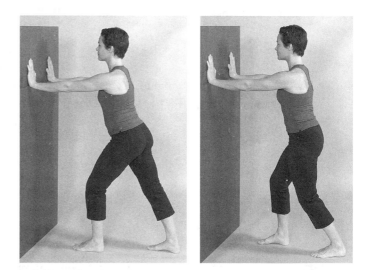

Quadriceps stretch

While standing, hold on to a sturdy chair back, a counter, or a railing with one hand. Bend one leg and, with the hand on that side, pull your foot up gently behind you, keeping your abdominal muscles pulled in and your knees close together. Maintain the position for at least 30 seconds. Repeat with the other leg.

Calf stretch

Stand about 2 to 3 feet from a wall and place your palms on the wall. Step forward with one foot. Keeping both feet flat on the floor and your toes pointing straight ahead, bend the forward leg at the knee and lean forward, keeping your back leg straight (left). Maintain the position for at least 30 seconds. Repeat with the other leg. Now do a set bending rather than straightening the back leg (right); maintain the position for at least 30 seconds.

How to fit exercise into your life

Sure, you're busy. But that's no excuse not to exercise. The key is to build some of it into the things you already do so you don't have to devote a lot of extra time to it. Here are some of the most common obstacles to physical activity and how to overcome them to make exercise a normal part of your life. Write down the top two or three obstacles that you face, and then jot down solutions you think will work for you.

Obstacle

- Between work, family, and other demands, I'm just too busy to exercise.

Solutions

- **Make physical activity a priority.** Carve out some time each week to be active and put it on your calendar. Wake up half an hour earlier to go for a walk, schedule lunchtime workouts, or take an evening fitness class.
- **Build physical activity into your routine chores.** Rake the yard, wash the car, or do energetic housework. That way, you're doing what needs to be done and you're being active at the same time.
- **Make family time physically active.** Plan weekend hikes, family softball games, or after-dinner walks around the block.

Obstacle

- By the end of a long day, I am just too tired to work out.

Solutions

- **Break your workout into three 10-minute segments each day.** Three short walks during the day may be easier to fit in and less tiring than one 30-minute walk, and still provide the health benefits.
- **Find another time during the day to work out.** If evening workouts are not for you, try a bike ride before breakfast or a walk at lunchtime.
- **Sneak physical activity into your days.** Take the stairs instead of the elevator, park farther away in parking lots, and walk in place, lift hand weights, or do mat Pilates exercises while you're watching TV.

Obstacle

- My weight is fine, so why should I exercise?

Solutions

- **Think about the other health benefits.** Regular physical activity can help improve your cholesterol levels and blood pressure. It also reduces your risk of developing heart disease, type 2 diabetes, and some cancers. Overweight people who are active and fit tend to live longer than people who are not overweight but are inactive and unfit. Physical activity can also lift your mood and boost your energy level.
- **Do it just for fun.** Play a team sport, work in the garden, or go for bike rides with your kids to have fun while you're getting fit.
- **Train for a charity event.** This is a good way to help others while you are helping yourself.

Obstacle

- The treadmill and stationary bike have gotten boring.

Solutions

- **Meet a friend for workouts.** If a buddy is on the next bike or treadmill, your workout will be more enjoyable and the time will go faster.
- **Watch TV or listen to music, a book on tape, or a foreign language CD while you walk or pedal indoors.** Check out music or books on DVD from your local library, or trade them with friends.
- **Change the scenery.** A change in scenery can relieve boredom. When the weather is nice, take your workout outdoors. Any change in routine can help respark your enthusiasm.

Obstacle

- I'm afraid I'll get injured.

Solutions

- **Start slowly.** If you are starting a new exercise routine, go slowly at first. Even if you are resuming an activity that you once did well, start up again slowly to make sure you don't get injured.
- **Choose moderate-intensity physical activities.** You're not likely to hurt yourself by walking 30 minutes a day. You can get hurt from

doing vigorous physical activities, however, especially if you're not used to doing them.

- **Take a class.** A knowledgeable group fitness instructor can teach you how to move using the right form, to lower your risk for injury. The instructor can observe your movements and tell you if you're doing them correctly.

- **Work out in the water.** Whether you swim laps or do water aerobics, working out in the water is easy on your joints and helps limit sore muscles and injury.

- **Work with a personal trainer.** A certified personal trainer can show you how to warm up, cool down, use fitness equipment like treadmills and weight-training machines, and use proper form to help you stay injury-free. Personal training sessions may be costly, so find out about fees before making an appointment.

Obstacle

- I'm just not athletic.

Solutions

- **Find a physical activity you enjoy.** You don't have to be an athlete to benefit from physical activity. Think of what you enjoy doing. Try yoga, tai chi, hiking, gardening, biking, or swimming.

- **Choose an activity you'll be able to stick with.** Walking is one of the best exercises you can do. Just put one foot in front of the other, and use the time to relax, talk with a friend, or simply enjoy the scenery.

Obstacle

- I don't want to spend a lot of money to join a gym or buy exercise equipment.

Solutions

- **Choose free activities.** Take your children to the park to play, go for a walk with a friend, or ride your bike to do errands.

- **Find out if your employer offers any discounts on gym memberships.** Some companies get lower membership rates at fitness or community centers or pay for part of an employee's membership fee. More and more employers are providing on-site fitness centers for their workers.

- **Check out your local park district or community center.** These centers often cost less than private gyms, fitness centers, or health clubs.

- **Choose physical activities that don't require any special gear.** Walking requires only a pair of sturdy shoes. To dance, just turn on some music.

Obstacle

- I don't have anyone to watch my kids while I work out.

Solutions

- **Do something physically active with your kids.** Kids need physical activity, too. No matter what age your kids are, find an activity you can do together. Teach them how to dance. Take a walk. Run around the park. Play softball, basketball, volleyball, or soccer together. Go for bike rides.

- **Take turns with other parents.** One of you takes care of the kids while the other one works out. Get together with other families in the neighborhood and start a babysitting co-op.

- **Hire a baby-sitter.** Sometimes you need to make exercise a priority. Consider it an investment in your health and fitness. It's worth it to get some time to yourself.

- **Look for a fitness or community center that offers child care.** Cost and quality vary, so get all the information up front.

Obstacle

- My family and friends are not physically active.

Solutions

- **Don't let that stop you. Do it for yourself.** Enjoy the rewards you get from working out—better sleep, a happier mood, more energy, and a stronger, more fit body.

- **Join a class or sports league where people count on you to show up.** If your teammates or dance partner count on you, you won't want to miss a workout, even if your family and friends are not involved.

Obstacle

- The winter is too cold and the summer is too hot to be active outdoors.

Solutions

- **Walk around the local mall.** You don't have to buy anything. Just window shop as you walk. Be sure to take advantage of any stairs in the mall. You can also walk up and down the escalators.
- **Join a fitness or community center.** Find one that lets you pay only for the months or classes you want, instead of the whole year.
- **Exercise at home.** Work out to fitness videos or DVDs. Check out a different one from the library every week for variety. Use the bottom step of a stairway in your house and improvise your own step class.

Obstacle

- I don't feel safe exercising by myself.

Solutions

- **Join or start a walking group.** You can enjoy added safety and company as you walk.
- **Take an exercise class at a nearby park district or community center.** You'll be with other people who have the same wellness goals.
- **Work out at home.** You don't need a lot of space. Turn on the radio and dance or follow along with a fitness show on TV.

Obstacle

- I have a health problem (or injury) and I don't want to make it worse.

Solutions

- **Talk about it with your doctor.** Exercise actually helps many health problems, including diabetes, heart disease, asthma, and arthritis. If you have an injury or health problem, find out what physical activities you can do safely and follow your doctor's or physical therapist's advice about the length and intensity of your workouts.
- **Start slowly.** Take it easy at first and see how you feel before trying more challenging workouts. Stop if you ever feel out of breath, dizzy, faint, or nauseated, or if you have any pain.

THE 10,000 STEPS PROGRAM

The 10,000 Steps Program began in Japan in the mid 1960s. Alarmed by the rising rates of obesity in his country, Dr. Yoshiro Hatano wondered how many calories a person could burn by walking briskly. His investigations showed that the average person takes between 3,500 and 5,000 steps a day in the course of daily activities. Boosting that tally to 10,000 steps per day should lead to improved health and reduced weight, he theorized. At the same time, Japanese technicians were inventing the pedometer, and the walking craze was born. Pedometer use spread rapidly across Japan as people took to the sidewalks.

Adding 3,000 to 4,000 more steps each day translates into about 30 minutes of additional daily activity, depending on the speed of walking. Working up to 10,000 steps should provide about 15 more minutes of exercise, or 45 minutes in all—a respectable amount. Setting a goal of 10,000 steps a day gives you the option of choosing either minutes per day in activity or steps per day. Just as exercising for longer than 30 minutes a day brings added benefits, so does walking additional steps very day. The more steps you take, the more health benefits you gain.

But if you're sedentary and are just starting a walking program, you should set your sights on an 8,500-step goal at first and then work up to 10,000 steps. The number of steps recommended for children is even higher—about 12,000 steps—because children need more activity than adults and because they are generally more active than adults to begin with.

How far would you have to walk to reach 10,000 steps? Considering that the average person's stride length is about 2½ feet long, you'd have to walk about 2,000 steps to complete 1 mile. This means that 10,000 steps is the equivalent of walking nearly 5 miles a day. That sounds like a lot, but you can accomplish this goal gradually. Try increasing the average number of your daily steps by 500 each day. That's less than a city block. Continue to increase the number of steps or time you walk each week, and you should be averaging 10,000 steps by the end of about 14 weeks.

CHOOSING THE RIGHT EXERCISE EQUIPMENT

Which type of exercise is best? The one you're going to stick with over the long term. For some people, that means working out at home on exercise equipment. If you're considering buying exercise equipment, evaluate advertising claims for fitness products carefully. Be skeptical of claims that you will lose several pounds, inches, or pant sizes in a short time. For example, don't fall for any product that claims it can help you lose "seven inches in seven days." It's impossible for most people to achieve such major changes in appearance in a few days or weeks. When sizing up exercise equipment, be sure to:

- Ignore claims that an exercise machine or device can provide long-lasting no-sweat results in a short time. You can't achieve the benefits of exercise unless you exercise.

- Question claims that a machine can burn fat off a certain part of the body such as the buttocks, hips, or abdomen. Achieving a major change in appearance requires sensible eating and regular exercise that works the whole body.

- Read the ad's fine print. The advertised results may be based on more than just using a machine; they also may be based on restricting calories.

- Be skeptical of testimonials and before-and-after pictures from "satisfied" customers. Their experiences may not be typical. Just because one person had success with the equipment doesn't mean you will.

- Do the calculations when you read statements such as "three easy payments of" or "only $29.95 a month." The advertised cost may not include shipping and handling fees, sales tax, and delivery and set-up fees. Find out the details before you order.

- Get all of the information on warranties, guarantees, and return policies. A "30-day money-back guarantee" may not be too good if you have to pay to ship back a bulky piece of equipment.

- Check out the company's customer and support services. Call the advertised toll-free numbers to get an idea of how easy it is to reach a company representative and how helpful the person is.

The exercise paradox

Alarming news reports of the sudden deaths of renowned runner and fitness expert Jim Fixx and a series of basketball stars (including Hank Gathers, Reggie Lewis, and Pete Maravich) have puzzled people who are interested in staying healthy through exercise. If exercise is so good for you, why does vigorous exercise increase the risk for sudden death?

A couple of explanations have emerged that are aimed at two different age groups: people over age 40 and young people. In people over age 40, the cause is usually what doctors call plaque rupture. Plaques are deposits of fatty material that can build up in the lining of arteries. The theory is that unstable collections of plaque become activated during vigorous exercise and form a blood clot. If the blood clot blocks an artery leading to the heart, the result is a heart attack. Most people who have a heart attack while exercising have had existing heart disease for some time—and they may not have known they had it.

Regular exercise and appropriate fitness dramatically reduce the risk that you will have a problem during an episode of vigorous exercise. The people who get into trouble most often are those who have been physically inactive and suddenly engage in a vigorous activity. Most important, beware of shoveling snow if you are not exercising regularly.

The explanation is very different for younger people who die suddenly during physical activity. Sudden death of young athletes during exercise usually results from congenital (present at birth) abnormalities in the structure of their heart. These young athletes were born with an inherited heart defect that, in combination with vigorous physical exertion, caused the heart to stop suddenly. In many cases, they were not aware that they had the heart abnormality. Some of these congenital heart abnormalities can be detected with a thorough physical examination.

Whatever your age, the most important step you can take to protect yourself from having a heart attack during physical activity is to exercise regularly. The exercise doesn't have to be vigorous. Regular walking will move you out of the least fit, least active, high-risk category. If you have been sedentary for a long time, you should avoid vigorous physical activity (such as racquet sports, squash, or snow shoveling) you're not used to. Always warm up and cool down before and after exercising. And learn the warning signs of a heart attack—chest pain or pressure, light-headedness, dizziness or fainting, heart palpitations, pain in the left arm or jaw, shortness of breath, or anxiety.

If you exercise regularly, however, your risk is minimal compared with a person who is inactive and then suddenly does something strenuous. The risk goes up only slightly in people who exercise regularly—and regular exercise reduces the overall risk of dying. The

Exercising when you're not feeling well

If you're not feeling well and your symptoms are above the neck—such as a runny nose, sneezing, or sore throat—you can go ahead and exercise. But if your symptoms are below the neck—chest congestion or tightness, a deep cough, or upset stomach—you should postpone your activity. Also, avoid exercising when you have a fever.

risk is highest for sedentary people who perform a vigorous activity they are not accustomed to doing. The bottom-line message is: Don't be a weekend athlete who plays a wild basketball game once a week, month, or year, and does little other strenuous activity at any other time. Make an effort to fit physical activity into every day.

And don't underestimate the importance of diet. It won't do your heart much good if you exercise regularly and then reward yourself with a glazed doughnut or cheeseburger and fries. Avoid eating artery-clogging foods that are high in saturated and trans fats (and probably calories). It's also a good idea to consume heart-protecting fish oil (see page 8), either by eating 3 servings of fatty fish per week or by taking a fish oil supplement. Keeping the arteries clear enables them to deliver the extra oxygen-rich blood your heart needs to sustain regular physical activity.

Wearing the right shoes

Everyone's feet have a unique size and shape. But size and shape are not the only things to consider when looking for the proper athletic shoe. You also need to consider the type of activity you'll be doing most often and buy a shoe that fits the activity. If you plan mostly to walk, but also want to play some basketball in the driveway with your kids now and then, look for an all-purpose cross-training shoe. But if you perform a specific sport or activity three or more times a week, you should wear shoes designed just for that activity because wearing the right shoe can help prevent injuries, such as knee pain, shin splints, or ankle sprains.

If you jog or run, invest in a shoe with plenty of impact-absorbing cushioning. Walkers need shoes that have heels with added shock absorption and soles with rounded toes for a good push-off. People who play basketball, squash, or racquetball require shoes that support the ankle as they move from side to side.

When shopping for the proper shoe, consider your arch. Is it high, medium, or low? A highly arched foot needs a well-cushioned shoe, while a flatter foot requires something called a motion-control shoe, which prevents the inward rolling of the ankle known as pronation. People with medium arches should ask for a stability shoe, which is more bendable than a motion-control shoe but still gives good support. You can assess your arch by stepping on a towel or rug as you get out of the shower and examining your footprint. If you can see a lot of your instep in the middle of your footprint, you have a lower arch. If you see very little of your instep in your footprint, you have a higher arch.

√ **How many steps in a mile?**

One mile equals 5,280 feet. On average, it takes about 2,000 steps to walk a mile. Of course, everyone's stride varies, but the average stride is roughly 2 to 3 feet in length. So it might take you between 1,700 and 2,600 steps to complete a mile. Each step will take you closer to your health and wellness goals.

Never buy vinyl or plastic shoes, because they don't stretch or breathe. When buying shoes, make sure they feel comfortable from the start and have enough room for your toes, especially if you have calluses or bunions. Follow these recommendations for getting a good fit:

- Measure your feet at the end of the day or after a workout, when they're at their largest.

- Wear the same type of socks you'll be wearing during exercise.

- Measure both feet; one foot is often longer than the other.

- Make sure there is a thumb's width of space from your longest toe to the end of the shoe.

Preventing muscle soreness

Muscle soreness can be a problem for every recreational and professional athlete, but you can prevent much of the pain—and still gain—by educating yourself about muscle soreness and taking steps to prevent it. Two kinds of exercise-related muscle soreness commonly occur. One is the soreness you feel during or immediately after exercise. This type of muscle soreness usually reflects simple fatigue caused by a buildup of chemical waste products in the muscles after exercise. The discomfort often subsides after a minute or two of rest. Once the soreness goes away, you can usually keep exercising without any more pain. If the discomfort persists after a rest period, stop your activity and rest the part of the body that hurts. Don't start moving again until you can exercise that area without pain.

The other kind of muscle soreness is the delayed-onset type that develops 12 hours or longer after you work out. This type of muscle soreness is pretty common after a workout, especially if you aren't used to the activity. For example, if you haven't exercised in 6 months, and then you suddenly walk 3 miles and do some push-ups and sit-ups, you may feel sore over much of your body the next morning. You might also notice muscle stiffness and weakness. These symptoms are a normal response to the unusual exertion, part of an adaptation process that makes you stronger once your muscles recover. The soreness generally feels the worst within the first 2 days after starting an activity and subsides over the next few days.

There are a couple of things you can do to avoid delayed soreness, or at least keep it to a minimum. One step is to warm up before your workout and cool down afterward. To warm up, stretch the muscles you'll be using and do a few minutes of light, low-impact aerobic activity, such as walking or biking. It's also important to give your muscles time to adapt to your activity. For example, if you've been inactive and your ultimate goal is to walk 3 miles in 45 minutes, start by walking a mile or so, and then add another quarter- to half-mile at each workout until you can comfortably walk 3 miles. Then you can begin to increase your walking speed to achieve your 45-minute goal.

These principles apply to any activity, but they're especially useful for weight training because you don't want to overtax your muscles at the very beginning. Nor do you want to overtax your heart. Don't jump into exercise at your utmost effort, because doing so places extra strain on your heart. This is another reason to warm up and cool down. Warm-ups give your heart time to get accustomed to the increased activity and workload; cool-downs slowly ease the heart back into its normal rate.

Remember—your body doesn't like sudden changes. Any unaccustomed activity can cause delayed soreness, so avoid making sudden, major changes in the type of exercise you do or how long you do it.

Sticking with it

Once you've gotten into an exercise routine, you may find that you go off course once in a while as your motivation starts to lag. Here are some proven strategies to rekindle your interest and keep you going:

- Ask someone to be your exercise buddy. Many people feel that having someone to exercise with helps keep them motivated.
- Set a goal, and decide on a reward when you reach it.
- Alternate the types of exercise you do. Walk one day and swim the next. If you work out at a gym, use the stair machine one day and work out with weights the next day.
- Keep a record of what you do and of your progress. Understand that

there will be times when you don't show rapid progress but are still benefiting from your exercise.

- Plan ahead for travel, bad weather, and house guests. For example, an exercise video can help you exercise indoors when the weather is bad.

- Don't let other people distract you. Tell everyone about your exercise time and remind them that they should respect it. Better yet, invite others to come along.

- Be patient with yourself. On certain days, you just won't be as motivated. Exercise less or do something different. When you're sick or injured, or have too many demands, go easy on yourself. A short break from exercising isn't a disaster.

- Have fun exercising. Do an activity you like. Try reading, listening to recorded books, watching TV, or listening to your favorite music while you exercise—it makes the time go faster.

3

WEIGHT, PREVENTION, AND WELLNESS

DOCTORS AND MEDICAL RESEARCHERS are rethinking their notions of weight and health. Not too long ago, doctors might not have commented on their patients' weight for fear of making them feel bad. Or overweight patients might have been told not to worry about their excess weight until they developed a risk factor such as high cholesterol or high blood pressure. But being overweight is now seen as an independent risk factor for heart disease, stroke, and type 2 diabetes. Being overweight takes its toll on the heart, and it does so long before a person's blood pressure or cholesterol levels indicate that anything is wrong.

Nearly 65 percent of all American adults between ages 20 and 74 are overweight—a 20-percent increase from 1960 to 2002. During the same time, obesity—defined as having a BMI (body mass index; see page 85) of 30 or higher or being 20 percent over ideal weight—more than doubled among American adults, with most of the increase occurring in the past 20 years. And the epidemic is not limited to adults: the percentage of young people who are overweight has more than doubled in the last 20 years. Nearly one out of five children and adolescents between the ages of 2 and 19 years is obese. People who are obese have a significantly increased risk for heart disease, high blood pressure, type 2 diabetes, arthritis-related disabilities, and some cancers.

Overweight vs. obese

What's the difference between being overweight and being obese? Overweight refers to a moderate excess of body weight—less than 20 percent over

---

METABOLIC SYNDROME: ARE YOU AT RISK?

Doctors have developed a new way to understand a person's risk of having long-term health problems by evaluating a set of conditions or laboratory findings that tend to cluster together and indicate increased health risks. Individually, these features increase a person's risk for cardiovascular (heart and blood vessel) disease and type 2 diabetes; having three or more is defined as the metabolic syndrome, and this increases the risk even more. Metabolic syndrome increases the likelihood of early death not only from heart disease, but from all causes. The syndrome is extremely common, affecting about one in three people between ages 40 and 60.

A diagnosis of metabolic syndrome is made when a person has at least three of the following five conditions:

1. Increased waist circumference (over 40 inches in men and 35 inches in women)
2. High levels of triglycerides in the blood (150 or higher)
3. Low levels of beneficial HDL cholesterol (under 40 in men and under 50 in women)
4. High blood pressure (130/85 or higher)
5. Elevated fasting blood glucose (100 or higher)

Doctors think that lifestyle factors, especially being overweight, play a major role in the development of metabolic syndrome. You can reduce your risk by consuming a low-fat, high-fiber diet that includes plenty of fresh vegetables and fruits, legumes, and whole grains; making an hour of physical activity part of your daily routine; and losing weight if you are overweight. Just maintaining a stable weight throughout young adulthood into middle age is linked to a substantially lower risk of developing metabolic syndrome, regardless of how heavy you are.

the normal range for your height or a body mass index (BMI; see page 85) of between 25 and 29.9. Obesity is weighing 20 percent or more over your ideal weight or having a BMI of 30 or higher. When a person is obese, the excess body weight is usually from body fat, not muscle. So a person can be overweight without being obese, but many people who are overweight are also obese.

Doctors use a number of methods to find out whether someone is overweight or obese. Some are based on the relationship between height and weight; others are based on measurements of body fat. BMI, the most commonly used method, is an evaluation of how much weight a person carries in proportion to his or her height, and it is correlated with body fatness. Having a high BMI can raise your risk for serious health problems. Check the BMI chart on page 85. If the chart tells you that you are overweight or obese, you may be at risk for the following disorders:

- Type 2 diabetes
- Heart disease and stroke
- Some cancers
- Sleep apnea
- Osteoarthritis
- Gallbladder disease
- Fatty liver disease

A high BMI has been linked to higher death rates from cancers of the esophagus, colon and rectum, liver, gallbladder, pancreas, and kidney in both men and women. The same is true for cancers of the stomach and prostate in men and cancers of the breast, uterus, cervix, and ovary in women. Women who gain more than 20 pounds from age 18 to midlife double their risk for breast cancer, compared with women whose weight remains stable during that time.

People who are obese have a 10 to 50 percent increased risk for death from all causes, compared with people who are at a healthy weight (having a BMI of 18.5 to 24.9). Obesity causes about 112,000 excess deaths per year in the United States, mostly from heart disease. There is some controversy about whether being overweight (but not obese) increases the risk for premature death. But everyone agrees that being overweight is associated with the following health risks, all of which can be reduced by losing as little as 10 to 20 pounds.

- **Type 2 diabetes**   You can lower your risk of developing type 2 diabetes by losing weight and increasing your physical activity. If you already have type 2 diabetes, losing weight and becoming more physically active can help you control your blood sugar levels.

- **Heart disease and stroke**   Losing 5 to 10 percent of your weight can lower your risk of developing heart disease or having a stroke. If you weigh 200 pounds, this means losing as little as 10 pounds.

- **Atrial fibrillation**   Having a high BMI often accompanies enlargement of the left atrium of the heart. This condition sets the stage for atrial fibrillation, an abnormal heart rhythm in which the atria (upper chambers of the heart) beat chaotically instead of rhythmically.

- **Cancer**   Being overweight can raise your risk of developing several types of cancer, including cancers of the colon, esophagus, and kidney. Men who are obese are at increased risk of developing cancer of the prostate. Obese women are at increased risk of developing cancer of the gallbladder, uterus, cervix, or ovaries. Gaining weight during your adult life increases your risk of developing several types of cancers; avoiding weight gain as you age can prevent a rise in your cancer risk.

- **Sleep apnea**   A person who is overweight often has excess tissue around his or her neck. This extra tissue can block the airway during sleep and make breathing difficult or loud, or stop altogether. Excess fat stored throughout the body can also produce substances that cause inflammation, which is a risk factor for sleep apnea.

- **Osteoarthritis**   This is the type of arthritis that's caused by wear and tear on the joints. Extra weight puts extra pressure on the joints and cartilage, causing them to wear away faster. Weight loss can alleviate stress on the knees, hips, and lower back.

- **Fatty liver disease**   People who are overweight or have diabetes or prediabetes (a condition in which blood sugar levels are higher than normal but not in the range for a diagnosis of diabetes; see page 201) are at increased risk of having fatty liver disease (characterized by an accumulation of fat in the liver). It is not yet known why some people who are overweight or have diabetes develop fatty liver disease while others don't, but it is known that losing weight can help reduce the buildup of fat in the liver and prevent further damage. (People with fatty liver disease should avoid drinking alcohol.)

Body mass index

Doctors use BMI to screen for both overweight and obesity in adults. BMI is a calculation based on height and weight. BMI does not directly measure the percent of body fat, but it's a more accurate indicator of overweight and obesity than weight alone. BMI is calculated by dividing a person's weight in kilograms by the square of their height in meters. The mathematical formula is "weight (kg)/height (m^2)." But you don't have to do the math. Just look up your BMI on the table below. To use this table, find your height in the left-hand column. Move across to your weight. The number at the top of the column is the BMI at that height and weight. Pounds have been rounded off.

A healthy BMI is between 18.5 and 24.9. You are considered underweight if your BMI is less than 18.5, overweight if your BMI is between 25 and 29.9, and obese if your BMI is 30 or higher. Risks are increased further in men who have a waist circumference of 40 inches and in women who have a waist circumference of 35 inches.

BMI	19	20	21	22	23	24	25	26	27	28	29	30	31	32	33	34	35	36	37	38	39	40
Height (Inches)											Weight (Pounds)											
58	91	96	100	105	110	115	119	124	129	134	138	143	148	153	158	162	167	172	177	181	186	191
59	94	99	104	109	114	119	124	128	133	138	143	148	153	158	163	168	173	178	183	188	193	198
60	97	102	107	112	118	123	128	133	138	143	148	153	158	163	168	174	179	184	189	194	199	204
61	100	106	111	116	122	127	132	137	143	148	153	158	164	169	174	180	185	190	195	201	206	211
62	104	109	115	120	126	131	136	142	147	153	158	164	169	175	180	186	191	196	202	207	213	218
63	107	113	118	124	130	135	141	146	152	158	163	169-	175	180	186	191	197	203	208	214	220	225
64	110	116	122	128	134	140	145	151	157	163	169	174	180	186	192	197	204	209	215	221	227	232
65	114	120	126	132	138	144	150	156	162	168	174	180	186	192	198	204	210	216	222	228	234	240
66	118	124	130	136	142	148	155	161	167	173	179	186	192	198	204	210	216	223	229	235	241	247
67	121	127	134	140	146	153	159	166	172	178	185	191	198	204	211	217	223	230	236	242	249	255
68	125	131	138	144	151	158	164	171	177	184	190	197	204	210	216	223	230	236	243	249	256	262
69	128	135	142	149	155	162	169	176	182	189	196	203	210	216	223	230	236	243	250	257	263	270
70	132	139	146	153	160	167	174	181	188	195	202	209	216	222	229	236	243	250	257	264	271	278
71	136	143	150	157	165	172	179	186	193	200	208	215	222	229	236	243	250	257	265	272	279	286
72	140	147	154	162	169	177	184	191	199	206	213	221	228	235	242	250	258	265	272	279	287	294
73	144	151	159	166	174	182	189	197	204	212	219	227	235	242	250	257	265	272	280	288	295	302
74	148	155	163	171	179	186	194	202	210	218	225	233	241	249	256	264	272	280	287	295	303	311
75	152	160	168	176	184	192	200	208	216	224	232	240	248	256	264	272	279	287	295	303	311	319
76	156	164	172	180	189	197	205	213	221	230	238	246	254	263	271	279	287	295	304	312	320	328

Calculating BMI is simple, quick, and inexpensive—but it has some limitations. One problem is that very muscular people, such as athletes, may fall into the overweight category when, in reality, they are healthy and fit. Another problem is that people who have lost muscle mass, such as the elderly, may fall into the healthy weight BMI category (BMI 18.5 to 24.9) when they are actually overweight based on percent of body fat. So BMI is useful as a screening tool for individuals and as a general guideline to monitor trends in the population, but doctors don't use it by itself to determine a person's overall health status.

Why are we getting bigger?

The answer to that question is easy: We consume more calories than our body burns. (Yes, calories still count.) But although the answer may be easy, doing something about it can be difficult. Many weight-loss programs focus on getting inactive overweight people to be more active, because exercise is essential for any successful weight loss strategy. But little attention has been paid to the reduction of sedentary activities. What's everyone's favorite sedentary activity? You guessed it: watching TV. Studies show that, on average, adult men spend about 29 hours a week watching TV; adult women spend 34 hours a week. Recent decades have seen a steady increase in the number of homes with multiple TV sets, DVD players, cable TV, and remote controls—as well as an increase in the number of hours spent watching TV. It's no coincidence that these figures match the increasing rates of obesity.

BREAKING NEWS **Obesity may be contagious**

You may be able to catch obesity from your overweight friends. Researchers have found that the chances of a person becoming obese are 57 percent higher if a friend has also become obese. The chance of one brother or sister becoming overweight is also higher if the other has already become overweight. The same goes for married couples. Of course, you can't actually "catch" obesity from friends or family members, but you can be strongly influenced by them, which is what the study demonstrates. Another message from the study: If you want to slim down, you're likely to be more successful if you do it with a friend or in a group rather than on your own.

Waistlines: A growing problem

Doctors want to know not only how much fat you have on your body, but also where the fat is located on your body. Women typically collect fat in their hips and buttocks; men tend to build fat in the abdominal area. Excess abdominal fat is an important, independent risk factor for a number of health conditions including high blood pressure, unfavorable blood cholesterol, and type 2 diabetes, all of which are major risk factors for heart disease and stroke.

Because waist circumference is directly related to abdominal fat, doctors use waist measurement to help determine a person's health risks. If you carry fat mainly around your abdomen, you are more likely to develop obesity-related health problems. Women with a waist measurement of more than 35 inches and men with a waist measurement of more than 40 inches are more likely to have weight-related health risks than people with lower waist measurements.

Even if your weight is normal, your risk of developing these disorders is elevated if you carry more weight in the abdominal area than around your hips and thighs. How can you tell if your waist circumference is too high? Use a tape measure to measure your waist. Place the tape measure just above the top of your hip bone (the bone on the side of your abdomen), at about the level of your belly-button, and wrap it around your middle, keeping the tape snug (but not tight) and parallel to the floor. Read the measurement as you relax your abdominal muscles and exhale. Ask your doctor to measure your waist at your next visit.

Who needs to lose weight?

Doctors generally agree that people who have a BMI of 30 or higher can improve their health through weight loss. This is especially true for people with a BMI of 40 or higher, who are considered extremely obese. Preventing additional weight gain is essential if you have a BMI between 25 and 29.9. Obesity experts recommend that you try to lose weight if you have two or more of the following conditions:

- **Family history of certain diseases.** If you have close relatives who have had heart disease or type 2 diabetes, you are more likely to develop these problems if you are obese.

- **Obesity-related health conditions.** High blood pressure, a high LDL (bad) cholesterol level, low HDL (good) cholesterol, high triglycerides (another type of blood fat), and high blood sugar (glucose) are all warning signs of some obesity-related diseases.
- **Large waist circumference.** Men who have a waist circumference greater than 40 inches, and women who have a waist circumference greater than 35 inches are at increased risk for type 2 diabetes, dyslipidemia (abnormal amounts of fat in the blood), high blood pressure, and heart disease.

A weight loss of just 5 to 10 percent of your body weight can do much to improve your health by lowering your blood pressure and other risk factors for obesity-related diseases. In addition, a 5 to 7 percent weight loss brought about by a moderate diet and regular exercise can delay or possibly prevent type 2 diabetes in people who are at high risk for the disease.

Choosing a weight-loss program

Choosing a weight-loss program can be tough. You may not know what to look for in a program or even what questions to ask. There's a lot of conflicting and inaccurate information out there, so the most important thing you can do is to talk to your doctor. He or she can help you decide which program is best for you. If you feel uncomfortable talking about your weight with your doctor, remember that he or she is there to help you get healthy and can give you reliable information.

Your doctor will probably recommend a weight-loss program that includes a sensible eating plan that is balanced, nutritious, and easy to follow, along with increasing your physical activity. Safe and effective weight-loss programs often include the following:

- Healthy eating plans that cut calories but don't eliminate specific foods or food groups
- Tips for how to increase your level of physical activity
- Guidelines on healthy behavior changes
- Slow and steady weight loss—not plummeting weight loss
- Medical care, if you plan to lose weight by following a special-formula diet, such as a very-low-calorie diet

- And most important, a strategy to help you keep the weight off once you lose it

COMMERCIAL WEIGHT-LOSS PROGRAMS

Some people look to commercial weight-loss plans after trying unsuccessfully to lose weight on their own. Others just like the support of a structured program. Before you sign up for a weight-loss program, check it out to make sure it's sensible and right for you. Remember, quick weight-loss methods don't produce lasting results. Weight-loss methods that rely on diet aids like drinks, prepackaged foods, or diet pills don't work in the long run.

Always keep in mind that calories count more than the types of food in your diet. Overweight people on a reduced-fat, high-glycemic-index diet lose just as much weight—about 8 percent of their original weight—as people on a low-carbohydrate, low-glycemic-index diet. So it's mostly about calories.

Whether you lose weight on your own or with a group, keep in mind that the most important changes are long term. No matter how much weight you have to lose, modest goals and a slow course will boost your chances of both losing the weight and keeping it off.

Tips for healthy weight loss

When you're trying to lose weight, you need all the help you can get. Work with your doctor to come up with healthy strategies designed to change not only what you eat, but also the way you eat. The following tips can help you lose weight and keep it off.

- **Set goals.** People who successfully lose weight choose two or three goals at a time that are specific, attainable, and flexible (because no one is perfect). "To exercise more" is not specific enough. "Walk five miles a day" is specific and measurable, but is it attainable if you're just starting out after being inactive for a very long time? "Walk 30 minutes every day" is more attainable, but what happens if it rains all day? "Walk 30 minutes five days each week" is specific, attainable, and flexible. In short, a good goal. (You can work out to an exercise video on rainy or snowy days.)

- **Eat slowly.** Changing the way you eat can make it easier to eat less without feeling deprived. It takes at least 15 minutes for your brain to get the message that you've been fed. Slow eating will give your brain time to receive those signals of fullness by the end of the meal.

- **Use smaller plates.** Smaller portions won't look so small on a salad plate.

- **Don't listen to fast music.** Studies show that listening to fast music while eating makes you eat faster, so you ultimately take in more calories.

- **Watch your cues.** Learn what things in your day encourage you to eat when you're not hungry, and then change those cues. For example, you may be more likely to overeat while watching television, or whenever treats are on display at work. Try to break the association between eating and those cues. Don't eat while watching TV. Leave the coffee-break room right after you pour your coffee.

- **Never reward yourself with food.** Your grade school teachers knew that candy is a powerful motivator, but don't fall into the same trap. If you need to reward yourself for your weight-loss successes, do so by taking a leisurely bath, having a cup of herbal tea, or buying a magazine.

- **Don't skip meals.** Delaying eating or skipping a meal can make you overeat later in the day. Instead, eat three small meals a day and snack on cut-up vegetables, low-fat popcorn, or a piece of fruit if you get hungry between meals.

- **Eat more fiber.** Adding more whole grains, beans, and lentils to your diet will make you feel fuller. Fiber also slows the rate at which glucose (blood sugar) enters your bloodstream. Serve bean burritos or enchiladas on whole-grain tortillas for dinner, toss some beans into a salad, or order lentil soup at lunch.

- **Make healthy substitutions.** Use fat-free sour cream and low-fat cheeses instead of the high-fat variety. Drink water, iced tea, or low-sodium tomato juice instead of sugary soft drinks. Replace those snack chips with a piece of fruit.

- **Indulge, only once in a while.** Go ahead and have a small dish of ice cream (but make it low-fat or reduced-fat) with chocolate sauce on top a couple of times a month. It'll give you something to look forward to and won't upset your healthy eating plan too much.

FIVE STEPS TO POSITIVE LIFESTYLE CHANGE

Researchers have identified five stages of readiness that people go through when faced with the decision to make a healthy change in lifestyle or behavior, such as losing weight or quitting smoking. Known as the Transtheoretical Model of Behavior Change, it is based on the idea that making a change for the better is a shifting state rather than a fixed decision. According to the theory, a person who needs to lose weight, stop smoking, or get more exercise may go back and forth between being highly motivated to change and being unmotivated. Once you have identified your current state of change readiness, you can take the actions that are appropriate for that stage.

Although the following stages are presented step by step, people don't necessarily progress from one stage to the next in order. Some people go to the next stage, some stay in one place for a while, and others slip back to a previous stage. Changing a behavior that you've lived with for decades is extremely difficult. Expect to have setbacks, make mistakes, and start over again.

Here are the five steps:

1. **Precontemplation**   During this stage, you probably have little interest in making a lifestyle change—in fact, you may have no intention of doing so—but perhaps your doctor has told you that you need to lose weight for the sake of your health. This is a good time to gather information about making a change. For example, if you need to lose weight, find out the health benefits and different ways of accomplishing this change. Learn more about how a weight problem affects your health and self-image.

2. **Contemplation**   You may be seriously considering how to lose those extra pounds during this stage. Write down the benefits and challenges of losing weight to help identify your personal weaknesses, so you're not blindsided by the stumbling blocks you will surely encounter along the way. Over time, the cons of weight loss—eating "unappetizing" foods or fielding complaints from family members about changes in meals—become less and less important. Try to imagine how you would look and feel if you successfully dropped the weight.

3. **Preparation**   In this stage, you make a specific plan to lose weight over a reasonable time period—say, the next six months—although you may not know which weight-loss method to try. Now is the time to make small changes, such as turning down dessert, and set realistic goals so you can celebrate the victories instead of feeling frustrated when you can't reach an impractical goal.

4. **Action**   This stage encompasses the first six months of change. Make your behavior changes more concrete: Keep junk food out of the house. Avoid fast food. Walk for 30 minutes a day. During this time, you will probably make some progress but you may also go off track at times. Seek out help and encouragement from your doctor, your family, and your friends so you can prevent a relapse, but also pick yourself up and start over if you've strayed from the plan.

5. **Maintenance**   After the first six months, your new lifestyle habits will become almost second nature. Keep working on preventing a setback and appreciate the achievements you've made so far.

The downside of weight loss

Losing weight is never easy and some pitfalls are likely to await you on your way to a healthy weight. For example, weight loss has been linked to some medical conditions, such as gallstones. Quitting smoking becomes more difficult when you have to contend with a possible weight gain that happens to many people who quit. Yo-yo dieting (losing and gaining back weight) also poses some health risks. This section will help you evaluate the overall risks and benefits of weight loss and avoid these potential problems.

WEIGHT LOSS AND GALLSTONES

Gallstones are clusters of solid material that form in the gallbladder. The most common type of gallstone is made mainly of cholesterol. Gallstones can develop as one large stone or as many small ones. They vary in size and can be as large as a golf ball or as small as a grain of sand

Dieting can increase your risk of developing gallstones. People who lose a large amount of weight quickly (at a rate of more than 3 pounds a week) are at greater risk for gallstones than are those who lose weight more slowly (at a rate of 2 pounds or less a week). The problem seems to develop when dieting shifts the balance of bile salts and cholesterol in the gallbladder: cholesterol levels rise and the amount of bile salts goes down. Following a diet that is too low in fat or going for long periods without eating—skipping breakfast, for example, which is a common practice among dieters—may also cause the gallbladder to contract so infrequently that it can't empty out the bile, increasing the probability that gallstones will form.

There are a number of things you can do to reduce your risk of developing gallstones while you lose weight. Most important is to lose the weight gradually. Depending on your starting weight, lose no more than ½ to 2 pounds per week. Your food choices can also affect your risk for gallstones. Include enough healthy fats (see page 7) in your diet to stimulate gallbladder contracting and emptying; about 20 to 30 percent of your total calories should come from fat. Getting more fiber and calcium may also reduce the likelihood of gallstones. In addition, regular physical activity can lower your risk for gallstones. Aim for about 60 minutes of moderate- to vigorous-intensity activity most days of the week to manage your body weight and prevent unhealthy weight gain. To keep the pounds off, you'll have to get at least 60 to 90 minutes of daily moderate-intensity physical activity.

Although you can't change your genetic makeup, you can work on changing your eating and exercise habits and other environmental factors. Try these helpful tips:

- Eat smaller portions of nutritious meals that are lower in fat and sugar and higher in fiber.
- Slow down when you're eating! You will end up feeling just as full but you'll be eating fewer calories.
- Learn to recognize and control environmental cues (such as the cookie jar or TV) that make you want to eat when you're not hungry.
- Get at least 30 minutes of moderate-intensity physical activity (such as brisk walking) on most days of the week.
- Take a walk—do anything active—instead of watching TV.
- Eat meals and snacks at the table, not in front of the TV.
- Keep records of your food intake and physical activity.

THE UPS AND DOWNS OF YO-YO DIETING

Yo-yo dieting, also known as weight cycling, is the frequent loss and regaining of body weight. This cycle often happens to people who frequently go on weight-loss diets. How much weight do you have to lose and gain for it to count as yo-yo dieting? The cycle applies to losing and regaining as little as 5 to 10 pounds, but some people's weight can change by 50 pounds or more while dieting.

The jury is still out as to whether weight cycling leads to serious health problems, but some studies suggest a link to high blood pressure, abnormal blood cholesterol, gallbladder disease, and other conditions. Studies have shown that women who yo-yo diet tend to gain more weight over time than women who don't lose and regain weight. Binge eating (when a person eats a lot of food at one time while feeling out of control; see next page) has also been linked to women who weight cycle.

Even more serious is the finding that yo-yo dieting may damage your immune system. People who have weight cycled more than five times have fewer of the type of immune system cells (known as killer cells) that fight viruses. These are the immune system cells that may also play a role in fighting cancer. The highest levels of these cells are found in people whose weight has stayed the same for a number of years.

Yo-yo dieting can also affect your mental health. People who weight cycle often feel frustrated and depressed about their inability to keep the weight off. If your weight keeps going up and down, don't make yourself feel bad. Try to focus on making healthy permanent changes in your eating and exercise habits (see page 91). Trying to stay positive can help you stay focused.

Some people worry that weight cycling can put more fat around their abdominal area—a legitimate concern, because having excess fat in this area can increase the risk for heart disease, abnormal blood fats, type 2 diabetes, and some other health problems. It is not clear if or how weight cycling causes this phenomenon, but studies are ongoing to determine if this is the case.

To avoid yo-yo dieting, be ready to make lifelong lifestyle changes. A healthy diet and physical activity are the keys to your efforts. Focus on making healthful food choices, such as eating more high-fiber foods like fruits and vegetables and cutting down on foods that are high in saturated or trans fats. Walking, jogging, or other physical activities can help keep you active and feeling good.

Eating disorders

The unrealistic ideal of thinness in our society has made many women—and men—feel uncomfortable about their body. People with a poor body image are more likely to struggle with weight loss. Nearly half of all women in this country are on a diet at any given time and, for some people, dieting can easily cross over into an eating disorder. Taken to an extreme, eating disorders can lead to the following serious health problems, some of which can be life-threatening: irregular heartbeat, heart failure, kidney or liver damage, loss of bone mass, malnutrition, and depression.

Binge eating

Most people overeat from time to time. Maybe you feel that you all too often eat more than you should. But eating a lot of food doesn't necessarily mean that you have a binge eating disorder. Doctors generally agree that people with a serious binge eating problem often eat an unusually large amount of food and feel that their eating is out of control. People with binge eating disorder also display the following behaviors:

- Eating much more quickly than usual during binges
- Eating until they are uncomfortably full
- Consuming large amounts of food even when they are not hungry
- Eating alone, because they are embarrassed about the amount of food they eat
- Feeling disgusted, depressed, or guilty after overeating

Binge eating also occurs in another eating disorder called bulimia (see page 98). But people with bulimia usually purge, fast, or exercise excessively after they binge eat. Purging means vomiting or abusing diuretics (water pills) or laxatives to keep from gaining weight after binge eating; fasting is not eating for at least 24 hours. Strenuous exercise, in this case, means exercising for longer than an hour after binge eating. Purging, fasting, and exercising excessively are dangerous ways to try to control weight.

Binge eating disorder is the most common eating disorder. About 2 percent of adults in the United States (as many as 4 million Americans) have binge eating disorder. Many people with the problem are either overweight or obese, but normal-weight people also can have the disorder. The problem affects up to 15 percent of people who are mildly obese and who try to lose weight on their own or through a commercial weight-loss program. The disorder is even more common in people who are severely obese. People who are obese and have binge eating disorder often become overweight at a younger age than those without the problem. They often lose and gain back weight (yo-yo dieting; see page 93). Binge eating disorder is slightly more common in women than in men.

No one knows for sure what causes binge eating but as many as half of all people with the problem have depression or have had depression in the past. It is not known if depression causes binge eating disorder or if binge eating disorder causes depression. Binge eaters tend to report more health problems, including stress, trouble sleeping, and suicidal thoughts than other people. They may feel so bad about themselves that they skip work, school, or social activities to binge eat.

Most people who binge eat, whether they are obese or of normal weight, feel ashamed or embarrassed and try to hide their problem from family and friends. Studies suggest that people who binge eat may have trouble handling their emotions. Many binge eaters say that being angry, sad, bored, worried, or stressed can cause them to go on an eating spree. Some behaviors and emotional problems seem to be more common in people with

THE FEMALE ATHLETE TRIAD

The benefits of physical activity almost always outweigh the risks. But some women who exercise excessively or train intensively for athletic competition and do not consume enough calories to compensate for their increased activity level risk developing a disorder known as the female athlete triad. This disorder is a cluster of three conditions—eating disorders (see page 94), lack of periods, and the bone-thinning disorder osteoporosis (see page 325)—that can occur together.

The prevalence of the female athlete triad is difficult to assess because many women with an eating disorder are secretive about their eating habits, but estimates range from 15 to 62 percent of all female college athletes. Among the contributing factors are pressure by coaches and parents to win at all costs, frequent weigh-ins that penalize athletes for weight gain, and society's preference for a thin body, especially in women. The girls and women most at risk of developing the condition are those in activities such as gymnastics, figure skating, distance running, ballet, and swimming.

The female athlete triad can put you at risk for some potentially serious health problems. The lack of periods indicates inadequate production of the female hormone estrogen, which is essential for the maintenance of bone strength. If you miss your period for more than four months because of excessive exercise, you will begin to lose bone mass, which can lead to frequent stress fractures and bone thinning (osteoporosis). Failing to keep your body weight at a normal level can also have harmful effects on your heart, hormone system, and digestive system. In addition to the lack of periods, common symptoms of the female athlete triad include:

- Fatigue
- Anemia
- Depression and other psychological problems
- Stress fractures
- Inability to concentrate
- Intolerance to cold; having cold hands and feet
- Constipation
- Dry skin
- Light-headedness
- Slow pulse
- Low blood pressure
- Downy hair growth on the face and body

Having your periods stop is not a normal consequence of intense training. It is a sign that your body is not getting enough nourishment and, to help protect you from starving, your body has shut down your reproductive system. If you exercise vigorously on a regular basis and your periods have stopped, see your doctor right away so you can prevent further bone loss. He or she will encourage you to gradually gain some weight and cut back on your training, enough to restart your periods. Your doctor may also prescribe estrogen replacement therapy (possibly in the form of birth-control pills) to prevent bone loss until your body weight returns to normal.

Eat three nutritious meals a day and have a couple of healthy snacks to adequately stoke your body's furnace. Get plenty of rest. Sleep a full eight hours and take at least one day off from your sport each week to let your body heal. Resist pressure from your coach, parents, or peers to obsess about winning or your weight because your long-term health is more important than any temporary victory.

binge eating disorder, including alcohol abuse, impulsive behavior, feeling a lack of control, not feeling part of the community, and inability to identify and talk about their feelings.

Researchers are looking into how brain chemicals and metabolism (the way the body uses calories) can affect binge eating disorder. Some studies suggest that genes may be involved in binge eating, because the disorder often occurs in several members of a family, but this research is still in the early stages.

Anorexia

People with anorexia see themselves as overweight even though they are underweight—often even dangerously thin. The process of eating becomes an obsession. They develop unusual eating habits, such as avoiding food or meals, picking out a few foods and eating them in small quantities, or carefully weighing and portioning food. People with anorexia often check their body weight repeatedly, and many use other tactics to control their weight, such as intense and compulsive exercise, or vomiting and abuse of laxatives, enemas, and diuretics. Most people who have anorexia fail to eat enough to maintain their body functions. The condition affects both males and females, but is much more common among females. Doctors theorize that the condition has something to do with a person's need to feel in control.

The outlook for a person with anorexia varies from person to person. Some people recover fully after a single episode, some experience a fluctuating pattern of weight gain and relapse, and others undergo a deteriorating course of illness over many years. Anorexia can be fatal. The most common causes of death from severe anorexia are cardiac arrest and an imbalance of electrolytes (minerals involved in regulating many body processes).

The following factors are characteristic of people who have anorexia:

- Resistance to keeping body weight at or above a normal weight for age and height
- Intense fear of gaining weight or becoming fat
- An unrealistic view of one's body shape and weight, excessive emphasis on body weight or shape, and denial of the health risks of having an extremely low body weight
- Infrequent or absent menstrual periods in girls and women

Bulimia

Bulimia is characterized by recurrent episodes of uncontrollable binge eating (consuming massive quantities of food). To compensate for the bingeing and to prevent weight gain, the person tries to eliminate the eaten food by self-inducing vomiting or misusing laxatives, diuretics (water pills), enemas, or other medications. This elimination phase is known as purging. The person might also fast or exercise excessively. People with bulimia often perform the behaviors in secret, feeling ashamed when they binge but relieved after they purge. For a diagnosis of bulimia, the bingeing and purging occur at least twice a week for at least three months.

Up to 4 percent of college-age women have bulimia, and half of all people who have anorexia (see previous page) also have bulimia. People with bulimia usually weigh a normal amount for their age and height, but they may fear gaining weight, want to lose weight, and feel strongly dissatisfied with their body. People with bulimia often have problems with impulse control; they may be sexually promiscuous or abuse drugs or alcohol. Many have underlying feelings of depression, loneliness, or shame, although, on the surface, they appear confident and are often fun to be with.

HOW TO PREVENT EATING DISORDERS

The societal pressures to be thin, especially for women, are so great that it is not surprising that most girls and young women accept dieting as part of growing up. But dieting and restricting calories can have serious psychological and physical consequences, including the inability to focus at school, being tired, and depression. Schools are developing programs to promote awareness of eating disorders as well as healthy attitudes about body image. Also, a national effort is being made to offer screening for eating disorders to adolescents and young adults so they can get help early. Health professionals and researchers are looking for effective ways to prevent eating disorders. Here are some things you can do to reduce your risk:

- **Know your family health history.** Eating disorders tend to run in families. If you have a family member with an eating disorder, you are at increased risk of also developing one. If you know your family's health history (see page 179), you may be able to more easily see the signs in yourself.

- **Watch your family dynamics.** Living in a family that overvalues appearance or makes disapproving remarks about a child's looks and weight can set the stage for a body image problem.

- **Get a handle on your feelings.** Talk to your doctor or find a therapist you can talk to about the strong emotions you are having trouble dealing with.

- **Don't be a perfectionist.** Many people with an eating disorder are very driven and hardworking. Avoid placing too much pressure on yourself to get perfect grades or to excel in sports, playing a musical instrument, or any other activity. Children who feel inadequate and powerless may try to take control of their lives by controlling what they eat.

- **Ignore media messages.** Don't pay attention to media messages that connect popularity or success to being thin. Most ultrathin fashion models are severely underweight.

- **Avoid repeated dieting.** Constantly dieting or thinking about dieting teaches you unhealthy attitudes toward food and can lead to unhealthy eating behaviors.

- **Ease into life transitions.** Some people develop anorexia or bulimia when they start a new job, enter a new school, get married or divorced, or break up with a boyfriend or girlfriend. During these transitional times, which can be stressful for anyone, make sure you have a strong social support network to turn to.

If you think you might have an eating disorder, it is important to know that you're not alone. Most people who have an eating disorder have tried, but failed, to control it on their own. It's usually essential to get professional help. Talk to your doctor about the kind of treatment that would work best for you. The good news is that most people with eating disorders do well in treatment and are able to overcome the problem.

STRESS, REST, AND RELAXATION

YOUR KIDS ARE FIGHTING over the TV remote, your boss asked you to work overtime, your spouse wants to know what's for dinner, and your elderly father just called because he can't figure out the Medicare form. Stress often attacks from every angle at once, leaving you breathless, with your heart pounding and mind racing. When the chaos subsides, your hormones switch off the stress response and your body returns to normal.

But in modern society, stress doesn't always let up. Many people experience constant anxiety and worry about daily events and relationships. High levels of stress hormones wash through their system, staying in the blood and tissues. The body's stress response gave ancient people the speed and endurance to quickly escape life-threatening peril. But today, it can be switched on and remain on in people who experience chronic stress. Such long-term activation of the body's stress-response system can have a damaging effect on the body, increasing the risk for obesity, heart disease, depression, and a number of other health problems. Learning how to cope with stress in a positive way can help you stay healthy and well.

How stress affects your health

People talk about stress as if it's all bad, but that's not the case. Some stress is good for you. If you didn't feel some tension before a job interview, for example, you might come across as unenthusiastic or uninterested. You don't need to eliminate stress completely—in fact, that's impossible to do—because life is full of stressful situations. You just need to learn how to respond to it in a healthy way.

While some stress is good, too much stress can be harmful. Everyone responds to stress in a unique way, influenced partly by heredity and partly by the environment. But some people have an overly sensitive response to stress. They have a nervous system that is on overdrive, alert, and ready to deal with a threat, even when no threat is present.

It is thought that major stresses in early childhood, such as being neglected by parents or physically or sexually abused, can make the stress response increase with each new stressful experience. By adulthood, a child in this situation can have an extremely sensitive stress response. In life-threatening situations—such as living in a dangerous neighborhood—this exaggerated response can help the person survive. But in everyday life, it can make a person overreact emotionally to relatively nonthreatening, commonplace situations. People who undergo severely stressful experiences in childhood appear to respond normally to stress, but seem to be unable to turn off the stress response, keeping them in a state of prolonged stress arousal. Such prolonged stress can have harmful effects that could result in illness.

Stress and the immune system

When you have an infection, your immune system sends out infection-fighting cells to battle the invading microorganisms. Doctors now know that signaling molecules from the immune system can also activate the part of the brain that controls the stress response (the hypothalamus). Through a cascade of hormones released from the pituitary and adrenal glands, the hypothalamus causes blood levels of the hormone cortisol to rise. Cortisol is the flight-or-fight stress hormone that enables us to get through difficult or threatening situations. The brain uses cortisol to suppress the immune system during times of stress because the immune system's response to stress produces inflammation in the body.

This complex communication system enables the immune system to talk to the brain, and the brain to talk back and shut down the immune system's response when it's no longer needed. When you think about this two-way communication, you can begin to understand the kinds of disorders that might develop if too much or too little communication takes place in either direction.

If you're constantly under pressure, the part of your brain that controls the stress response is going to continually pump out stress hormones like cortisol. These hormones bathe the immune system's infection-fighting cells in a sea of instructions that tell them to stop fighting. This means that, when you're under constant stress, your immune system is less able to respond to a disease-causing invader like a bacterium or virus.

This theory explains in part why people under persistent stress—such as caregivers of relatives with Alzheimer's disease, medical students taking exams, military recruits undergoing basic training, and couples having marital problems—may be more susceptible to infections. People in these situations may also become vulnerable to more serious disorders, such as infertility, delayed growth and development in children, digestive problems such as Crohn's disease, depression, anxiety disorders, anorexia, type 2 diabetes, and heart disease. Long-term stress can also have an impact on other risk factors for disease, including high blood pressure, unfavorable cholesterol levels, smoking, physical inactivity, and overeating.

Stress and chronic disease

Having to deal with long-term stress can cause cortisol (the stress hormone) levels in the body to rise and remain elevated. This process can produce physiological changes that can increase the risk for a number of common chronic disorders, including those described below.

TYPE 2 DIABETES

The flow of hormones such as cortisol that are released during stressful times can raise blood sugar levels. Elevated cortisol levels can also cause fat to accumulate around the abdomen; fat cells in the abdominal area are less responsive to the effects of insulin than cells in other parts of the body. When cells do not respond sufficiently to insulin, they don't take in glucose from the bloodstream. An elevated level of glucose in the blood is the hallmark of diabetes.

HEART DISEASE

Stress has not been officially named a risk factor for heart disease, but it can worsen risk factors for heart disease—including high blood pressure, lack of exercise, and overeating. It is known that during stress, blood flow to the heart is reduced and blood clots form more easily. People who are under chronic stress, whose body is always on alert, tend to have more blockages in their arteries than people who are not under continuous stress.

CANCER

Stress-induced changes in the immune system do not directly cause cancer. However, studies looking at whether stress reduction can strengthen the immune system and possibly slow the progression of cancer are under way. Researchers think that stress might repress the immune system cells needed to destroy cancer cells. They are also trying to learn if a healthy immune system can actually protect people from cancer.

Stress and underlying health problems

The way your nervous system responds to stress can also worsen any health problems you may have. A variety of unrelated health problems can flare up when a person experiences increased life stress. The following medical conditions could be aggravated by stress:

- **Asthma**   A weakened immune system caused by stress can make you more susceptible to colds and the flu, which make breathing more difficult when you have asthma. Strong emotions can also cause adverse changes in breathing.

- **Stomach ulcers**   Most ulcers are caused not by stress but by the bacterium Helicobacter pylori. But stress can definitely make ulcers worse. Stress triggers the body to produce higher amounts of stomach acid, which can inflame ulcers that already exist.

- **Heartburn**   The same stomach acid that exacerbates ulcers can worsen heartburn.

- **Multiple sclerosis**   Life stressors seem to make symptoms of multiple sclerosis worse and may even bring on new symptoms. The reasons for this are not fully understood.

- **Arthritis**   When you get stressed out, your body tenses up, potentially causing joint pain to get worse.

- **Acne**   Stress may trigger the release of hormones known to worsen acne by boosting production of oily substances from glands in the skin. Stress may also increase production of chemicals that can cause inflammation in the skin.
- **Wound healing**   Stress has been shown to reduce wound healing by up to 40 percent.

Sleep and stress

When you sleep, your brain goes through distinct stages that alternate throughout the night. Different things happen during each stage. Some stages of sleep help you feel rested and energetic the next day; other stages help you learn or make memories. In short, many important things occur during sleep, which help you stay healthy and allow you to perform at your best while you're awake. Americans have been sleeping less and less with each passing decade. At the turn of the 20th century, people slept an average of nine hours each night. By 1970, nightly sleep had gone down to about seven and a half hours. Today, many people sleep only six hours a night—and some sleep even less.

Lack of sleep can affect your mood and your ability to think clearly, and also your health. In fact, sleep deprivation can be downright dangerous: you are more likely to be involved in a car accident if you drive when you are drowsy.

Lack of sleep and health problems

Insufficient sleep has been linked to an increased risk for type 2 diabetes. Sleep deprivation seems to affect diabetes risk in two ways: by promoting weight gain and by worsening insulin resistance (the cells' response to the hormone insulin, which allows cells to take in the sugar glucose for energy.) Lack of sleep causes weight gain by reducing the nightly production of growth hormone. During the deepest level of sleep, known as slow-wave sleep, the body repairs tissues. One way it does this is by producing growth hormone, which triggers both the manufacture of protein in muscle and the breakdown of stored fat. This process regulates the body's proportion of muscle to fat. A chronic deficit of slow-wave sleep can lower the amount of growth hormone available, causing greater accumulation of fat stores and lower muscle mass, which, when combined with other risk factors such as unhealthy eating and physical inactivity, can lead to obesity. Obesity is the most important risk factor for type 2 diabetes (see page 245). Sleep loss can also lower the levels of a blood protein known as leptin, which controls appetite.

Not sleeping enough can also interfere with the body's normal use of carbohydrates and glucose. Healthy people without diabetes who sleep less than four hours a night show signs of developing impaired glucose intolerance (blood sugar levels that are higher than normal, but lower than those indicating diabetes), a marker of prediabetes. Their blood sugar levels rise higher and return to normal more slowly when they don't get enough sleep. Their body also secretes less insulin. People who routinely fail to get sufficient sleep—six and a half or fewer hours per night—also often develop insulin resistance.

Sleep deprivation has been linked to an increased risk for high blood pressure, heart disease, and other common chronic disorders. The steady release of stress hormones caused by sleep deprivation can affect the immune system, increasing susceptibility to colds and other infections. Also, because the immune system helps the body fight cancer, reduced immune system function from insufficient sleep can increase the risk for cancer.

A chronic lack of sleep may accelerate the aging process. When you don't get enough sleep, your brain doesn't make normal amounts of hormones, mimicking the hormone levels of a much older person. But getting a full night's sleep can return hormone levels to normal, reversing the aging effect.

How much sleep is enough?

Sleep needs vary from person to person, and they change throughout life. Most adults need eight hours of sleep each night. Newborns, on the other hand, sleep between 16 and 18 hours a day, and children in preschool sleep between 10 and 12 hours. School-aged children and teens need at least nine hours of sleep nightly.

Some people think that adults need less sleep as they get older, but there is no evidence to show that older people can get by with less sleep than younger people. As people age, however, they often do sleep less, or they spend less time in the deep, restful stages of sleep. Older people are also more easily awakened. Insomnia is a major symptom of menopause, and many older women report difficulty falling asleep or waking for long periods during the night, or experiencing both problems.

Why sleep is good for you

Does it really matter if you get enough sleep? Yes indeed. Not only does the quantity of your sleep matter, but the quality of sleep is important as well. People whose sleep is interrupted repeatedly or is cut short (parents of infants, for example) might not be getting enough time in certain stages of sleep. In other words, how well rested you are and how well you function the next day depend not just on your total sleep time, but also how much of the various stages of sleep you get each night. Here's what happens when you do and when you don't get enough sleep:

- **General health**   During deep sleep, the body produces many hormones that are essential for proper functioning of the body. Sleep deprivation has been shown to weaken the immune system, increasing a person's susceptibility to infections and other illnesses. Lack of sufficient sleep may also contribute to obesity (see page 82), which increases the risk for related health problems.

- **Performance**   You need sleep to think clearly, react quickly, and create memories. The pathways in the brain that help you learn and remember are very active when you sleep. People faced with mentally

---

BREAKING NEWS   **Napping may cut your risk of dying from a heart attack**

No need to feel guilty any longer about that catnap you take in the middle of the day, because it's good for your health. A large study tracking more than 20,000 people found that those who took an afternoon nap lasting at least 30 minutes, 3 times or more a week had an almost 40 percent drop in their risk of dying from heart disease compared to those who stayed awake all day.

Of those studied, working men who napped experienced a 64 percent lower risk of death from a heart attack and other heart-related conditions than those who did not nap. The effect didn't seem to hold true for women.

The scientists decided to study this issue because deaths from heart disease tend to be low in countries where people generally take afternoon siestas. The working hypothesis is that napping is a great stress-reliever and rejuvenator.

challenging tasks do better after a good night's sleep. Sleep also seems to be essential for creative problem solving. Skimping on sleep has a price. Although you might not notice, cutting back by even one hour can make it tough to focus the next day and can slow your response time. When you lack sleep, you're more likely to make bad decisions and take more chances, jeopardizing your job or school performance and increasing your risk for accidents. Driving while drowsy can be just as dangerous as driving drunk because you can't react quickly to potentially hazardous situations.

- **Mood**   Insufficient sleep can make you irritable and is linked to poor behavior and trouble with relationships, especially among children and teens. People who chronically lack sleep are also more likely to experience depression.

Could you have a sleep disorder?

People vary in their need for—and satisfaction with—sleep. If you spend enough time in bed and still wake up tired or feel sleepy during the day, you may be one of the estimated 40 million Americans with a sleep disorder. The most common sleep disorders are insomnia, sleep apnea (sleep-disordered breathing; see page 110), restless legs syndrome, and narcolepsy.

INSOMNIA

Insomnia is the inability to fall asleep or to stay asleep throughout the night. The condition isn't defined by the number of hours you sleep or how long it takes you to fall asleep. It refers to difficulty falling asleep, or frequently waking during the night and being unable to go back to sleep.

Insomnia can cause problems—including fatigue, lack of energy, difficulty concentrating, and irritability—during the day. Insomnia can be short term, intermittent, or constant. Short-term insomnia lasts from a single night to a few weeks. Insomnia that occurs from time to time is said to be intermittent. Chronic insomnia occurs on most nights and lasts a month or more. The following factors can make insomnia more likely:

- Being older age (insomnia occurs more frequently in people over age 60)
- Being a woman, especially during menopause
- Having depression

- Having stress or anxiety
- Having a medical problem, or taking some medications

Insomnia has many causes. Short-term and intermittent insomnia usually result when a person experiences one or more irritating circumstances such as the following:

- Environmental noise
- Extreme temperatures
- Change in the surrounding environment
- Sleep/wake schedule problems such as jet lag or shift work
- Medication side effects

Chronic insomnia is more complex, often stemming from a combination of factors, including underlying physical or emotional disorders. For example, one of the most common causes of chronic insomnia is depression. Other underlying causes can include arthritis, kidney disease, heart failure, asthma, sleep apnea, narcolepsy, restless legs syndrome, Parkinson's disease, and hyperthyroidism (an overactive thyroid gland). Lifestyle factors, including the misuse of caffeine, alcohol, or other substances; disrupted sleep/wake cycles from shift work or other nighttime activities; and chronic stress can also contribute to chronic insomnia.

CAUTION WITH SLEEP MEDICATION

Doctors generally prescribe sleep-promoting medications only after other strategies have failed, and only as part of a long-term sleep program. Hypnotics (including sedatives, tranquilizers, and antianxiety drugs) are among the most frequently prescribed sleep medications. Hypnotics induce sleep by depressing the central nervous system. All sleep medications have potential side effects and should be used only under the guidance of a health professional. Many sleep medications are addictive or habit-forming or may require increasingly larger doses to have the same effect. For this reason, when doctors prescribe sleep medication, they usually prescribe it at the smallest dose possible and for only a short time. The dosage of some sleep medications must be gradually reduced as they are discontinued. To avoid problems such as withdrawal symptoms, make sure you work with your doctor to gradually stop any sleep medication you are taking. Complete withdrawal can take several weeks.

SLEEP APNEA

Sleep apnea is a condition in which regular breathing stops repeatedly or gets very shallow during sleeping. Each pause in breathing lasts at least 10 seconds, and pauses can occur dozens of times an hour. Sleep apnea is a common sleep disorder, especially among obese men, and, in severe cases, can be life-threatening. Although sleep apnea occurs more often in people who are overweight, thin people can also have it.

The most common type of sleep apnea is obstructive sleep apnea, when excess tissue in the neck area obstructs breathing. When this occurs, air temporarily stops flowing into the lungs through the mouth and nose, and the amount of oxygen in the blood can drop dangerously low. Affected people typically stop breathing, then struggle to restart breathing for several seconds until they awaken just enough to open up their airway. Normal breaths then start again with a loud snort or choking sound. Sleep apnea prevents restful sleep because an affected person partially awakens multiple times during the night, which results in poor-quality sleep.

People with sleep apnea often snore loudly, although not everyone who snores has sleep apnea. Some people with sleep apnea don't even realize they snore, and most people with the condition don't know they have it or that they're having problems breathing while sleeping. A family member or bed partner may be the first to notice the signs of sleep apnea.

Untreated, sleep apnea can increase your risk of developing high blood pressure and even of having a heart attack or stroke. The disorder can also increase your risk for type 2 diabetes and make you more prone to having work-related accidents and driving accidents. If you think you may have sleep apnea, see your doctor right away. The condition can be treated successfully.

RESTLESS LEGS SYNDROME

Restless legs syndrome (RLS) is a nervous system disorder characterized by unpleasant sensations in the legs and an uncontrollable urge to move the legs to relieve those feelings. The sensations are often described by people as burning, creeping, tugging, or like insects crawling inside the legs. The sensations range in severity from uncomfortable to irritating to painful.

The most unusual aspect of RLS is that lying down and trying to relax activates the symptoms. As a result, most people with RLS have difficulty falling asleep and staying asleep. Left untreated, the condition causes exhaustion and daytime fatigue. Many people with RLS report that their job, personal relations, and activities of daily life are affected negatively because of their exhaustion. They often are unable to concentrate, have impaired memory, or fail to accomplish daily tasks.

RLS affects as many as 12 million Americans, but some experts estimate a much higher occurrence because RLS is thought to be underdiagnosed and, in some cases, misdiagnosed. Some people with RLS refuse to seek medical care, believing they will not be taken seriously, that their symptoms are too mild, or that their condition is not treatable. Some doctors attribute the symptoms to simple nervousness, insomnia, stress, arthritis, muscle cramps, or aging.

RLS occurs in both men and women, but the incidence may be slightly higher in women. Although the syndrome may begin at any age, even as early as infancy, most people who are severely affected are middle-aged or older. The disorder seems to get worse with age; older people experience symptoms more frequently and for longer periods of time.

More than 80 percent of people with RLS also experience a more common condition known as periodic limb movement disorder (PLMD). PLMD is characterized by involuntary leg twitching or jerking movements during sleep that typically occur every 10 to 60 seconds, sometimes throughout the night. The symptoms make the person wake up repeatedly, severely disrupting sleep. The movements caused by PLMD are involuntary—people have no control over them. The cause of RLS and PLMD is unknown.

Many doctors recommend lifestyle changes to reduce or eliminate symptoms. Avoiding caffeine, alcohol, and tobacco may provide some relief. Iron, folic acid (a B vitamin), and magnesium supplements in appropriate amounts may also be helpful. Taking a hot bath, massaging the legs, and using a heating pad or ice pack are other measures that may provide relief.

NARCOLEPSY

Narcolepsy is a chronic nervous system disorder caused by the brain's inability to regulate sleep-wake cycles normally. At various times throughout the day, people with narcolepsy experience fleeting urges to sleep. If the urge becomes overwhelming, affected people fall asleep for a few seconds to several minutes. In rare cases, people remain asleep for an hour or more.

In addition to excessive daytime sleepiness, the other major symptoms of narcolepsy include the sudden loss of voluntary muscle control; vivid hallucinations when falling asleep or awakening; and brief episodes of total paralysis at the beginning or end of sleep. The cause of narcolepsy remains unknown. The condition probably involves many factors that interact to cause the sleep disturbances.

INSOMNIA AND MENOPAUSE

During menopause (including perimenopause, menopause, and post-menopause), many women have sleep disturbances caused by hot flashes and night sweats, common symptoms during this time. But because female hormones act like a sleep aid, much of the sleep loss that occurs during menopause happens because estrogen and progesterone levels are going down. Hormone replacement therapy (HRT; see page 520) can be given for menopause-related sleep loss, but the benefits of treatment have to be weighed against its risks (which include an increased risk for breast cancer, heart disease, blood clots, and stroke). Women who have no risk factors for these disorders can consider taking low-dose HRT for short periods of time to relieve symptoms.

Other options for treating sleep loss during menopause are prescription sleep medications and foods containing soy, such as tofu and soybeans. Soy products have phytoestrogen, a hormone-like substance that mimics estrogen, but soy foods haven't been shown to help reduce menopausal symptoms very much.

✓ Don't drink alcohol to fall asleep

Alcohol consumed just before bedtime may help you fall asleep faster, but it also disrupts your sleep during the night. The alcohol wakes you up during the middle of the night and hampers your ability to fall back asleep. The more you drink, the more disrupted your sleep, and the more likely you are to feel tired and sleepy the next day. The problem is even worse for older people because they retain higher levels of alcohol in the blood than younger people after drinking the same amount. Bedtime alcohol consumption can also make older people unsteady if they have to walk to the bathroom during the night, significantly increasing the risk for falls and injuries.

Getting help for sleep problems

Although sleep disorders can negatively affect your health and safety, they can be treated. Talk to your doctor if you have any of the following signs of a sleep disorder:

- You consistently take more than 30 minutes to fall asleep at night.
- You wake up several times each night and then have trouble falling back to sleep, or you wake up too early in the morning.

- You often feel sleepy during the day, take frequent naps, or fall asleep at inappropriate times during the day.

- Your bed partner says that when you sleep, you snore loudly, snort, gasp, or make choking sounds.

- You have creeping, tingling, or crawling feelings in your legs or arms that are relieved by moving or massaging them, especially in the evening and when trying to fall asleep.

TIPS FOR IMPROVING YOUR SLEEP

Like eating a nutritious diet and being physically active, getting a good night's sleep is vital to your health and well-being. The following steps can boost your chances of getting a good night's sleep. Try these tips, and record your sleep and sleep-related activities in a sleep diary. If you still have problems sleeping, bring your diary with you to the doctor. The more information your doctor has, the easier it will be to recommend a solution to the problem.

Follow a regular sleep schedule: go to bed and wake up at the same times as often as you can, including on weekends.

- Exercise at the same time each day, but not within three hours of bedtime. (Exercise raises your heart rate and alertness, making you less sleepy.)

- Get some natural, outdoor light every day.

- Avoid caffeine late in the day. The stimulating effects of caffeine in coffee, colas, teas, and chocolate can take as long as eight hours to wear off fully.

- Don't drink alcohol to make you sleep. It can disrupt your sleep instead.

- Don't smoke. Nicotine is a stimulant.

- Avoid large meals late at night. A large meal can cause indigestion that interferes with sleep. Drinking too many fluids at night can make you wake up to use the bathroom.

- If possible, avoid medications that delay or disrupt sleep. Some commonly prescribed heart, blood pressure, and asthma medications, as well as some over-the-counter and herbal remedies for coughs, colds, or allergies, can disrupt sleep patterns.

- Don't take naps after 3 p.m. Naps can boost brain power (and may cut your risk of dying from a heart attack) but late afternoon naps can make it harder to fall asleep at night. Keep naps shorter than an hour.

- Create a safe and comfortable place to sleep. Make sure it's dark, quiet, well-ventilated, and neither too dry nor too humid. Keeping the temperature in your bedroom on the cool side can help you sleep better.

- Develop a nighttime routine that helps you slow down and relax.

- If you're having trouble falling asleep within about 15 minutes, get up, do a quiet activity, and return to bed when you're sleepy.

- Your bed partner notices that your legs or arms jerk often during sleep.

- You have vivid, dreamlike experiences while falling asleep or dozing.

- You have episodes of sudden muscle weakness when you are angry or afraid, or when you laugh.

- You feel as if you can't move when you first wake up.

Children display many of the same signs when they have a sleep disorder, but they often don't act sleepy during the day. Instead, they may seem overactive and have difficulty focusing or performing well in school.

Ways to lower stress

The human body has an amazing ability to heal itself. This section will point out ways to reduce and control the stress in your life. Probably the single most important way to minimize and manage the stress in your life is to follow a healthy lifestyle, which includes eating a nutritious diet, being physically active, learning positive coping skills, enjoying life, and getting support from family and friends when you need it. One of the most effective on-the-spot strategies for relieving stress is meditation, which can immediately change your mental state and relax you.

Eat a nutritious diet

A healthy diet (see chapter 1) not only provides nutrition for your body, it also fuels your mind. When your body is well-nourished, you are better able to cope with both the day-to-day stresses in your life as well as the difficult situations that arise. Here are a few tips for helping you cope with stress in a healthier way:

- Eat a balanced diet. A balanced, nutrient-dense diet will give you the energy you need to think rationally and clearly and may improve your ability to deal with potentially stressful situations.

- Limit your intake of caffeine and sugar. Caffeine and sugar can give you a temporary "high" but can also make you jittery and nervous. Avoiding caffeine will help you feel more relaxed and less nervous, and your sleep will improve.

- Avoid self-medicating with alcohol or drugs. Alcohol and other drugs cannot make your problems and stress go away and, in fact, can often make them worse. While under the influence, you are not able to deal with your problems with a clear mind.

Be physically active

One of the best ways to turn off your stress alarm is to exercise. Exercise rebalances the body's hormones and chemical messengers, enhances your overall health and well-being, and provides some specific stress-busting benefits. Here's how exercise can help you deal in a positive way with stress at work and at home. (See chapter 2 for a fuller discussion of the benefits of exercise.)

- **Exercise serves up endorphins.** Exercising for at least half an hour triggers brain chemicals known as endorphins (which bring on a sense of mild euphoria and well-being and relieve pain).
- **Exercise helps you release tension.** Exercise helps ease daily tensions. A strong body increases your ability to cope with the troublesome things that come at you every day.
- **Exercise is active meditation.** The repetitive motion of running, swimming, hiking, or biking combined with rhythmic breathing can help you get in touch with your body and may even put you into a meditative state, especially if you exercise outdoors.
- **Exercise makes you feel better emotionally.** Regular exercise has been shown to reduce mild depression and anxiety.
- **Exercise makes you sleep better.** Working your body physically makes it easier for you to let go and relax. You'll fall asleep faster and sleep more soundly.

GOOD STRESS-BUSTING EXERCISES

What types of exercise are best for reducing stress? Here is a short list of the characteristics of the kinds of exercise that are best for helping relieve stress:

- **Noncompetitive** Trying to beat your tennis partner isn't always the best way to unwind. Besides, if you lose, you may be too hard on yourself or even get resentful of the winner. Stick to activities that don't involve winning or losing, like walking, jogging, or swimming.

- **Enjoyable**   If you pick an activity you like, you're more likely to stay with it and have a good time, releasing stress at the same time.

- **Aerobic**   Activities that use the large muscle groups will help you let go of tension better than strength-training exercises, which actively use muscle tension. (Stretching is also a good way to loosen muscles.)

- **Informal**   Don't choose an activity that draws too much attention to your performance. For example, if you play golf with buddies who try to outdo one another, it could actually increase your stress level.

- **Regular**   Exercise regularly—every day if you can—to reduce stress on a regular basis.

Yoga

If the stress in your life is getting to you, take a yoga class. Yoga is a Hindu religious practice that combines a variety of postures and controlled breathing exercises to attain serenity in body and mind. As a bonus, yoga also increases flexibility and body tone. Yoga has become hugely popular in the United States as a way of reducing stress—millions of Americans regularly practice it. The tradition's calm and careful poses focus the mind away from a hectic day so you can be more "in the moment" as you move your body into positions that require precise balance and concentration.

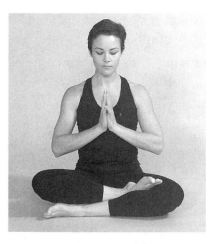

Yoga is based on a system of thought involving the central nervous system, channels of energy, and chakras (centers of energy located throughout the body where nerves come together). In traditional Hindu belief, the body has seven major chakras. The purpose of yoga is to awaken something called kundalini, a bundle of energy that lies dormant at the base of the spine. When awakened, kundalini rises up through six of the centers to the seventh chakra at the top of the head, bringing balance and health to the mind and body as well as spiritual awareness.

Many health clubs and fitness centers offer yoga classes and some employers conduct on-site yoga classes in response to the demand. Check with your local community center, park district, or employer to see if they offer a conveniently timed yoga class near you. But keep in mind that maintaining yoga postures represents very-low-intensity exercise compared with strength training or aerobic activities. Use yoga as a supplement to aerobic exercises like brisk walking, jogging, biking, swimming, or stair climbing, not as a substitute, so you can keep your heart and lungs strong.

Although yoga seems so serene that it must be safe, injuries can occur if you push yourself too far in trying to attain a correct posture. The best advice is, if it hurts, pull back. Common yoga injuries are caused by over-stretching of the neck, shoulders, spine, legs, and knees. If you have a pre-existing medical condition, talk to your doctor before participating in a yoga class. Following these guidelines can help you get the most out of yoga:

- Check your instructor's credentials.
- Do some warm-up exercises before class to limber up your muscles and joints.
- Wear loose clothing.
- Start slowly if you're a beginner.
- Ask the instructor if you're not sure how to do a posture.
- Don't stretch your joints to the point where they hurt.
- Drink plenty of water.
- Stop if you feel pain or exhaustion.

Tai chi

Initially developed in China 2,000 years ago as a martial art, tai chi is a graceful form of exercise that has become extremely popular worldwide. Health advantages include stress reduction, improved balance, and increased flexibility, especially in older people. Tai chi involves moving the body slowly and gently while breathing slowly and meditating mindfully. Many people who do tai chi believe that it helps the flow of a vital energy called qi (pronounced "chee") throughout the body. Qi is a fundamental principle of Chinese medicine.

You can practice tai chi on your own or in a group. The graceful movements make up what practitioners call forms (or routines). Some movements are named for the motions made by animals or birds, such as "White Crane Spreads Its Wings." The simplest form of tai chi uses 13 different movements. More complex styles can incorporate dozens.

In tai chi, each movement flows into the next. Your entire body is always in motion, performing the movements gently and at a consistent speed. To ensure the smooth flow of qi, you need to keep your posture straight and your body, especially your upper body, upright. Many tai chi practitioners imagine a string running from the top of the head into the sky, which allows the body's weight to sink down into the soles of the feet.

In addition to movement, two other important elements of tai chi are breathing and meditation. In tai chi practice, it is important to pay attention to what you are doing and to put aside distracting thoughts. You also breathe in a deep, relaxed, and focused way. This focused breathing combined with full attention is believed to improve health in the following ways:

- Promoting the exchange of gases in the lungs
- Improving the functioning of the digestive system
- Increasing calmness and awareness
- Improving balance
- Lowering blood pressure

Tai chi movements are less jarring even than low-impact exercises, so the system is perfect for people who have arthritis. Again, aerobic exercise is the best type of physical activity for your heart, so you should practice tai chi along with, not in place of, regular aerobic exercise such as walking.

Stay connected

Staying connected and talking about your problems and feelings with people you trust can reduce stress, keep you healthy, and help you solve your problems. When you talk out a difficult situation or problem with someone else, you see your problem in a different way. And friends are good medicine. Studies have found that people who have a large social network with ties to friends, family, work, and community have fewer respiratory infections than people who have fewer connections with other people. Get support wherever you can—from a friend, family member, coworker, doctor, teacher, counselor, member of the clergy, or support group.

Be positive

Being optimistic seems to provide a buffer against negative consequences from stress and may help people live longer and healthier. People who are optimistic do not blame themselves or feel negatively about themselves when faced with stress or setbacks. They tend to believe that things will go well for them and they have confidence that they can handle problems that come their way. Compared with people who are pessimistic, optimists tend to have fewer infections, are in better general health, and tend to live longer. Optimists are less likely to have depression, and if they have cancer, they seem to have better outcomes than people with cancer who are pessimists.

But there is hope for people who tend to think negatively about things. You can learn about techniques that can help you look at your situation differently. For example, instead of saying "I can't do this" or "I'm not prepared," you can remind yourself that "I'm well prepared and ready for this." Before situations in which we are anxious or sad, we tend to have unrealistically negative or distorted thoughts. But you can learn to adjust these distorted thoughts and remind yourself of your positive qualities. This can help you relax and enable you to conquer the challenge or deal with a difficult situation.

Instead of ignoring your accomplishments and focusing on what you see as your faults and failures, try to concentrate on your achievements and seek out supportive and nurturing personal contacts. Instead of assuming the worst will happen and not considering possible positive outcomes, be hopeful about your ability to meet challenges and the gratification you will get from a positive outcome such as doing a job well. Even people who have depression can learn to readjust their negative thinking patterns; when given counseling to help them be more aware of their thoughts and adjust their thinking and coping patterns into more realistic or appropriate ones, they are able, with practice, to maintain these positive thinking patterns over the long term and handle future setbacks more effectively.

Laugh

Having a sense of humor and being able to laugh are essential components of stress management. In fact, the act of laughing itself produces physical changes that help the body fight stress in a number of ways:

- **Laughing provides a physical workout.** A hearty laugh contracts the abdominal muscles, exercises the diaphragm, works the shoulders, and even gives the heart a workout.
- **Laughing improves hormone levels.** Laughter reduces the level of stress hormones such as cortisol, which can be harmful if elevated for long periods of time. At the same time, laughter raises the level of

health-boosting hormones such as the feel-good endorphins. It also boosts the immune system, potentially reducing susceptibility to infections and other illnesses.

- **Laughing connects you with other people.** When you laugh, people tend to laugh with you. Bringing laughter into other people's lives instantly provides a bond between you. And when you make other people feel better emotionally, their stress levels are lowered and they also reap the health benefits of reduced stress.

- **Laughing changes your perspective.** Humor can give you a more upbeat perspective and enable you to see situations as less threatening. When you view situations as challenges rather than threats, you can deal with them more easily and in a positive way. Also, laughter provides immediate distraction from any negative emotions you are feeling, including anger or guilt—instant stress relief.

Get more humor and laughter into your life by watching hilarious TV shows and movies, seeing a comedy show with a friend (you'll both laugh more), and trying to see humor even in the frustrations or setbacks in your life.

WHEN TO GET HELP

Sometimes, overwhelming stress can cause symptoms similar to those of depression. To help you determine if your feelings are more than a temporary setback or low mood and may be a sign of depression that requires professional help, talk to your doctor if you experience any of the following:

- Your low mood feels severe and painful and you feel it will never end.
- You often feel sad and tearful and that life is not worth living.
- You feel so desperate that you think about quitting your job, running away, taking a drug overdose, or injuring yourself.
- Your low mood is accompanied by symptoms such as loss of appetite, trouble sleeping, loss of sexual desire, or inability to concentrate or make decisions.
- You are dealing with your stress by drinking alcohol, binge eating, sleeping more than usual, or using recreational drugs.
- You no longer enjoy activities that you formerly found pleasurable.
- You have feelings of worthlessness, helplessness, hopelessness, or guilt.

Enjoy life

It's when your life is so full with work and the demands of family and home and you feel you don't have a free moment that it is essential to take a break and do something enjoyable. Too much work or study can lead to burnout and is actually inefficient. Taking time out for yourself can give you a needed refresher and boost your energy. Do things that make you feel happy: take a walk with a friend, meet a friend for lunch or dinner, go to a movie, take a warm bath, or read that book you've been wanting to read for a long time.

Meditate

Meditation is one of the most commonly practiced mind-body interventions. It can be described as a conscious mental process that induces a pre-set series of changes in the body known as the relaxation response. Meditation is used so often for health purposes that medical researchers became interested in finding a scientific explanation for the beneficial effects of meditation on the body. Researchers used such techniques as magnetic resonance imaging (MRI) to identify the parts of the brain that become active during meditation. They found that the parts of the brain that are normally activated during periods of attention and those that control the autonomic nervous system (responsible for body functions, such as breathing and heartbeat, which are not under conscious control) come into play during meditation. Meditation has been shown to produce considerable increases in activity in parts of the brain linked to positive emotional states. Studies have found that meditation can boost the effectiveness of the influenza vaccine, suggesting a potential improvement in immune function.

There are many types of meditation, most of which originated in ancient religious and spiritual traditions. While meditating, a person uses specific techniques, such as focusing attention, for example, on a word (called a mantra by meditation practitioners), an object, or the breath; a specific posture; and an indifferent attitude toward distracting thoughts and emotions. People meditate for many reasons. Some people do it to increase physical relaxation, mental calmness, and psychological balance. Others try it to cope with stress or a medical condition, or just for overall wellness. Some people say they are trying to achieve a "heightened state of awareness."

WHAT IS MEDITATION?

The term "meditation" refers to a group of techniques used in Eastern religious or spiritual traditions. These techniques have been used by many different cultures throughout the world for thousands of years. Today, many people use meditation outside of its traditional religious or cultural settings, primarily for health purposes.

While meditating, a person learns to focus his or her attention and to draw attention away from the automatic stream of thoughts that normally occupy the mind. The practice induces physical relaxation, mental calmness, and emotional balance. Practicing meditation can actually change how you relate to the usual flow of emotions and thoughts in your mind. You can practice meditation alone or with other mind-body techniques such as yoga (see page 116) or tai chi (see page 117).

Most types of meditation use the following four elements to bring about the meditative state:

- **Quiet location**   Choose a quiet place with as few distractions as possible; this is especially helpful for beginners. People who have been practicing meditation for a long time sometimes develop the ability to meditate in public places.

- **Comfortable posture**   Depending on the type of meditation you engage in, you can do the practice while sitting, lying down, standing, walking, or in other positions.

- **Attention focus**   Focusing your attention is a big part of meditation. For example, you might focus your attention on a mantra (a specially chosen word or set of words), on an object, or on your breathing.

- **Open attitude**   Having an open attitude during meditation means letting distractions come and go naturally without thinking about them. When distracting or wandering thoughts occur, don't try to suppress them; instead, gently bring your attention back to your self-chosen focus. In some types of meditation, you'll learn to observe the rising and falling of thoughts and emotions as they occur spontaneously.

THE RELAXATION RESPONSE

The medical community has been using relaxation techniques for years to treat chronic pain and insomnia. There is strong evidence that relaxation techniques and hypnosis can relieve the pain caused by cancer. Relaxation may also improve insomnia, but the extent of the improvement in sleep onset and duration doesn't seem to be very great.

The Relaxation Response was developed by Herbert Benson, M.D., of Harvard Medical School. The technique is a straightforward practice that takes only 10 to 20 minutes a day. It involves systematically relaxing your muscles while becoming aware of your breathing. The following instructions are from Dr. Benson's book *The Relaxation Response*, which was originally published in 1975:

1. Sit quietly in a comfortable position.

2. Close your eyes.

3. Deeply relax all your muscles, beginning at your feet and progressing up to your face. Keep them relaxed.

4. Breathe through your nose. Become aware of your breathing. As you exhale, say the word ONE silently to yourself.

5. Continue this practice for 10 to 20 minutes. When distracting thoughts occur, try to ignore them by not dwelling upon them and return to repeating ONE.

6. When you finish, sit quietly for several minutes, at first with your eyes closed and later with your eyes open. Don't stand up right away.

7. Don't worry about whether you were successful in achieving a deep level of relaxation. Maintain a passive attitude and permit relaxation to occur at its own pace. With practice, the response should come with little effort.

8. Practice the technique once or twice a day, but not within two hours after a meal because the digestive process seems to interfere with the Relaxation Response.

MEDITATION TO IMPROVE YOUR HEALTH

Meditation used for health purposes is a type of mind-body medicine that attempts to improve health by focusing on the interactions that occur between the brain and the rest of the body, the mind, or a person's behavior. It also tries to influence the ways in which emotions, the mind, spirituality, and behavior can directly affect health. Doctors may recommend meditation to their patients for a variety of health problems, including the following:

- Anxiety
- Pain
- Depression
- Mood and self-esteem problems
- Stress
- Insomnia
- Physical or emotional symptoms arising from serious illnesses and their treatment, such as heart disease, HIV/AIDS, and cancer

It's common for people to use meditation as a way of coping with health problems. A large national survey found that nearly 8 percent of the participants had used meditation specifically for health reasons during the year before the survey. If you are considering using meditation for a medical condition, be sure to talk to your doctor first, to see if it fits into your overall treatment plan.

5

REDUCING YOUR HEALTH RISKS

EVERY DAY, YOU MAKE CHOICES that can be good for your health or bad for you. Some of these choices may involve potentially dangerous behaviors. The behaviors that are most likely to increase your health risks are smoking, drinking alcohol excessively, using drugs, and practicing unsafe sex. This chapter can help you understand the impact of risky choices on your health and that of your family.

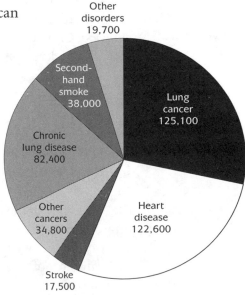

Other disorders
19,700

Second-hand smoke
38,000

Lung cancer
125,100

Chronic lung disease
82,400

Other cancers
34,800

Heart disease
122,600

Stroke
17,500

Deaths from cigarette smoking

This chart uses figures from the Centers for Disease Control and Prevention to show the number and causes of deaths attributed to smoking each year in the United States. Of the more than 440,000 smoking-related deaths, four out of five result from lung disease (especially lung cancer and emphysema), heart disease, and stroke.

The health risks of tobacco use

Cigarette smoking is the single most preventable cause of death in the United States, causing premature death in more than 440,000 people in this country each year. Smoking has harmful effects on the whole body. Lifelong smokers have a 50 percent chance of dying from a smoking-related disease. Smoking cuts years off the end of your life and increases your risk for lung cancer and other diseases of the respiratory system, heart disease, and high blood pressure. Secondhand smoke can cause lung cancer and heart disease in nonsmokers and increase respiratory illnesses such as asthma in children.

When you smoke, your bloodstream absorbs nicotine rapidly and the chemical travels to your brain in seconds. Nicotine is a highly addictive substance, which is why people have a hard time quitting smoking. In fact, nicotine's addictive quality has been found to be even stronger than that of heroin and cocaine. At first, when you smoke, nicotine, a stimulant, makes you feel good, so you want to smoke more. But your body needs increasingly more nicotine in order to feel good—so you smoke more.

Tar is the sticky brown residue that forms when tobacco is burned. It's made up of many harmful chemicals, including hydrocarbons, known cancer-causing substances. Tar raises the risk for lung cancer, emphysema, and other respiratory disorders. But tar is only the beginning of the story. Tobacco smoke contains thousands of other chemicals—about 60 of which cause cancer—including arsenic, ammonia, formaldehyde, lead, benzene, and vinyl chloride. Cigarette smoke also contains carbon monoxide, which increases your risk of developing heart disease or of having a heart attack or stroke.

Smoking's effects on health

Smoking damages nearly every major organ of the body. Most people think of lung cancer when they consider the health hazards of smoking. But smoking is a major factor in the development of other disorders as well. If you smoke, you have a substantially increased risk of having a heart attack—the No. 1 killer in the United States. Smoking also contributes to bone thinning and many digestive disorders. The risk of developing smoking-related diseases increases with total lifetime exposure to cigarette smoke, defined as the number of cigarettes a person smokes each day, the intensity of smoking (the size and frequency of puffs), the age at which smoking began, the number of years a person has smoked, and his or her exposure to second-hand smoke.

SMOKING AND THE RESPIRATORY SYSTEM

Smoking is the major cause of lung cancer; an estimated nine out of 10 cases of lung cancer are the result of smoking. Lung cancer is the No. 1 cancer killer of both men and women in the United States. In fact, lung cancer causes more deaths each year than the next three most common cancers combined—cancers of the colon, breast, and prostate. Tobacco smoke contains more than 60 known cancer-causing agents that directly damage cells in the lungs, making them more likely to become cancerous.

The poisons in tobacco smoke cause the airways to produce excessive amounts of mucus, which clogs the airways. The air passages begin to swell and, over time, smokers have more and more trouble clearing mucus from their airways. They often develop a cough that won't go away. Sometimes this cough turns into a lung disease called chronic bronchitis.

Tobacco smoke destroys the cells that clear debris from the lungs and paralyzes the hairlike projections that line and protect the airways. Over the long term, smoking can cause the tiny air sacs in the lungs to burst and merge, forming fewer but larger air sacs. These larger air sacs reduce the surface area of the lungs, making them less able to transfer oxygen into the bloodstream and making it harder and harder for you to breathe normally. This is how emphysema develops. Emphysema is a disease that is almost always the result of smoking.

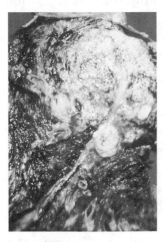
Lung with cancer

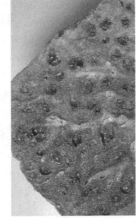
Lung with emphysema

How smoking affects the lungs

Smoking is the major cause of lung cancer and emphysema (a chronic lung condition in which damage to the tiny air sacs in the lungs makes breathing difficult). Chronic inflammation of lung tissue from cigarette smoke and tar residue left by the smoke triggers a cascade of changes in cells in the lungs that can lead to cancer or emphysema, or both. In this cross-section of a lung with cancer (left), the white area in the upper lobe is cancerous tissue and the blackened areas are deposits of tar. The lung with emphysema (right) has multiple cavities (caused by the destruction of air sacs) that are surrounded by black deposits of tar.

SMOKING AND HEART DISEASE

Smokers face a substantially higher risk of dying from heart disease than nonsmokers. Smoking increases the tendency of blood to clot, and can promote the buildup of fatty deposits called plaques in artery walls (atherosclerosis; see page 218). Smoking increases the risk for atherosclerosis by lowering the levels of helpful HDL cholesterol, which removes cholesterol from the arteries. A plaque can enlarge and be covered with a cap of smooth muscle cells. Over time, the muscle cap can rupture and form an open wound that attracts red blood cells to the site to form a clot to seal off the rupture. However, the clot can eventually grow and block the artery. If the artery feeds blood to the heart, the result is a heart attack. If the artery feeds blood to the brain, the result is a stroke. Heart disease is more likely to recur in a smoker after bypass surgery than in a nonsmoker. Women over age 35 who smoke and take birth control pills are at substantially increased risk for blood-clot formation that can lead to a heart attack or stroke.

Smoking can also promote the buildup of plaque in the arteries that carry blood to the arms and legs. This can cause painful cramping of the leg muscles while walking (a condition called intermittent claudication). Smoking also raises blood pressure, another powerful risk factor for heart attack and stroke. Smoking lowers your endurance and tolerance for exercise, further increasing your risk for heart disease and high blood pressure.

IT'S NOT JUST CIGARETTES THAT AREN'T SAFE

Some people think smokeless tobacco (chewing tobacco and snuff), pipes, and cigars are safe—but they're not. Using smokeless tobacco can cause cancer of the mouth, precancerous sores known as oral leukoplakia, nicotine addiction, and cancer of the vocal cords and esophagus (the muscular passage between the throat and stomach). Tobacco products also cause gum problems (periodontal disease; see page 430), now recognized as a risk factor for heart disease. Pipe and cigar smokers can develop cancers of the mouth, lip, throat, voice box, esophagus, and bladder. Those who inhale are also at increased risk for lung cancer.

SMOKING AND CANCER

Cigarette smoking is responsible for about 30 percent of all cancer deaths in the United States each year. Cigarette smoking causes nearly 9 out of 10 lung cancer deaths and is responsible for most cancers of the mouth, throat, voice box, and esophagus. If you smoke and also drink alcohol, your risk for mouth and throat cancers is multiplied to a risk far greater than that incurred by either activity alone; in fact, the combination of heavy smoking and drinking is attributed to about three out of four cases of mouth cancer and throat cancer.

Smoking is a major cause of bladder cancer in both men and women. Although bladder cancer is much more common in men, it can be especially harmful to women. Women smokers seem to face a higher risk of developing bladder cancer than male smokers, and they are twice as likely as males to die from it. Part of the explanation for this disparity may be that bladder cancers in women are generally diagnosed at a more advanced stage than in men. Another reason may be physiologic: the relative thinness of the female bladder and the presence in females of more aggressive, rare cell types that are more likely to become cancerous.

Smoking is also a risk factor for cancers of the kidney, pancreas, cervix, and stomach, as well as one form of leukemia. The risk of developing any of the smoking-related cancers is dose-related—the more cigarettes you smoke, the younger you start smoking, and the more years you smoke, the greater your risk. But it's not just smokers who are at risk: secondhand smoke causes an estimated 3,000 lung cancer deaths among nonsmokers in the United States each year.

Cigar smokers are at increased risk for cancers of the mouth, throat, voice box, and esophagus. These risks are similar to the risks from cigarette smoking. Smokeless tobacco users have an increased risk for cancers of the mouth, especially cancers of the cheek and gum, and cancers of the voice box and esophagus.

SMOKING AND BONE HEALTH

Cigarette smoking has been shown to be a risk factor for osteoporosis (see page 325) and bone fractures. Osteoporosis is a condition in which the bones weaken and are more likely to break. Fractures from osteoporosis cause pain, disability, and loss of independence, and they can be fatal. Osteoporosis is a major health threat for an estimated 44 million older Americans, most of whom are women.

Cigarette smoking was first identified as a risk factor for bone loss and osteoporosis more than 20 years ago, but it can be hard to tell whether a decrease in bone density has been caused by smoking itself or by other factors common among smokers. For example, many smokers are thinner than nonsmokers, tend to drink more alcohol, may be less physically active, and often consume less-nutritious foods. Women who smoke are also likely to go through menopause at an earlier age than nonsmokers. (Loss of the bone-preserving female hormone estrogen at menopause is responsible for this effect.) All of these are risk factors for osteoporosis apart from tobacco use.

However, most studies on the effects of smoking on the bones suggest that smoking itself increases the risk of having a fracture. For example, studies have found that the longer a person smokes and the more cigarettes he or she smokes, the greater his or her risk for fractures later in life. Smokers who have fractures take longer to heal than nonsmokers and experience more complications while healing. Women who smoke often produce less estrogen, which may lead to increased bone loss. Quitting smoking seems to reduce the risk for low bone mass and fractures, but it may take several years to achieve this benefit.

SMOKING AND THE DIGESTIVE SYSTEM

Smoking has harmful effects on all parts of the digestive system and plays a role in the development of heartburn and peptic ulcers. Smoking increases the risk for the inflammatory bowel disease Crohn's disease, gallstones (which form when liquid stored in the gallbladder hardens into pieces of stone-like material), and liver damage.

Heartburn

Heartburn is very common—more than 50 million Americans have it at least once a month and about 15 million have it daily. Heartburn is a symptom of a condition called gastroesophageal reflux disease (GERD), which occurs when the acidic digestive juices in the stomach flow backward, up into the esophagus (the tube that connects the mouth to the stomach), causing inflammation. Stomach acid helps break down food. While the stomach is naturally protected from acidic juices, the esophagus doesn't have the same protection. Normally, a muscular valve at the lower end of the esophagus keeps the acids inside the stomach and out of the esophagus. But smoking weakens the valve, allowing stomach acid to flow into the esophagus, which then becomes injured or damaged from inflammation, producing GERD.

Peptic ulcers

A peptic ulcer is a sore in the lining of the stomach or the first part of the small intestine. One in 10 people develops a peptic ulcer at some time in life. A common cause of peptic ulcers is the bacterium Helicobacter pylori (H. pylori), which can burrow into the protective lining of the stomach or small intestine, attach to underlying cells, and release chemicals that further harm the lining, exposing the cells to damage from stomach acids. Another possible cause of peptic ulcers is the long-term use of nonsteroidal anti-inflammatory medications such as aspirin and ibuprofen, which can interfere with the stomach's natural ability to protect itself from stomach acid and other digestive juices.

People who smoke cigarettes are more likely than nonsmokers to develop an ulcer. If they continue smoking, the ulcer may not heal, or it may take longer than usual to heal. The chances for an ulcer to heal are greater if you quit smoking than if you continue to smoke and take medication. Smoking also weakens the immune system, increasing the risk for an H. pylori infection that can lead to an ulcer.

Another way that smoking may promote ulcer formation is by temporarily reducing the amount of sodium bicarbonate in the body; sodium bicarbonate is a substance made by the pancreas to aid digestion by neutralizing any acid from food that is not absorbed by the stomach. Cigarette smoking may intensify the amount of acid secreted by the stomach over time.

Crohn's disease

Crohn's disease is an inflammatory disorder that causes swelling deep in the lining of the intestine, causing pain and diarrhea. The disease usually affects the small intestine, but it can arise anywhere in the digestive tract. Current and former smokers have a higher tendency to develop Crohn's disease than nonsmokers. In people with Crohn's disease, smoking is linked to a higher rate of relapse, a recurring need for corrective surgery, and the need for drug treatment—especially among affected women. Doctors aren't sure why smoking boosts a person's risk of developing Crohn's disease, but some researchers think that smoking may limit blood flow to the intestines or cause immune system changes that result in inflammation. Inflammation is the major factor in the development of Crohn's disease.

Liver disease

The liver is an organ that performs many vital tasks. One of its more important functions is to process drugs, alcohol, and other toxins and remove them from the body. Smoking reduces the liver's ability to perform this task. Sometimes, if the liver has been damaged from cigarette smoking, the dose of medication needed to treat an illness may have to be adjusted. Smoking can also worsen the kind of liver disease that results from drinking too much alcohol (see page 353).

The effects of smoking during pregnancy

Smoking is especially harmful during pregnancy (see page 494) and can have long-lasting effects on the health of the fetus. For example, smoking during pregnancy can cause permanent damage to a fetus's arteries, raising the risk for the development of heart disease and stroke in adulthood. The children of mothers who smoked during their pregnancy have more evidence of atherosclerosis later in life than children whose mothers did not smoke during pregnancy. The arteries of children who were exposed to smoke before birth have thicker walls, a finding that becomes apparent by young adulthood. Children of mothers who smoked during their pregnancy are also at increased risk of developing asthma and of having an attention deficit disorder or learning disability.

Smoking during pregnancy doubles the chances that a baby will be born with a low birth weight, which has been linked to an increased risk of developing type 2 diabetes later in life. However, doctors do not fully understand exactly how low birth weight and type 2 diabetes are related. Smoking during pregnancy also increases the risk for an ectopic pregnancy, miscarriage, stillbirth, and other pregnancy-related complications, and sudden infant death syndrome (SIDS).

SMOKING'S EFFECTS ON THE EYES

The toxic chemicals in tobacco smoke can damage the eyes and cause or worsen several eye disorders such as cataracts and age-related macular degeneration, and may lead to blindness.

Cataracts

Cataracts (a condition in which the lens of the eye loses its transparency; see page 408), if untreated, can lead to loss of vision. In many people, cataracts develop as a normal part of aging. But in some cases, cataracts can be prevented. Smoking is a major risk factor for cataracts, especially a type of cataract called a nuclear cataract. People who smoke 20 or more cigarettes a day are more than twice as likely to develop cataracts as people who never smoked. The risk increases the more a person smokes, and heavy smokers develop more serious cases than light smokers.

Although the exact mechanism by which smoking causes cataracts is not fully understood, it may be that tobacco smoke destroys antioxidants (which help maintain the transparency of the lens) and other micronutrients that are essential for keeping the eyes healthy.

Age-related macular degeneration

Age-related macular degeneration (AMD: see page 413) affects the small central area of the retina at the back of the eye (the macula), which is responsible for clear, central vision. AMD is the most common cause of blindness in people over age 55. Smoking is the major preventable risk factor for AMD. Smokers are two to three times more likely than nonsmokers to develop any form of AMD and are more likely to experience relapses after laser treatment for AMD.

Diabetic retinopathy

Smoking can accelerate or worsen diabetic retinopathy (see page 416), an eye complication of diabetes in which the blood vessels that supply the retina in the back of the eye are damaged by high blood sugar levels. Like excess blood sugar, smoking may worsen the condition by damaging blood vessels in the eye. Smoking may also damage the retina by reducing the amount of oxygen that reaches it.

Thyroid eye disease

Thyroid eye disease, a complication of Graves' disease, is four times more likely to develop in a person with Graves' disease who smokes than in a nonsmoker who has Graves' disease. The more heavily a person smokes, the greater the risk. Why this occurs is unclear but doctors think it may be because smoking impairs the immune system.

Optic neuropathy

Smokers are more likely than nonsmokers to develop a condition called anterior ischemic optic neuropathy (an eye disease that results in a sudden, painless loss of vision that can lead to permanent blindness) and to develop it at younger ages than nonsmokers. The condition occurs when blood flow to the arteries of the eyes is blocked, usually by atherosclerosis (the buildup of fatty deposits in artery walls; see page 218). Smoking is a major risk factor for atherosclerosis.

WHY YOU'RE HOOKED

Researchers have discovered why smokers have such a hard time quitting. Normally, the brain releases dopamine (a chemical that produces feelings of pleasure) when you perform a rewarding behavior, such as eating when you are hungry. The brain then quickly releases another chemical, called acetylcholine, which stops the release of dopamine.

When you smoke, nicotine triggers the release of dopamine but prevents the brain from turning it off by blocking the release of acetylcholine. As a result, the brain continues pumping out dopamine, making you feel better and better. After nicotine levels in the bloodstream fall, dopamine production declines. The brain, recalling the good feelings, wants more dopamine, producing cravings for another cigarette. These processes take place inside a part of the brain scientists call the reward center.

Secondhand smoke

Ninety percent of nonsmokers are exposed to smoke from someone else's cigarette, pipe, or cigar, and a significant percentage of people are constantly exposed to secondhand smoke in the workplace or at home. Secondhand smoke can be harmful to nonsmokers, causing an estimated 38,000 deaths each year—about 35,000 from heart disease and 3,000 from lung cancer. The people most susceptible to the harmful effects of secondhand smoke are those who live or work with smokers: constant exposure to smoke at home or in the workplace nearly doubles the risk of having a heart attack.

Smoke emitted from the burning end of a cigarette contains higher concentrations of many toxins, including nicotine, than the smoke inhaled from a cigarette by a smoker. Secondhand smoke contains at least 250 chemicals known to be toxic, including more than 50 that can cause cancer.

Inhaling secondhand smoke is especially dangerous for someone with asthma, other lung conditions, or heart disease, and for children. One in three American children 18 years old or younger lives with at least one smoker. Exposure to secondhand smoke increases a child's risk for bronchitis, pneumonia, asthma, and frequent ear infections, and may be linked to

SIDS (sudden infant death syndrome). Exposure to secondhand smoke during childhood may also increase a child's risk of developing heart disease later in life.

These health risks are just a few of the many good reasons for a parent or grandparent or other household member to think about quitting smoking. Never smoke indoors around people of any age. Don't allow anyone to smoke in your home and, if you are in the home of a smoker, politely ask the person if he or she could go outside to smoke.

How to quit smoking

It's never too late to quit smoking. Quitting smoking makes a big difference right away. Your ability to taste and smell food improves. Your breath smells better. Your cough may go away. These welcome effects occur in men and women of all ages, regardless of how long they have been smoking. And quitting smoking incurs even more benefits over time including the following:

- Quitting smoking cuts your risk for lung cancer and several other cancers, other lung and respiratory disorders, and heart disease and stroke.

- One year after quitting, your risk of heart disease drops by half. Fifteen years after you stop, your health risk equals that of a person who never smoked.

- Ex-smokers experience fewer days of illness, fewer health complaints, and less bronchitis, pneumonia, and other respiratory problems than current smokers.

- Quitting smoking saves money. A pack-a-day smoker can expect to save more than $1,000 every year. As the price of cigarettes continues to rise, so will the economic rewards of quitting.

The first few weeks after quitting are the hardest. Some people who give up smoking have withdrawal symptoms from nicotine's powerful addictive qualities. You may become irritable, hungry, or tired. You may have headaches, feel depressed, or have problems sleeping or concentrating. A few lucky people don't experience any withdrawal symptoms, but you should expect to feel at least uncomfortable—maybe even very distressed—for some period of time after you quit smoking.

THE HEALTH BENEFITS OF QUITTING

Even if you have been smoking for years, when you quit, your body begins a series of changes to repair the damage caused by smoking and restore health to your cells and organs.

Time since last cigarette	Health benefit
20 minutes	Blood pressure decreases. Pulse rate drops. Circulation increases, making hands and feet feel warmer.
8 hours	Breathing gets easier because carbon monoxide (which depletes the body of oxygen) in the blood decreases and oxygen increases.
24 hours	Risk for heart attack decreases.
48 hours	Senses of smell and taste start to return. Nerve endings begin to grow back.
2 weeks to 3 months	Circulation continues to improve. Walking gets easier. Lung function increases.
1 to 9 months	Symptoms such as coughing, sinus congestion, fatigue, and shortness of breath subside.
1 year	Risk for heart disease is cut in half.
5 years (to 15 years)	Risk for stroke decreases to that of a person who has never smoked.
10 years	Risk for lung cancer decreases up to 50 percent. Risk for cancers of the mouth, throat, esophagus, bladder, kidneys, and pancreas drops.
15 years	Risk for heart disease is the same as that of a person who has never smoked. Risk of dying from any smoking-related cause is nearly the same as that of a person who has never smoked.

Breaking the addiction

Smoking is a strong addiction for both the body and mind. That's why it's so hard to stop. But many people succeed. Since 1965, more than 40 million Americans have quit smoking. Help is available. Try these tips to get the help you need:

- Get as much information as you can. Read self-help books and brochures; call 1-800-QUIT NOW (1-800-784-8669); call your state "quitline."
- Attend individual or group counseling.
- Be active. Exercising, even for just five minutes, can help reduce the craving for a cigarette.
- Join a smoking-cessation support group.
- Ask a friend to quit with you.
- Talk to your doctor about nicotine-replacement therapy or medication (see page 139) to ease your withdrawal symptoms.

Each person is different, so you need to find what works best for you. In many cases, combining several smoking-cessation methods is the key. Although some people can stop on their own, others may need help from a doctor, a clinic, or an organized smoking-cessation program.

The first step is to make a firm decision to quit smoking. Then choose a date to stop smoking, and pick one or more ways to quit. Before your stop date, try changing your smoking habits. For example, if you smoke a cigarette after each meal, increase the time after a meal before you have a cigarette. If you smoke while reading the newspaper, try chewing gum instead. Changes in habits such as these may help make the process of quitting a little easier.

On the day you quit, get rid of all your cigarettes. Throw away your ashtrays. Try changing your routine. When you eat your meals, sit in a different place at the table. While you have coffee, read a book or listen to music to distract you from the desire to have a cigarette. When you get the urge to smoke, do something else instead. Carry other things with you to put in your mouth, such as gum, hard candy, carrot sticks, or a toothpick. Eat healthy snacks such as raw fruit and vegetables to keep your mouth occupied. Reward yourself at the end of the day for not smoking. See a movie, take a walk, or play cards with friends.

HOW TO CONTROL YOUR WEIGHT WHEN YOU QUIT SMOKING

Many people gain weight when they quit smoking. Still, the most important single step you can take to improve your health is to quit smoking. Stop smoking first, and then try to reach and stay at a healthy weight for the rest of your life. And remember, not everyone gains weight when they stop smoking. Of those who do, the average weight gain is between 6 and 8 pounds. Only 10 percent of people who stop smoking gain a large amount of weight (30 pounds or more).

If you do gain a few pounds when you quit, don't get down on yourself. Instead, feel proud of yourself that you have been able to quit. Think about all the following benefits quitting smoking will give you:

- More energy and endurance
- Whiter teeth
- Fresher breath
- Fresher smelling clothes and hair
- Fewer wrinkles and healthier-looking skin
- A clearer voice

Regular exercise will help you avoid large weight gains when you quit smoking. It may also boost your mood and help you feel more energetic. You'll probably be able to breathe easier during physical activity. Start out with at least 30 minutes of moderate-intensity physical activity on most days of the week, preferably every day. You can accomplish this by breaking it up into shorter sessions—it doesn't need to be done all at once. After you quit smoking and are ready to lose weight, you'll need to increase the amount of physical activity to at least 60 to 90 minutes a day to achieve your weight loss goals.

You may be tempted to eat more snacks and drink more alcohol to make up for the lack of cigarettes, but these compensations are likely to lead to weight gain. The tips below can help keep you from gaining weight as you quit smoking:

- Don't go too long without eating. Hunger can compel you to make unhealthy food choices.
- Eat enough at mealtimes to satisfy you, but don't overeat. Eat slowly so you can pick up on your body's signals that tell you when you are full.
- When you're hungry between meals, choose healthy snacks, such as fresh, canned, or dried fruit; air-popped popcorn; or fat-free yogurt.
- Instead of an alcoholic drink, choose an herbal tea, hot cocoa made with fat-free milk, fruit juice, or sparkling water with lemon.
- When you crave a cigarette, chew on cut-up vegetables and fruit to help keep your mouth occupied.

GETTING HELP TO QUIT

Keep in mind that you're trying to break an addiction. When you quit, you may need extra help to cope with your body's strong desire for nicotine. Talk to your doctor about using a nicotine replacement product such as a nicotine patch, nicotine gum, nicotine nasal spray, nicotine inhaler, or nicotine lozenges, or a prescription medication such as bupropion or varenicline to help you quit (see box). Nicotine replacement products, which provide nicotine but not the other harmful chemicals in tobacco, can help relieve some of the symptoms of physical dependence. At the same time, it's essential to address your psychological dependence on smoking because

STOP-SMOKING AIDS

A number of over-the-counter and prescription nicotine replacement products and prescription medications are available to help you quit smoking. Over-the-counter nicotine replacement products include the nicotine patch, nicotine gum, and nicotine lozenge. Prescription products include the nicotine nasal spray and nicotine inhaler. As with all medications, it is important to follow your doctor's instructions, use the products only as prescribed, and follow the directions on the package.

The nicotine patch releases a constant amount of nicotine into the body; most of the patches are worn all day and changed every 24 hours. Nicotine gum delivers nicotine to the brain more quickly than the patch but several minutes less quickly than the smoke from a drag on a cigarette, making the "hit" less intense. The recommendation is 10 to 15 pieces of gum a day but no more than 30 a day and for no longer than three months. The nicotine lozenge, in the form of a hard candy, releases nicotine as it slowly dissolves in the mouth over about 20 to 30 minutes. The recommendation is no more than 20 lozenges per day.

The nicotine nasal spray, which is dispensed from a pump bottle similar to a decongestant spray, quickly relieves cravings for a cigarette because the nicotine is rapidly absorbed through the nasal membranes and reaches the bloodstream faster than with the other nicotine replacement products. The nicotine inhaler is a plastic cylinder containing a cartridge that delivers nicotine when you puff on it. The inhaler delivers nicotine into the mouth (not the lung) and enters the body much more slowly than the nicotine in cigarettes. You use the inhaler when you have a craving for a cigarette, up to (but no more than) 16 cartridges a day for up to 12 weeks.

The prescription medication bupropion, which is also prescribed for depression, seems to help lessen the discomforts of nicotine withdrawal, making quitting more manageable. Using it (for up to three months) in combination with a nicotine replacement product increases the chances for long-term success. Another prescription medication, varenicline, works in two ways—cutting the pleasure of smoking and reducing withdrawal symptoms. Varenicline is used for three months for quitting, and can then be used for another three months to help you stay off cigarettes.

you are giving up a habit, which requires a major change in behavior.

Pairing nicotine replacement with a program that helps change behavior, addressing both the physical and psychological dependence on nicotine, can double your chances of successfully quitting. Ask your doctor to recommend a stop-smoking program. You can also contact the American Cancer Society (1-800-ACS-2345), American Lung Association (1-800-LUNG USA), the smoking quitline (1-800-QUIT NOW; 1-800-784-8669), or your local health department to find smoking-cessation classes in your area.

The harmful effects of alcohol

Alcohol is the most commonly abused drug in the United States. Three out of 10 American adults engage in at-risk drinking patterns. Excessive consumption of alcohol can cause short-term, acute problems and have harmful, long-lasting effects on organs and tissues throughout the body. For example, long-term heavy drinking can damage the liver, inflame the pancreas, and cause high blood pressure, heart failure, dementia, and vitamin deficiencies and malnutrition. Chronic alcohol use is the third-leading cause of cancer in the United States. Excessive drinking can interfere with every aspect of your life, including your relationships and responsibilities at work or school.

WHAT IS MODERATE DRINKING?

When it comes to drinking alcohol, adults should heed doctors' recommendations: if you drink, limit your drinking to no more than two drinks a day for men and one drink a day for women. One drink is usually defined as 12 ounces of beer or a wine cooler, 5 ounces of wine, or 1.5 ounces of distilled spirits. All of these drinks contain 15 grams of alcohol. This level of consumption is considered moderate use. Moderate drinking has been shown to reduce the risk for heart disease in some people, but doctors don't recommend drinking alcohol as a way of preventing heart disease because of the potentially devastating harm from drinking too much. Keep in mind that social drinking can quickly escalate into problem drinking; it doesn't take much alcohol over the moderate levels to significantly increase your risk for alcohol-related problems.

Alcohol use disorders

Most people who drink alcohol do so responsibly and sensibly. But about three in 10 American adults drink at levels that increase their risk for health problems and trouble with relationships, work, or school. Men who have five or more drinks in a day (or fifteen or more in a week) and women who have four or more drinks in a day (or eight or more in a week) are at increased risk for alcohol-related problems. Responses to alcohol can vary from person to person, depending on factors such as age, underlying health problems, and some medications a person is taking. The following terms are used to describe various degrees of alcohol use.

INTOXICATION

Alcohol intoxication occurs when the amount of alcohol a person drinks exceeds his or her tolerance for alcohol and impairs his or her mental and physical abilities. He or she may experience moodiness, irritability, slurred speech, poor coordination, and memory loss (blackout). These effects usually wear off when the person stops drinking. However, if a person continues to drink more and more, the results can be life-threatening. Intoxication can produce the following impairments in this order:

1. Loss of normal social inhibitions (such as talking more than usual)
2. Loss of memory
3. Confusion
4. Disorientation
5. Lack of coordination
6. Increasing sluggishness
7. Coma
8. Death (when excess alcohol shuts down the respiratory system)

ALCOHOL ABUSE

Alcohol abuse is defined as an unhealthy pattern of alcohol use that can lead to the next, most serious alcohol use disorder, alcohol dependence. If your drinking has *repeatedly* caused or contributed to one or more of the following situations in the past 12 months, you probably have alcohol abuse and you should get help right away:

- You have risked physical harm by, for example, driving, operating machinery, or swimming after drinking.
- You have had problems with relationships with your family or friends.
- Your drinking has interfered with your obligations and responsibilities at home, work, or school.
- You have had run-ins with the law (such as an arrest or other legal problems).

ALCOHOL DEPENDENCE

Alcohol dependence is the most serious alcohol abuse disorder. A person who has alcohol dependence usually experiences a heightened tolerance for alcohol and withdrawal symptoms. Tolerance is a need to substantially increase the amount of alcohol to achieve intoxication or the desired effect. Withdrawal occurs when drinking is stopped or decreased. People who are dependent on alcohol generally feel compelled to drink, spend a lot of time drinking and obtaining alcohol, continue to drink in spite of having physical or mental problems from alcohol, and have severe problems resulting from their drinking.

If you have experienced three or more of the following in the past 12 months, you probably have alcohol dependence and you should get help right away:

- You have not been able to stick to drinking limits, and have repeatedly gone over them.
- You have not been able to cut down or stop drinking, or have made repeated attempts that failed.
- You have more tolerance for alcohol—you need to drink more alcohol to get the same effect.
- When trying to quit or cut back on your drinking, you have experienced symptoms of withdrawal, including tremors, sweating, nausea, or insomnia.
- You have continued to drink despite recurring physical or psychological problems.
- You have spent a lot of time drinking, anticipating drinking, or recovering from drinking.
- You have spent less time on activities or pursuits that used to be important or pleasurable to you.

PEOPLE WHO SHOULD NEVER DRINK

For most adults, drinking moderate amounts of alcohol (two drinks a day for men and one drink a day for women) poses few health risks and may even be healthy, but some people should never drink alcohol. Do not drink if you:

- Have a health condition (such as liver disease) that could be made worse by drinking. Ask your doctor if you have a condition that could be worsened by drinking.
- Are pregnant or are trying to become pregnant (alcohol can severely injure a developing fetus).
- Are a recovering alcoholic (which puts you at risk for a relapse).
- Take certain over-the-counter or prescription drugs such as some sleep medications, antianxiety medications, antidepressants, or anticonvulsants, which can interact with alcohol to cause problems.
- Are under age 21 (because your brain and nervous system are still developing and could be harmed by excessive alcohol intake).
- Plan to drive or use high-speed machinery (alcohol can impair your judgment and slow your reactions).

Acute effects of alcohol

You don't have to be an alcoholic to experience problems from alcohol. In the short term, alcohol intoxication can cause conditions such as gastritis (inflammation of the stomach), alcoholic hepatitis, pancreatitis, and heart arrhythmias. Being intoxicated also impairs judgment; interferes with the ability to perform at work or school; and raises the risk of being involved in a car collision, violence, or arrests or other run-ins with legal authorities.

ALCOHOL AND THE BRAIN

All you have to do is watch a person who has had too much to drink try to walk across a room to see that alcohol affects the brain. Some impairment can be noticeable after only one or two drinks but it is usually temporary, stopping when the effects of the alcohol wear off.

Large quantities of alcohol, especially when consumed quickly and on an empty stomach, can cause a person to black out—to be unable to later recall events that occurred while intoxicated. Drinkers who experience blackouts

Drinking alcohol and taking medication can be a bad combination. Alcohol can interact with medications either by interfering with how the body (primarily the liver) processes the medication or by strengthening the effects of the medication (particularly on the central nervous system). Even many over-the-counter medications and herbal preparations can cause negative side effects when taken with alcohol. If you are taking any kind of medication—prescription, over-the-counter, herbal remedies, or vitamin or mineral supplements—make sure your doctor knows. He or she can tell you whether any of them have potentially harmful effects when combined with alcohol. The following are some common classes of prescription drugs that can interact with alcohol in a harmful way:

- Antibiotics
- Antihistamines
- Barbiturates
- Benzodiazepines
- Histamine H2 receptor agonists
- Muscle relaxants
- Nonopioid pain medications
- Anti-inflammatory agents
- Opioids
- Warfarin

typically drink too much too quickly, which causes the alcohol level in the blood to rise rapidly. Drinking too much can affect judgment and increase a person's risk of doing things he or she would not do while sober. Some people learn later that while they were under the influence they engaged in potentially dangerous activities such as taking illegal drugs, engaging in unprotected sex, or driving.

GASTRITIS

Drinking a large amount of alcohol can irritate and cause inflammation of the stomach lining, a condition called gastritis. Gastritis can cause abdominal discomfort, persistent pain between the lower ribs and navel, nausea, poor appetite, and bloating. The condition can be avoided by stopping drinking or drinking only moderately.

FATTY LIVER DISEASE

The damage done to the liver by excessive alcohol consumption generally progresses in three stages: from fatty liver disease to alcoholic hepatitis (see below) to cirrhosis. Drinking heavily for even a few days can cause fatty liver disease, the most common alcohol-induced liver disorder. The condition is marked by an excessive buildup of fat inside liver cells. Fatty liver disease can be reversed by stopping drinking.

ALCOHOLIC HEPATITIS

Alcoholic hepatitis (see page 353) is inflammation of the liver induced by excessive drinking. If a person continues to drink heavily, alcoholic hepatitis can lead to chronic liver disease and cirrhosis. However, alcoholic hepatitis can often be reversed over time if a person stops drinking before the condition has progressed to liver disease and cirrhosis. If a person who already has cirrhosis develops alcoholic hepatitis, the cirrhosis can progress rapidly to liver failure and death.

ACUTE PANCREATITIS

Acute pancreatitis is a sudden, severe inflammation of the pancreas. Most cases of acute pancreatitis are caused by alcohol abuse. If a person does not stop drinking, the condition can lead to chronic pancreatitis; even one attack of acute pancreatitis, if it damages cells in the pancreas and causes scarring, can sometimes trigger the development of chronic pancreatitis.

Alcohol's effects

Alcohol can have devastating short-term and long-lasting effects on the body, from the skin to the muscles to the liver, brain, and heart. Chronic heavy drinking is a major cause of death in the United States.

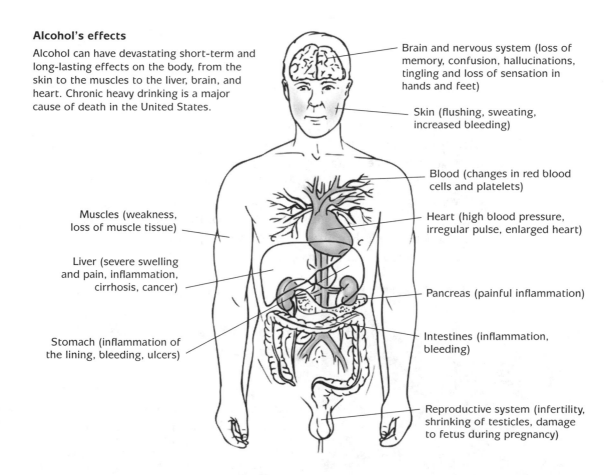

Brain and nervous system (loss of memory, confusion, hallucinations, tingling and loss of sensation in hands and feet)

Skin (flushing, sweating, increased bleeding)

Blood (changes in red blood cells and platelets)

Heart (high blood pressure, irregular pulse, enlarged heart)

Pancreas (painful inflammation)

Intestines (inflammation, bleeding)

Reproductive system (infertility, shrinking of testicles, damage to fetus during pregnancy)

Muscles (weakness, loss of muscle tissue)

Liver (severe swelling and pain, inflammation, cirrhosis, cancer)

Stomach (inflammation of the lining, bleeding, ulcers)

HEART ARRHYTHMIAS

Arrhythmias (see page 241) are irregularities in the natural rhythms of the heart, which can be mild or severe. A sudden, very rapid or very slow arrhythmia can reduce blood flow to the brain and may cause fainting or dizziness. Excessive intake of alcohol is a risk factor for arrhythmias.

Alcohol's long-term effects

Heavy consumption of alcohol over a long time can have lasting harmful effects on the body. Chronic heavy drinking can damage organs and tissues throughout the body, including the liver, the heart, the brain and nervous system, and the bones.

ALCOHOL AND LIVER DISEASE

The liver is one of the largest and most complex organs in the body. It stores energy and nutrients, manufactures proteins and enzymes needed for good health, protects the body from disease, and breaks down and helps remove harmful toxins such as alcohol from the body. Because the liver is the organ most responsible for processing alcohol in the body, it is especially vulnerable to injury from alcohol. As few as three drinks at one time can have toxic effects on the liver when combined with some over-the-counter medications, such as those containing acetaminophen.

Drinking heavily over a long period can eventually lead to the next stage of liver disease—a severe, potentially fatal condition called alcoholic hepatitis (see page 144), a type of inflammation of the liver. Symptoms of alcoholic hepatitis include nausea, lack of appetite, vomiting, fever, abdominal pain and tenderness, and jaundice. If heavy drinking continues, this stage can lead to cirrhosis of the liver, in which healthy liver cells are replaced by scar tissue, leaving the liver unable to perform its vital functions. Cirrhosis of the liver is the 12th leading cause of death in the United States.

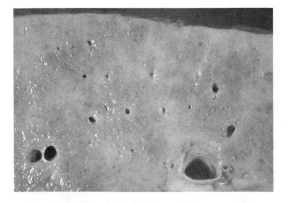

What alcohol can do to your liver
Heavy drinking over time puts excessive stress on the liver and can lead to cirrhosis and severe liver damage. Chronic exposure to alcohol can destroy liver cells and cause permanent scarring, as shown here.

Don't mix alcohol and acetaminophen

Using the over-the-counter pain reliever acetaminophen with alcohol on a regular basis can cause severe liver damage and liver failure. If you drink three alcoholic drinks a day, avoid using acetaminophen, a common ingredient in many nonprescription drugs. Overuse of acetaminophen is now the leading cause of liver failure in the United States.

Alcohol and the brain

Heavy drinking over a long period of time may produce brain deficits, or dementia, that can be permanent and debilitating. Alcohol-related dementia impairs mental functions such as memory and learning and can affect men and women of any age. Doctors are not sure if alcohol damages brain cells directly, or if the damage is caused by nutritional problems such as vitamin deficiencies, which are common in heavy drinkers, who often don't eat properly or have liver damage (which reduces nutrient absorption). Heavy drinking, especially when a person is not eating properly, can lead to malnutrition and vitamin deficiencies. A deficiency of the B vitamin thiamine (vitamin B1) is thought to play a major role in alcohol-related dementia because alcohol is known to have a direct effect on the absorption and use of thiamine in the brain.

Korsakoff's syndrome and Wernicke-Korsakoff syndrome are two forms of alcohol-related brain injury. At the early stages of these disorders, problems may be reduced or reversed if the person avoids alcohol, improves his or her diet, and takes thiamine supplements. Thiamine can help limit some of the toxic effects of alcohol.

Alcohol and the heart

While moderate drinking has been linked to a reduced risk for heart disease, heavy drinking, especially over a long period of time, can have harmful effects on the heart. Heavy drinking can damage the heart and lead to high blood pressure, stroke, alcoholic cardiomyopathy (enlarged and weakened heart), and congestive heart failure. Heavy drinking increases the level of potentially harmful fats called triglygerides.

Women and alcohol

Alcohol use disorders are more common in men than in women, but once alcohol becomes a problem for women, it worsens more rapidly than in men. Alcohol abuse or dependence can be especially harmful to women. The chemicals involved in breaking down alcohol differ between men and women. For example, the female body tends to have a higher percentage of fat than the male body, and fat cells tend to store alcohol for longer periods than other cells. Also, a woman's stomach may contain less of an enzyme needed for the initial breakdown of alcohol. This means that a woman's body breaks down alcohol at a slower rate than a man's, exposing her liver to higher blood alcohol concentrations for longer periods of time—a situation that is potentially toxic to the liver. Differences in how a woman's body breaks down and removes alcohol also may be linked to how much and how often she drinks, the fact that the female hormone estrogen is present in her body, and even the size of her liver.

For these reasons, women who drink excessive amounts of alcohol get intoxicated faster than men who drink the same amounts of alcohol. Regardless of the amount of alcohol consumed, women are also more likely than men to experience blackouts. Women who are heavy drinkers also develop alcohol-induced damage of the liver, heart muscle, and nerves after fewer years than heavy-drinking men.

Because of the devastating effects that drinking can have on a developing fetus during pregnancy, doctors recommend that all pregnant women and women of child-bearing age who are planning to become pregnant do not drink any alcohol.

Alcohol and bone health

Excessive drinking can increase the risk for the bone-thinning disorder osteoporosis (see page 325), especially in postmenopausal women. Excessive alcohol consumption can interfere with the metabolism of the mineral calcium, which is essential for bone health and strength. Alcohol can also disrupt the balance of calcium by interfering with the production of vitamin D, which is essential for calcium absorption by the bones.

The combination of bone loss and the effect of alcohol on balance and gait significantly increases the risk for falls and resulting fractures, especially in the hip and spine, posing an even greater health problem for people who are heavy drinkers.

Heavy drinking can cause hormone deficiencies in both men and women. Excess alcohol intake can reduce production of the male hormone testosterone (which is linked to production of osteoblasts, the cells that stimulate bone formation). In women, chronic drinking can cause irregular periods, reducing levels of the female hormone estrogen, which helps maintain bone health. Also, people with alcohol dependence tend to have elevated levels of the stress hormone cortisol, which decreases bone formation and increases bone breakdown. The good news is that stopping drinking can at least partly restore the activity of the bone-building cells and may even partially rebuild some lost bone.

Alcohol and cancer

Heavy drinking is considered a leading preventable cause of some kinds of cancer. The more a person drinks, the higher the risk for these cancers. Although the mechanism is not fully understood, researchers think that a suspected cancer-causing substance that forms as the body processes alcohol (called acetaldehyde) may have something to do with it. Natural compounds in the body called polyamines that are needed for cell growth react with the acetaldehyde from alcohol to trigger a series of reactions that damage DNA, a process that may lead to the formation of cancer.

Drinking alcohol is known to increase the risk for head and neck cancers—which include cancers of the mouth, throat (pharynx), voice box (larynx), and esophagus—in both men and women. If a person who drinks heavily also smokes cigarettes, the risk for these cancers increases exponentially—to a level much higher than the risk that smoking or drinking incurs on its own.

Long-term heavy drinking is indirectly linked to liver cancer because heavy drinking is a major cause of liver cirrhosis, which often leads to liver cancer. In women, alcohol may be a risk factor for breast cancer.

Teens and young adults and binge drinking

Alcohol is a major factor in all the leading causes of death in people under age 30. The news often brings reports of yet another alcohol-related tragedy involving a young person. Teens and young adults up to age 25 seem to be increasingly having problems involving alcohol (see page 140). Recent data show that about 70 percent of young adults in the United States—about 19 million people—consume alcohol.

It's not just that young people are drinking more but also the way they drink that puts them at increased risk for alcohol-related problems. Young people tend to drink the heaviest in their late teens and early- to mid-twenties and are especially likely to binge drink (having more than five drinks in a row at least once a month) and to drink heavily (consuming five or more drinks in a row on at least five occasions in one month).

Research shows that the brain continues to grow and develop throughout adolescence and up to about age 25. For this reason, alcohol affects the body and the brain in younger people differently than it does in adults. Many doctors are concerned that drinking during this critical developmental period may lead to lifelong impairment in brain function, especially in memory, motor skills, and coordination. Early alcohol use also usually signals a heightened risk for future drinking problems. Young people who begin drinking in their early teens not only have an increased risk of developing alcohol dependence later in life, but they also are prone to developing dependence more quickly and at a younger age and tend to develop chronic, relapsing dependence.

The most common source of alcohol for preteens and young teens is the home (either their own home or the homes of friends) and older kids (primarily siblings and other relatives). As a parent, you may have less direct influence on your children's drinking behavior than their peers do, but you can still play a major protective role. The example you set by your own drinking will affect your children's drinking throughout their life. Young people often model their drinking behavior after their parents' patterns of consumption and attitudes about alcohol use, so try to be aware of the messages you're sending through your behavior.

Strategies for cutting down on your drinking

Social drinking can quickly turn into problem drinking. If you think you may have a drinking problem, talk to your doctor or an alcohol treatment specialist. He or she can help you understand if your drinking pattern puts you at risk for problems or if you have an alcohol use disorder such as alcohol abuse or dependence. Depending on the evaluation, you may be able to successfully cut back on your own, or you may need to seek professional guidance to develop a safe plan for achieving sobriety.

If your drinking has not reached the stage of abuse or dependence, the following steps may help you cut down or keep your drinking at a sensible level. Try one or two strategies the first week and, as you succeed with those, add others:

- **Keep track.** Make a note of how much you drink. Use the system that is easiest for you: for example, carry an index card in your wallet, put check marks on a kitchen calendar, or use a personal computer.

- **Count and measure.** Know the standard drink sizes so you can count your drinks accurately. A drink is defined as a 12-ounce beer or wine cooler, 8 to 9 ounces of malt liquor, 5 ounces of wine, or 1½ ounces of hard liquor. If you are having a mixed drink in a bar or restaurant, ask the server or bartender how much liquor is in the drink.

- **Set goals.** Decide how many days a week you want to drink and how many drinks you'll have on those days. It's a good idea to have some days when you don't drink. Drinkers with the lowest rates of alcohol-use disorders (see page 141) stay within these limits: for men, no more than fourteen standard drinks a week and no more than four on any day; for women, no more than seven standard drinks a week and no more than three on any day.

- **Pace yourself.** Sip your drink slowly. Have no more than one drink with alcohol per hour. Alternate nonalcoholic drinks such as water, soda, or juice with drinks containing alcohol.

- **Eat when you drink.** Don't drink on any empty stomach. When you have some food as you drink, your body absorbs the alcohol more slowly.

Strategies for quitting drinking

If you have alcohol dependence and you want to stop drinking, don't do it alone. Sudden withdrawal from heavy drinking can cause dangerous side effects such as seizures. See your doctor or an alcohol treatment specialist who will work with you to develop a plan for quitting. Keep in mind that quitting drinking is not easy for anyone. It can take up to a year to successfully stop. The risk for relapse is highest in the first 6 to 12 months. But don't get discouraged. Having a relapse does not mean that you have failed, only that recovery is difficult. To give up drinking for good, for your health and the interests of your family, seek help as many times as you need to.

Your doctor or alcohol treatment specialist may recommend one or more of the following treatment strategies to help you quit. In most cases, a combination of these strategies is most effective.

- **Medication**   Medication for alcohol dependence, taken orally or by injection, has been shown to help people reduce their drinking, avoid a relapse into heavy drinking, achieve and maintain abstinence, or attain a combination of these goals. As with all medications, it is important to take it exactly as prescribed.

- **Counseling**   Knowledgeable doctors, nurses, and mental health professionals can provide effective behavioral support that can enhance your motivation to quit and, if you are taking medication to help you stop drinking, they can help you understand the reasons for and benefits of taking the medication. Even a few brief counseling sessions can be helpful.

- **Support**   Long-term participation in a mutual support group such as Alcoholics Anonymous (AA) can significantly increase your chances of successfully quitting drinking. These programs bring together people who are struggling with a drinking problem and support and encourage one another to stay sober. Learning about other people's drinking experiences and their coping strategies can help you sort out your own feelings and develop personal strategies for quitting.

In addition to the strategies above, the following tips can help you reach your goal of sobriety:

- **Avoid your drinking triggers.** What triggers your urge to drink? If certain people or places make you drink even when you don't want to, try to avoid them. If certain activities, times of day, or feelings trigger the urge, plan what you can do instead of drinking. If drinking at home is a problem, keep little or no alcohol there.

- **Plan ahead for handling urges.** Be prepared for times when you have the urge to have a drink. For example, it's always good to remind yourself why you're changing your drinking habits. Or try talking about it with a person you trust. Or get involved in a healthy activity that will distract you from the urge to drink. Or simply ride out the urge, knowing it will pass.

- **Know how to say "no" and mean it.** You will undoubtedly be offered a drink at times when you don't want one. Be prepared to say "no, thanks" quickly, politely, and convincingly. The faster you respond, the less likely you are to give in. Hesitating gives you time to think of excuses to accept the drink.

Preventing drug abuse

Drug abuse is using any drug for a purpose other than that recommended on the label or prescribed by a doctor, or using any drug for nonmedical use. Drug dependence (or addiction) is an uncontrollable physical craving for a drug. Drug abuse and addiction are difficult and serious problems world-wide. Many dangerous drugs that carry the potential for abuse are available both legally and illegally in the United States. Not everyone who takes an addictive drug becomes dependent on it. Some people are more susceptible to drug addiction than others for reasons that include both inherited and environmental factors. There are no reliable statistics on the total number of people who are dependent on drugs in the United States because many people who are addicted obtain their drugs illegally and many never seek treatment.

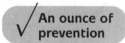

An ounce of prevention

The best way to prevent drug abuse is to never start using drugs. It's easiest to resist the temptation to use drugs before you've ever tried them.

The most dangerous drugs have traditionally been alcohol, heroin, and cocaine, but many newer drugs (such as the club drug ecstasy and the prescription pain relievers oxycodone and hydro-codone) can be just as harmful. In addition to costing the country billions of dollars a year in lost productivity and health-care costs, drug use has other high costs to society:

- Spread of infectious diseases such as HIV/AIDS and hepatitis C either through sharing of intravenous (IV) needles or unprotected sex
- Deaths due to overdose or other complications from drug use
- Effects on the fetus of pregnant drug users
- Other effects such as crime and homelessness

Illegal drugs

While alcohol is the most commonly used legal drug in the United States, marijuana, cocaine, and heroin are the most commonly used illegal drugs. About 80 percent of current illegal drug users use marijuana or hashish. Alcohol, tobacco, and marijuana are often referred to as "gateway drugs" because many people who end up using hard drugs often start out by using these substances. Each drug has specific effects on the brain and body. Some of the most common illegal drugs are discussed here, along with their short-term and long-term effects.

COMMONLY ABUSED DRUGS AND THEIR EFFECTS

The following information describes the effects, symptoms, and long-term risks of the most commonly abused drugs.

Type of drug	Effects	Symptoms	Risks
Amphetamines Speed or uppers. Prescribed for weight loss, narcolepsy, and attention deficit disorders.	Speed up physical and mental processes.	Weight loss, dilated pupils, insomnia, and trembling.	Psychosis and violent behavior.
Barbiturates Downers. Prescribed as sleeping pills and anticonvulsants.	Slow down physical and mental processes.	Slurred speech, confusion, lack of coordination and balance, extreme lethargy, and drowsiness.	Death (from overdose), especially when used with alcohol.
Benzodiazepines Prescribed as tranquilizers or sleeping pills or to reduce anxiety.	Sedate the mind and relax the muscles.	Calmness, lethargy, and drowsiness.	Confusion, coma, and death (from overdose).
Cannabis Marijuana and hashish.	Relaxes the mind and body and heightens perception.	Red eyes, dilated pupils, lack of coordination, lethargy, hunger, and mood swings.	Damage to brain, heart, lungs, and reproductive system.
Cocaine Can be snorted, injected, or smoked.	Stimulates the nervous system and produces heightened sensations and sometimes hallucinations.	Dilated pupils, trembling, apparent intoxication, agitation, rapid breathing, and elevated blood pressure.	Ulceration and perforation of nasal passages (if drug is snorted), itching (which can lead to open sores), seizures, and abnormal heart rhythms.
Opiates Opium, morphine, heroin, methadone, and synthetic pain relievers such as oxycodone and hydrocodone.	Relieve pain and produce temporary euphoria.	Weight loss, lethargy, mood swings, excessive sweating, slurred speech, sore eyes, and drowsiness.	Constipation, infection (if drug is injected), absence of periods in women, and death (from overdose).
Hallucinogens LSD, mescaline, and psilocybin mushrooms.	Unpredictable. Produce pleasant or frightening hallucinations.	Dilated pupils, excessive sweating, trembling, and fever and chills.	Long-term psychological problems and flashbacks.
Inhalants Fumes from glue, cleaning fluids, or aerosol cans.	Produce hallucinations, giddiness, and euphoria.	Confusion, dilated pupils, flushed face, and unconsciousness.	Damage to brain, liver, or kidneys, and death (from suffocation).
Club drugs Ecstasy, GHB (gamma hydroxybutyrate), flunitrazepam, ketamine, and nitrous oxide.	Ecstasy stimulates the nervous system and produces hallucinations. GHB depresses the central nervous system. Flunitrazepam has sedative effects. Ketamine produces dreamlike states and hallucinations. GHB, flunitrazepam, and ketamine are known as date rape drugs. Nitrous oxide depresses the nervous system, possibly causing unconsciousness.	Ecstasy causes confusion, depression, sleep problems, anxiety, paranoia, blurred vision, and fainting. GHB causes lethargy, seizures, and coma. Flunitrazepam causes sleepiness and amnesia. Ketamine impairs motor function and causes delirium and amnesia. Nitrous oxide causes slurred speech and lack of coordination and balance.	Ecstasy increases heart rate and blood pressure and can cause brain damage. GHB can cause coma and seizures. Flunitrazepam can be fatal when mixed with alcohol. Ketamine can be fatal (from respiratory failure). Nitrous oxide can cause unconsciousness from a depressed nervous system.

MARIJUANA

Marijuana, a drug that comes from the leaves of the Cannabis sativa (hemp) plant, is the most commonly abused illegal drug in the United States. It is a dry, shredded mix of flowers, stems, seeds, and leaves and is usually smoked but is also consumed in food or drinks. In a more concentrated, resinous form, it is called hashish and, as a sticky black liquid, hash oil. The main active chemical in marijuana is THC (delta-9-tetrahydrocannabinol), which binds to certain nerve cells in the brain and triggers a series of reactions that ultimately lead to the high that users experience.

When marijuana is smoked, its effects begin immediately after the drug enters the brain and last from one to three hours. When consumed in food or drinks, the short-term effects begin more slowly, usually in one half to one hour, and last longer, for up to four hours. Smoking marijuana deposits several times more THC into the blood than eating or drinking it.

Short-term effects

Within a few minutes after inhaling marijuana smoke, a person's heart begins beating more rapidly, the airways relax and become enlarged, and blood vessels in the eyes expand, making the eyes look red. Heart rate, normally 70 to 80 beats per minute, may increase by 20 to 50 beats per minute or, in some cases, even double. This effect can be stronger if other drugs are taken with marijuana.

As THC enters the brain, it produces a feeling of euphoria (the high) by acting on the brain's reward system, areas of the brain that respond to pleasurable stimuli such as food and drink as well as most drugs of abuse. THC activates the reward system in the same way that nearly all drugs of abuse do, by stimulating brain cells to release the feel-good chemical dopamine. A user may experience pleasant sensations, and time appears to pass very slowly. The drug can cause the mouth to feel dry, trigger sudden hunger or thirst, and make the hands tremble and turn cold. When the euphoria passes, the user may feel sleepy or depressed. Occasionally, marijuana use produces anxiety, fear, distrust, or panic.

Long-term effects

People who smoke marijuana regularly may have many of the same respiratory problems as tobacco smokers, such as a chronic cough and more frequent respiratory illnesses and infections. Regular marijuana smoking may also increase the risk for lung cancer and other cancers of the respiratory tract; marijuana smoke contains 50 percent to 70 percent more carcinogenic hydrocarbons than does tobacco smoke. Heavy, chronic marijuana use can impair critical skills related to attention, memory, and learning and can lead to loss of energy, ambition, and drive, and difficulty dealing with normal, everyday stress.

COCAINE

Cocaine, one of the oldest known drugs, is a powerfully addictive stimulant that directly affects the brain. The pure chemical form, cocaine hydrochloride, has been an abused substance for more than 100 years, and coca leaves, the source of cocaine, have been ingested for thousands of years. The powdered, hydrochloride salt form of cocaine can be snorted or dissolved in water and injected. Crack is cocaine that has not been neutralized by an acid to make the hydrochloride salt; crack comes in a rock crystal that can be heated and its vapors smoked. (The term "crack" refers to the crackling sound it makes when heated.)

Short-term effects

Cocaine's effects appear almost immediately after a single dose, and disappear within a few minutes or hours. Taken in small amounts (up to 100 milligrams), cocaine usually makes a person feel euphoric, energetic, talkative, and mentally alert (especially to the sensations of sight, sound, and touch), and can temporarily decrease the need for food and sleep. Some users find that the drug helps them perform simple physical and intellectual tasks more quickly, while others experience the opposite effect.

The short-term physical effects of cocaine include constricted blood vessels, dilated pupils, and increased temperature, heart rate, and blood pressure. Large amounts of cocaine (several hundred milligrams or more) intensify the high, but may also lead to bizarre, erratic, and violent behavior and may cause tremors, dizziness, muscle twitches, and paranoia. Cocaine-related deaths are often the result of cardiac arrest or seizures followed by respiratory failure. In rare cases, sudden death can occur on the first use of cocaine.

Long-term effects

Cocaine's stimulant and addictive effects are thought to result primarily from its ability to inhibit the reabsorption of dopamine by nerve cells. Over time, some people who use cocaine develop a tolerance for it and may increase their doses to intensify and prolong the euphoric effects. Other users become more sensitive to cocaine's anesthetic and seizure-promoting effects even without an increased dose; this increased sensitivity may explain some of the deaths that have occurred after apparently low doses of cocaine. Binge use of cocaine—taking the drug repeatedly and at increasingly high doses—can lead to a state of increasing irritability, restlessness, and paranoia. In severe cases, a person can lose touch with reality and experience auditory hallucinations (hearing voices).

METHAMPHETAMINE

Methamphetamine is a highly addictive drug with potent central nervous system stimulant properties. In the 1960s, methamphetamine was used widely in prescription medications and was commonly abused. In 1971, when regulators learned of its high potential for abuse, it was named a controlled substance and injectable forms of the drug were removed from the market. This led to a huge reduction in the abuse of the drug until a resurgence of methamphetamine abuse in the 1980s. Today, methamphetamine is considered a major drug of abuse—its widespread availability fueled mostly by illegal production in large and small hidden laboratories throughout the United States and illegal production and importation from Mexico. In many states in the West and Midwest, methamphetamine is second only to alcohol and marijuana as the drug used most frequently.

Short-term effects

Methamphetamine is a powerful stimulant that even in small doses can increase wakefulness and physical activity and decrease appetite. People who smoke or inject the drug experience a brief, intense sensation, or rush. Taking it by mouth or snorting it produces a long-lasting high that can continue for as long as half a day. Both the rush and the high are believed to result from the release of very high levels of dopamine into areas of the brain that regulate feelings of pleasure.

Methamphetamine has immediate toxic effects on the brain. In studies on animals, a single high dose of the drug has been shown to damage nerve terminals in the dopamine-containing areas of the brain. High doses of the drug can elevate body temperature to dangerous (and sometimes fatal) levels and can cause seizures.

Long-term effects

Long-term methamphetamine abuse leads to addiction and changes in the brain. Studies have found that as much as 50 percent of the dopamine-producing cells in the brain can be damaged after prolonged exposure to relatively low levels of methamphetamine. Chronic abuse can lead to psychotic behavior characterized by intense paranoia (which can produce homicidal and suicidal thoughts), visual and auditory hallucinations (seeing things that aren't there and hearing voices), and out-of-control rages that can trigger extremely violent behavior. Chronic abusers can also experience anxiety, confusion, insomnia, and mood disturbances.

Tolerance for methamphetamine can develop and, in an effort to intensify the desired effects, users may take higher doses, use the drug more frequently, or change their method of intake. In some cases, abusers forgo food and sleep while bingeing on methamphetamine—injecting as much as a gram of the drug every two to three hours over several days until they run out of the drug or are too disorganized to continue.

Although there are no physical manifestations of withdrawal when methamphetamine use is stopped, chronic users who stop taking the drug can experience depression, anxiety, fatigue, paranoia, aggression, and an intense craving for the drug.

HEROIN

Heroin is a highly addictive drug that is the most abused and the most rapidly acting of the group of drugs called opiates. Heroin is processed from morphine, a naturally occurring substance extracted from the seed pod of certain varieties of poppy plants. It is typically sold as a white or brownish powder or as a black sticky substance. Although purer heroin is becoming more common, most street heroin is combined ("laced") with other drugs or with substances such as sugar, starch, powdered milk, or quinine. Street heroin can also be combined with poisons such as strychnine. Heroin can be injected, smoked, or snorted. Injection is the most efficient way to administer low-purity heroin, but the availability of high-purity heroin and the fear of infection from sharing needles has made snorting and smoking the drug more common. All forms of heroin administration are addictive.

Because heroin abusers do not know the actual strength of the drug or its true composition, they are at risk for overdose or death. Heroin also poses special problems because of the transmission of HIV and other diseases that can occur from sharing needles or other injection equipment.

Short-term effects

People who inject heroin into a vein usually experience the euphoric feeling (rush) within 7 to 8 seconds; the onset of the rush is slower when heroin is injected into a muscle, taking 5 to 8 minutes. When heroin is sniffed or smoked, the peak effects of the drug are usually felt within 10 to 15 minutes. In addition to the initial feeling of euphoria, the short-term effects of heroin include a warm flushing of the skin, dry mouth, and a feeling of heaviness in the arms and legs. Heroin laced with fentanyl or poisons can cause death within hours.

Long-term effects

Addiction is one of the most significant effects of heroin use. With regular use, a person develops tolerance to the drug and must use more and more to achieve the same desired intensity or effect. As higher doses of the drug are used over time, a person becomes physically dependent on it.

Chronic heroin users may develop collapsed veins, infection of the heart lining and valves, abscesses, and liver disease. Lung complications, including various types of pneumonia, may result from the poor general health of many abusers, as well as from heroin's depressive effects on the respiratory system. In addition to the effects of the drug itself, street heroin may have additives that do not dissolve in the blood, potentially clogging the blood vessels that lead to the lungs, liver, kidneys, or brain; blockages in the blood vessels can cause infections or even kill small patches of cells in vital organs.

Withdrawal symptoms, which in regular heroin abusers may occur as early as a few hours after the last administration of the drug, can include drug craving, restlessness, muscle and bone pain, insomnia, diarrhea and vomiting, cold flashes with goose bumps, and kicking movements. Major withdrawal symptoms peak between 48 and 72 hours after the last dose and subside after about a week. Sudden withdrawal by heavily dependent users who are in poor health is sometimes fatal, although withdrawal from heroin is considered less dangerous than withdrawal from alcohol or barbiturates.

MDMA

MDMA (3,4-methylenedioxymethamphetamine) is a synthetic, psychoactive illegal drug that chemically resembles the stimulant methamphetamine and the hallucinogen mescaline. MDMA, known among users as ecstasy, acts as both a stimulant and a psychedelic, producing an energizing effect and distortions in time and perception and enhanced enjoyment from tactile experiences. Adolescents and young adults use it to promote euphoria, feelings of closeness and empathy, and sexuality, and to reduce inhibitions. It is considered a "party drug" and often is obtained at rave or techno parties and on college campuses.

Researchers have found that many ecstasy tablets contain not only MDMA but also a number of other drugs or drug combinations that can also be harmful, including methamphetamine, caffeine, the over-the-counter cough suppressant dextromethorphan, the diet drug ephedrine, and cocaine. As with many other drugs of abuse, MDMA is often used with other substances such as alcohol and marijuana.

Short-term effects

In high doses, MDMA can interfere with the body's ability to regulate temperature. On rare but unpredictable occasions, this can lead to a sharp increase in body temperature (hyperthermia) that can cause liver, kidney, and cardiovascular system failure, and death. Because MDMA can interfere with the body's ability to break down the drug, potentially harmful levels can be reached by repeated drug use within short intervals.

Users of MDMA face many of the same risks as users of other stimulants such as cocaine and amphetamines, including increases in heart rate and blood pressure (especially dangerous for people with circulatory problems or heart disease), muscle tension, involuntary teeth clenching, nausea, blurred vision, faintness, and chills or sweating. More than half of people who use MDMA report withdrawal symptoms, including fatigue, loss of appetite, depressed feelings, and trouble concentrating.

Long-term effects

Research in animals has linked MDMA exposure to long-term damage to brain cells involved in mood, thinking, and judgment. While similar brain damage has not been shown definitively in humans, the wealth of animal research showing MDMA's damaging properties suggests that MDMA is a dangerous drug.

LSD

LSD (lysergic acid diethylamide) was first synthesized in 1938 in Switzerland by a pharmaceutical chemist who was doing research on the possible medical applications of various lysergic acid compounds derived from ergot (a fungus that develops on rye grass). He created more than two dozen ergot-derived synthetic molecules. LSD is sold on the street in tablets, capsules, and, occasionally, in liquid form. It is an odorless and colorless substance with a slightly bitter taste that is usually taken by mouth. It is often added to absorbent paper, such as blotter paper, and divided into small squares, with each square representing one dose.

Short-term effects

The short-term effects of LSD are unpredictable, depending on factors such as the amount of the drug taken; the user's personality, mood, and expectations; and the surroundings in which the drug is used. The user typically feels the first effects of the drug within 30 to 90 minutes after taking it. These experiences last for extended periods of time and typically begin to clear after about 12 hours. The physical effects include dilated pupils, elevated body temperature, increased heart rate and blood pressure, sweating, loss of appetite, sleeplessness, dry mouth, and tremors. Sensations may seem to "cross over" for the user—that is, he or she may hear colors and see sounds. If taken in a large enough dose, the drug produces delusions and visual hallucinations (seeing things that are not there).

Long-term effects

LSD users often have flashbacks, during which they relive certain aspects of their LSD experience even long after they have stopped taking the drug. In addition, LSD users may develop long-lasting serious mental disorders, such as schizophrenia or

GETTING HELP

If you think you may be dependent on an illegal or prescription drug, get help. Asking for help is the first step toward overcoming your addiction. Talk to friends and family members first and ask for their support. You should also talk to your doctor or see a health professional who is trained in helping people who are addicted to drugs. Call local hospitals and ask if they have a substance abuse program.

The type of treatment you need will depend on the severity of your addiction. Treatment programs for drug addiction usually combine physical detoxification (the process of desensitizing the nervous system to the effects of the drug) with a rehabilitation program. Detoxification is usually done over a period of a week to 10 days in a hospital or treatment center, where your condition can be carefully monitored. In some cases, a less damaging drug such as methadone is substituted for a more dangerous drug such as heroin.

During and possibly after your rehabilitation program, you will participate in group therapy to help you deal with the psychological and social consequences of your past drug use and to show you how to make more positive life choices. No matter which program you go through, you may have a relapse at some point during your recovery, as many people do. Don't consider yourself a failure. Accept the fact and continue with your recovery. You will succeed eventually. To help you stay drug-free over the long term, get involved in an addiction-recovery program such as Narcotics Anonymous.

severe depression. LSD is not considered an addictive drug because it does not produce the compulsive drug-seeking behaviors that addictive drugs such as cocaine, heroin, and methamphetamine do. However, LSD users may develop tolerance to the drug and must consume progressively larger doses to experience the hallucinogenic effects they desire.

Prescription drug abuse

Prescription drug abuse is growing in the United States. It is estimated that more than 7 million Americans may use prescription drugs for nonmedical purposes. Doctors prescribe medications for specific health problems. Prescription drugs are effective when used properly, but some can be addictive and dangerous when misused. Although most people take their medications properly and addiction to prescription drugs is rare, three classes of drugs are frequently misused or abused:

- **Pain relievers**   Most commonly abused are opioid pain relievers such as oxycodone, hydrocodone, morphine, methadone, and combinations that include these drugs.
- **Tranquilizers and sedatives**   Most commonly abused are benzodiazepines prescribed for anxiety or sleep problems.
- **Stimulants**   Most commonly abused is methylphenidate prescribed for attention deficit hyperactivity disorder (ADHD), the sleep disorder narcolepsy, or obesity

These medications alter a person's mood, which is a major factor in why they are commonly abused. When people use these drugs for reasons other than those for which they were prescribed, they often take more than was prescribed. Taking the drugs in large doses can lead to physical and psychological dependence. If you abuse alcohol or are dependent on it, you are at increased risk of becoming addicted to another substance. Combining other drugs with alcohol can be life-threatening.

WHO IS AT RISK?

Some groups of people have a substantially higher risk of abusing or becoming addicted to prescription drugs than others. Adolescents are the No. 1 group to abuse prescription drugs (see page 469), especially painkillers, stimulants, barbiturates, and tranquilizers. Recreational use of the drug methylphenidate, prescribed for attention deficit hyperactivity disorder (ADHD), is also on the rise among adolescents and young adults. Oxycodone, often prescribed as a painkiller for cancer patients, has become a common street drug because it produces a long-lasting high. These drugs are usually either bought from a person for whom they were prescribed or stolen and then sold illegally.

Doctors prescribe drugs for older people three times as frequently as for the general population. An older person can sometimes receive an inappropriately high dose of a prescription medication (because the body's ability to process medications declines with age) or may mistakenly take higher-than-prescribed doses of a drug. Also, older people often have several health problems and many are taking over-the-counter medications and dietary supplements, increasing the potential for drug interactions. For these reasons, they are more likely to experience adverse consequences from misusing or abusing prescription medications. For example, commonly prescribed sedatives such as benzodiazepines can increase the risk for falls and vehicle accidents in older people and can cause physical dependence after as few as four months.

Women are much more likely than men to be prescribed a narcotic or addictive antianxiety medication, although men and women have similar rates of recreational prescription drug use. Also, people who work in the health professions may have an increased risk for prescription drug abuse and addiction because they have easy access to the drugs.

How to prevent prescription drug misuse and abuse

If your doctor gives you a prescription for a drug that can become addictive, ask the doctor if he or she can substitute a medication with a lower potential for dependence. Carefully follow your doctor's instructions to make sure you are taking the correct dose.

The following guidelines can help protect you and your family from prescription drug misuse or abuse:

- Tell your doctor about all the medications you're taking, including over-the-counter medications and dietary supplements such as vitamins.
- Take all medications only as prescribed.
- Read the package insert and the information your doctor or pharmacist provides before starting to take the drug.

- Ask your doctor or pharmacist about your medication, especially if you are unsure about its effects.

- Teach your children never to use any medication prescribed for someone else or share his or her prescription medication with friends—and don't do so yourself.

- Keep all medications out of the reach of children—even older children, who might be tempted to see what kinds of effects they can produce or share them with friends.

STRESS AND DRUG ABUSE

Stressful events are powerful triggers for the abuse of alcohol or other drugs. People under extreme stress often seek relief through alcohol or other drugs, or relapse into substance abuse after periods of abstinence. In fact, stress is the leading cause of relapse into drinking, drug abuse, and smoking.

Post-traumatic stress disorder (PTSD) is a mental disorder that can result from extreme stress, such as a terrifying event or series of events in which severe physical harm occurred or was threatened. PTSD can occur in anyone of any age who has witnessed or experienced a tragic incident such as a violent personal attack, a natural disaster such as a hurricane, war, or an accident. Symptoms can include reliving the trauma; avoiding people, places, and thoughts connected to the event; trouble sleeping; an exaggerated startle response; and hypervigilance (heightened alertness to potential threats).

A strong link exists between PTSD and substance abuse. In some cases, substance use begins after the traumatic event and the development of PTSD, making PTSD a risk factor for drug abuse. If you think you have experienced an event that puts you at risk for PTSD, see your doctor or a therapist, who can treat the illness and help you heal. They can also help you learn ways of coping with your strong emotions without having to resort to drug or alcohol use.

Anabolic steroids

Anabolic steroids, also known as androgenic steroids, are versions of the male hormone testosterone. The term "anabolic" means muscle-building; "androgenic" refers to enhanced masculine characteristics. Anabolic steroids are a class of drugs available legally only by prescription to treat conditions such as delayed puberty and some types of impotence that occur when the body produces abnormally low amounts of the male hormone testosterone. Doctors also prescribe anabolic steroids to treat body wasting in patients with AIDS or other diseases that cause loss of muscle.

Some men and boys and some women abuse anabolic steroids to improve their athletic performance and to enhance their physical appearance. Anabolic steroids can be taken by mouth (in pills or powder) or injected, typically in cycles of weeks or months (referred to as cycling), rather than continuously. Cycling involves taking multiple doses of steroids over a specific period of time, stopping for a time, and starting again. Users often combine several different types of steroids to maximize their effectiveness while trying to minimize negative effects, a practice referred to as stacking.

Abuse of anabolic steroids can lead to serious health problems, some of which are irreversible. The major side effects of abusing anabolic steroids are liver damage and cancer, jaundice (yellowish pigmentation of the skin), fluid retention, high blood pressure, and an increase in bad LDL cholesterol and a decrease in good HDL cholesterol. Other side effects include kidney tumors, severe acne, and trembling.

Some gender-specific side effects can also occur. For example, men can experience shrinking of the testicles, reduced sperm count, infertility, baldness, development of breasts, and an increased risk for prostate cancer. In women, steroids can stimulate the growth of facial hair, male-pattern baldness, changes in or cessation of the menstrual cycle, enlargement of the clitoris, and a deepened voice. People who share needles for injecting anabolic steroids also increase their risk of contracting or transmitting HIV/AIDS or hepatitis (which causes serious damage to the liver).

Adolescence is a key period of risk as young people try to make the most of their athletic potential. But anabolic steroids can halt growth prematurely by causing the skeleton to mature too soon and by accelerating puberty. This means that adolescents risk remaining short for the rest of their lives if they take anabolic steroids before the typical adolescent growth spurt.

Safer sex

Taking precautions during sex can reduce your risk of acquiring a sexually transmitted disease (STD) or transmitting an STD to your partner. STDs, which are also referred to as sexually transmitted infections (STIs), are transmitted during intimate sexual contact (including vaginal, oral, or anal intercourse) with someone who has the infection. Many of the organisms that cause sexually transmitted diseases live on the penis, vagina, anus, mouth, and the skin of surrounding areas.

Some STDs are transferred by direct contact with an infected sore on a person's genitals or mouth. However, most organisms are transmitted in body fluids without a visible sore during oral, vaginal, or anal intercourse. Some STDs such as HIV (the virus that causes AIDS) and hepatitis B can also be transferred by nonsexual contact with infected tissues or fluids, such as infected blood. Some STDs can be transmitted from a pregnant woman to her fetus during pregnancy, in breast milk to a nursing infant, and, rarely, through contaminated blood transfusions and blood products.

Sexually transmitted diseases

Every year, STDs affect more than 19 million Americans. Some STDs are much more common than others. Researchers have identified more than 20 different kinds of STDs, which fall into two main groups:

- **STDs caused by bacteria**   These infections can be treated, and often cured, with antibiotics. Common bacterial STDs include chlamydia and gonorrhea.

- **STDs caused by viruses**   These infections can be controlled, but not cured. If you acquire a viral STD, you might have it for life. Some viral STDs include HIV (the virus that causes AIDS), genital herpes, human papillomavirus (HPV), and hepatitis B.

CHLAMYDIA

Chlamydia infections are caused by the bacterium Chlamydia trachomatis and can be transmitted during vaginal, oral, or anal sexual contact with an infected partner. An estimated 2.8 million new cases of chlamydia occur each year among Americans; the highest rates are among 15- to 19-year-olds. Chlamydia often causes no symptoms—three out of four infected women and about half of infected men have no symptoms. When women have symptoms, they can include an abnormal vaginal discharge, pelvic pain, or a burning sensation when urinating. Symptoms in men include a discharge from the penis, a burning sensation when urinating, burning and itching around the opening of the penis, or, rarely, pain and swelling in the testicles. When the infection is spread during anal intercourse, symptoms can include rectal pain, discharge, or bleeding. Chlamydia can also affect the throat in men and women having oral sex with an infected partner.

Chlamydia infections can have serious short- and long-term consequences. In women, an untreated infection can spread into the uterus or fallopian tubes and cause pelvic inflammatory disease (PID). PID can cause permanent damage to the fallopian tubes, uterus, and surrounding tissues, which can lead to chronic pelvic pain, infertility, and a potentially fatal ectopic pregnancy (pregnancy outside the uterus). Women with a chlamydia infection are five times more likely than uninfected women to become infected with HIV if they are exposed to the virus. An untreated chlamydia infection during pregnancy may lead to premature delivery. Infected pregnant women can pass the infection to their babies during delivery, potentially causing eye and respiratory tract infections.

In men, complications from chlamydia infections are rare. However, if the infection spreads to the epididymis (a tube that carries sperm from the testicles), it can cause pain, fever, and, in rare cases, infertility.

To prevent the serious consequences of chlamydia, testing at least annually for the bacterium is recommended for sexually active women 25 years and younger. An annual screening test is also recommended for older women with risk factors such as a new sex partner or multiple sex partners. All pregnant women should have a screening test for chlamydia. Any man whose partner is infected should also seek treatment to avoid reinfecting his partner. Anyone who has been treated for chlamydia should notify all recent sex partners so they can see their health-care provider for treatment. People who are being treated for chlamydia should avoid sex until their treatment regimen is completed. If you are not sure if your partner has received treatment, see your health-care provider and be retested three to four months after your treatment is complete to make sure you have not been reinfected by your partner.

GONORRHEA

Gonorrhea is a curable STD that is caused by the bacterium Neisseria gonorrhoeae, which can grow and multiply in the warm, moist areas of the reproductive system, including the cervix (the opening to the uterus), the uterus, and fallopian tubes in women, and the urethra (the tube that carries urine out of the body) in both women and men. The infection is spread through contact with the penis, vagina, mouth, or anus, with or without ejaculation. Gonorrhea can also be spread from an infected mother to her baby during delivery.

An estimated 700,000 new cases of gonorrhea occur each year in the United States. Many people are unaware that they are infected because the infection usually does not produce symptoms, especially in women. When symptoms do occur, usually from 2 to 30 days after infection, in men they can include a burning sensation when urinating, or a white, yellow, or green discharge from the penis. In some cases, men can have painful or swollen testicles. In women, symptoms can include a painful or burning sensation when urinating, increased vaginal discharge, or vaginal bleeding between periods. Symptoms of rectal infection in both men and women include discharge, anal itching, soreness, bleeding, or painful bowel movements. Infections in the throat may cause a sore throat.

Untreated, gonorrhea can have serious and permanent consequences. In women, gonorrhea is a common cause of pelvic inflammatory disease (PID), which can lead to long-lasting chronic pelvic pain and can damage the fallopian tubes, causing infertility and an increased risk for ectopic pregnancy (pregnancy that develops outside the uterus). In men, untreated gonorrhea can cause epididymitis (a painful condition of the testicles), which can lead to infertility. Gonorrhea can also spread to the blood or joints, a condition that can be life-threatening.

People with gonorrhea can contract HIV more easily if they are exposed to HIV, and people who are infected with HIV and also infected with gonorrhea more easily transmit HIV to a sex partner.

Using latex condoms correctly and consistently can reduce the risk of transmitting gonorrhea. Anyone who is being treated for gonorrhea should tell any recent sex partners so that they can also seek treatment. This will help prevent reinfection and will help reduce the risk for serious complications. Anyone undergoing treatment for gonorrhea should avoid sex until they have completed their course of treatment.

SYPHILIS

Syphilis is a curable STD caused by the organism Treponema pallidum. With the development of antibiotics in the 1940s, the infection declined dramatically in the United States, but it now appears to be increasing, especially among young adults and men who have sex with other men. Two out of three new cases occur in men who have sex with other men. Untreated, syphilis can progress to more advanced stages and cause serious damage to the heart and central nervous system, which can be fatal. During pregnancy, the fetus of a pregnant woman with syphilis can become infected, which can lead to stillbirth or death shortly after birth. An infected newborn may not have signs or symptoms at birth but, without treatment, the infection can cause serious problems within a few weeks, including developmental delays or seizures, or death.

The first symptoms of a syphilis infection often go undetected. The initial symptom is usually a chancre, a painless open sore that usually appears on the penis or around or in the vagina. It can also occur in the anus or rectum. Because the sores can be hidden in these areas, it is not always obvious that a sex partner is infected.

Correct and consistent use of latex condoms can reduce the risk of spreading syphilis, but only if the infected area is protected (the sores are not always in areas protected by a condom). The presence of syphilis sores in an HIV-infected person increases the likelihood two to five times of transmitting HIV to a sex partner; at the same time, a person without HIV who has syphilis sores is two to five times more likely to acquire HIV from an HIV-infected partner. Because of this harmful combination, it is especially important for sex partners to know of each other's HIV status and history of other STDs in order to understand their risks and take preventive measures.

Effective treatment for syphilis is available and the infection is easy to cure in the early stages. For this reason, if your sexual behaviors put you at increased risk for STDs, you should get tested regularly for syphilis. Treatment will help you avoid the life-threatening complications that can result from untreated syphilis. People who are being treated for syphilis should contact their sex partners so they can be tested and seek treatment if necessary. A person can be infected with syphilis again even after successful treatment.

CRABS

Crabs, also known as pubic lice or crab lice, are tiny insects (about the size of the head of a pin) that are usually transferred from one person to another through sexual contact. (They can also be acquired through contact with infested clothing, bedding, or toilet seats.) Pubic lice tend to live in pubic hair and bite the skin to feed on blood. Although tiny, you can see them and their egg clusters, which cling to hair shafts. Their bites usually cause itching and irritation.

To avoid spreading pubic lice, all members of a household must undergo treatment at the same time (with an insecticidal lotion that kills both the lice and their eggs). All clothing and bedding must be washed in very hot water (exceeding 140°F) or dry-cleaned to kill the lice.

HUMAN PAPILLOMAVIRUS

An estimated 20 million Americans are currently infected with human papillomavirus (HPV), and more than 6 million new cases occur each year. At least half of all sexually active men and women acquire an HPV infection at some time in their life, and by age 50, at least 80 percent of women have acquired the infection. There is no cure for HPV infections but, in women, they usually clear up on their own.

HPV is a group of viruses that includes more than 100 different strains or types, some of which cause common skin warts and 30 of which are sexually transmitted. The sexually transmitted forms can infect the genital area, including the skin of the penis, the vulva in women, and the anus, and the linings of the vagina, cervix, and rectum.

HPV infections rarely cause symptoms but, even without symptoms, the virus can be easily spread to a sexual partner during vaginal, oral, or anal sex. Some types of HPV can cause genital warts (single or multiple growths or bumps that appear in the genital area). The warts can appear as soft, moist, pink, or flesh-colored swellings; raised or flat; single or multiple; small or large; and sometimes shaped like a cauliflower. In women, they can appear on the vulva, in or around the vagina or anus, or on the cervix; in men, they can appear on the penis, scrotum, groin, or thigh.

Of the 30 sexually transmitted forms of HPV, about 10 have been identified as having the rare potential to lead to cervical cancer or, less often, cancer of the vulva, vagina, anus, or penis. The single most effective way to prevent cervical cancer is for women to have regular Pap tests (see page 188) to detect abnormal, precancerous changes in cells in the cervix and receive treatment, if necessary, before the cells become cancerous.

Although you should always use condoms to avoid STDs, keep in mind that an HPV infection can occur in both males and females in genital areas that are not covered or protected by a condom. While the ability of condoms to prevent HPV is not clear, condom use is linked to a lower rate of cervical cancer.

HPV VACCINE MAY PREVENT CERVICAL CANCER

In 2006, the Food and Drug Administration approved the first vaccine to prevent cervical cancer, precancerous genital cell changes, and genital warts caused by the human papillomavirus (HPV). The vaccine may protect against four types of HPV, including the two responsible for 70 percent of all cervical cancer cases. Doctors expect that the vaccine may reduce the incidence of HPV-related diseases including cancer by 90 percent.

In tests, the vaccine was found to be effective for up to four and a half years and caused few side effects. Although the vaccine may prevent new HPV infections, it will not eliminate already existing HPV infections. Because women often get HPV infections soon after they become sexually active, the vaccine is most effective if it is given to girls before they start having sex. That's why many doctors recommend immunizing girls against HPV when they are 11 or 12 years old. But older girls and women can benefit, too—the vaccine is available anyone from ages 13 to 26.

Doctors are excited about the possibility that cervical cancer might be almost completely eliminated by widespread use of the vaccine, along with procedures such as the Pap test, HPV testing, follow-up testing of abnormalities in the cervix, and surgery to remove precancerous cells.

GENITAL HERPES

Genital herpes is an incurable viral infection that is very common in the United States. At least 45 million people ages 12 and older have been infected with genital herpes. The infection is more common in women than in men—one out of four women compared with one out of five men. Genital herpes is caused by the herpes simplex virus (HSV). There are two types of herpes viruses, and both can cause genital herpes. Type 1 HSV (HSV-1) most often causes blisters on the lips (known as fever blisters or cold sores), but it can cause genital infections as well. HSV-2 most often causes genital herpes, but it also can infect the mouth when it is transmitted during oral sex.

The infection may cause no symptoms or only mild symptoms. When symptoms occur, most often about two weeks after the first exposure, they usually appear as one or more blisters on or around the genitals or rectum; the blisters break, leaving tender sores that take two to four weeks to heal.

Some people may also have flu-like symptoms such as fever and swollen glands. Outbreaks can continue to occur—typically four or five in the first year—but they are usually less severe and don't last as long as the first one. The herpes virus stays in the body inside nerve cells indefinitely, but the outbreaks tend to decrease over several years.

Infected people can transmit HSV-2 even when they have no symptoms, and it is often transmitted by people who are unaware they are infected. Genital herpes can occur in both males and females in genital areas not covered by latex condoms. Therefore, while correct and consistent use of latex condoms can help reduce the risk of spreading the virus, it cannot guarantee full protection from the virus. People who have blisters should abstain from sexual activity (although they can also infect people when they do not have symptoms).

Because genital herpes can, in rare cases, cause potentially fatal infections in newborns, pregnant women need to be especially careful to avoid contracting the infection during pregnancy. If a woman has active genital herpes at delivery, a cesarean delivery is usually performed.

HIV/AIDS

HIV is the virus that causes AIDS, an infection that attacks cells of the immune system, leaving a person vulnerable to life-threatening infections and cancers. Without treatment, AIDS is usually fatal. The virus can be spread through sexual activity that involves contact with body fluids including semen, vaginal secretions, and blood. (It can also be spread nonsexually by sharing intravenous (IV) needles, from an infected pregnant woman to her fetus during pregnancy, and in breast milk to breastfeeding infants.) The virus cannot be spread by casual contact. Although there is no cure for AIDS, treatment is enabling more and more people with the virus to live long, productive lives.

In addition to consistently and correctly using latex condoms, an essential component of HIV prevention is early detection and treatment of other STDs. People who are infected with an STD other than HIV are two to five times more likely than uninfected people to acquire HIV if they are exposed to the virus through sexual contact. In addition, if a person who is infected with HIV is also infected with another STD, he or she is more likely to transmit HIV through sexual contact than other HIV-infected people. In short, having STDs other than HIV increases the likelihood of both transmitting and acquiring HIV. The reasons for this are twofold:

- **Increased susceptibility**   STDs that produce sores in the genital area—including syphilis and herpes—can cause breaks in the genital tract lining or skin that allow entry for HIV. STDs that do not produce genital sores—including chlamydia, gonorrhea, and trichomoniasis—seem to increase the concentration of cells in genital secretions that are targets for HIV.

- **Increased infectiousness**   Studies have found that when people who are infected with HIV are also infected with other STDs, they are more likely to have HIV in their genital secretions than are people who are infected with HIV but have no other STDs.

HEPATITIS B

A number of different viruses can cause hepatitis, and not all of them are sexually transmitted. Hepatitis B is the hepatitis virus that is most likely to be transmitted sexually. Of the 200,000 new hepatitis B infections in the United States each year, about half are transmitted through sexual activity. Some people develop a chronic hepatitis B infection that can cause severe complications, including cirrhosis of the liver and liver cancer (see page 269).

In many cases, a hepatitis B infection produces no symptoms. A person may be unaware of being infected and can spread the virus and not know it. When symptoms occur, they can include yellowing of the skin or whites of the eyes (jaundice), feeling tired, loss of appetite, nausea, abdominal discomfort, dark urine, gray-colored bowel movements, or joint pain.

The infection can be transmitted from an infected pregnant woman to her baby during birth. To prevent the spread of the virus, all pregnant women should have a blood test for hepatitis B during each pregnancy. Babies who are born to infected mothers are given a hepatitis B vaccination and another shot of hepatitis B immune globulin (HBIG) shortly after birth to prevent infection.

The most effective way to prevent hepatitis B is to have the hepatitis B vaccination. The vaccination is recommended for all infants, for children and adolescents who were not vaccinated as infants, and for all unvaccinated adults who are at risk for hepatitis B infection (such as health-care workers who handle blood and people who live with a person who has hepatitis B) as well as anyone who wants to be protected against hepatitis B. Using latex condoms correctly and consistently may help reduce the risk of hepatitis B transmission during sexual activity.

Bacterial vaginosis and trichomoniasis are two common infections that frequently occur in women. Although they are related to sexual activity, they can also be acquired without being sexually active.

Bacterial vaginosis

Bacterial vaginosis (BV) is the most common vaginal infection in women. It is a condition in which the normal balance of bacteria in a woman's vagina is disrupted, resulting in an overgrowth of certain bacteria. Not much is known about how women develop BV, but it seems to be linked to having a new sex partner or having multiple sex partners. The infection is uncommon in women who have never had intercourse, but it can occur without sexual activity.

BV may not cause any symptoms or it may cause an abnormal vaginal discharge with an unpleasant, fishlike odor, especially after intercourse. The discharge may be white or gray, and can be thin. Some women may also have burning during urination or itching around the outside of the vagina.

BV usually does not have complications, but the following are risk factors for complications in infected women:

- Increased susceptibility to being infected with other STDs, including HIV, chlamydia, and gonorrhea if exposed to them.
- Increased risk that an HIV-infected woman will pass HIV to her sex partner.
- Increased risk of developing pelvic inflammatory disease (PID), which can damage the fallopian tubes and cause infertility or a life-threatening ectopic pregnancy (pregnancy that occurs outside the uterus).
- Increased risk of complications during pregnancy.
- In pregnant women, an increased risk of premature birth or having a baby with a low birth weight (fewer than 5 pounds).

Because BV is not completely understood, it is unclear what are the most effective ways to prevent it. But the following measures can help reduce the risk of disrupting the natural balance of bacteria in the vagina and may help prevent BV:

- Avoid having sex.
- Limit the number of sex partners you have.

- Do not douche.
- If you are being treated for bacterial vaginosis, use all of the medication prescribed, even if you no longer have any signs or symptoms.

Trichomoniasis

Trichomoniasis is a curable STD caused by a single-celled protozoan parasite called Trichomonas vaginalis. More than 7 million new cases occur each year in the United States. In women, the vagina is the most common site of infection; in men, the urethra is the most common site. The infection is most often transmitted through penis-to-vagina intercourse and, in women having sex with women, vulva-to-vulva contact (the vulva is the genital area outside the vagina). The infection can sometimes be transmitted outside of sexual activity.

Most men with trichomoniasis have no symptoms, although some have temporary irritation inside the penis, a mild discharge, or slight burning after urination or ejaculation. Women with the infection can have a frothy, yellow-green vaginal discharge that has a strong odor. The infection can also make a woman uncomfortable during intercourse and urination, and cause irritation and itching in the genital area. In rare cases, lower abdominal pain can develop. Symptoms usually appear in women within 5 to 28 days of exposure to the parasite.

Using latex condoms consistently and correctly can reduce the risk of transmitting trichomoniasis. Anyone who is being treated for trichomoniasis should inform all sex partners so they can also seek treatment to avoid reinfections. Partners should avoid sexual contact until the treatment is complete and symptoms are gone.

How to prevent STDs

Abstinence is the only sure way to avoid STDs. The least risky way to have a sexual relationship is to be mutually monogamous with someone you know is free of any STD. Ideally, before having sex with a new partner, each of you should get screened for STDs and share the test results with each other. The following factors greatly increase your risk for STDs:

- Having sex without using a male or female condom.
- Not knowing whether a partner has an STD.

- Having more than one sexual partner. The more partners you have, the greater your risk of being exposed to an STD. Remember, you can't tell if someone has an STD just by looking at him or her.
- Having a partner with a past history of any STD.
- Having a partner who uses IV (intravenous) drugs.
- Having anal intercourse; some STDs are transmitted more easily during anal intercourse than other types of sexual activity.
- Using drugs or alcohol in a situation where sex might occur. Drinking alcohol or using drugs can increase the likelihood that a person will engage in unprotected or irresponsible sexual activity. In addition, some diseases can be transferred through the sharing of needles or other drug paraphernalia.

If you are sexually active, you should use a latex condom each and every time you have any type of sex to avoid contact with semen, vaginal fluids, and blood. Both male and female condoms dramatically reduce the risk that you will acquire or spread an STD. Some general guidelines:

- Use latex condoms for vaginal, anal, and oral intercourse.
- Use the condom from the beginning to the end of sexual activity and use a new one every time you have sex.
- Lubricants may help reduce the chance that a condom will break. Use only water-based lubricants, because oil-based or petroleum-type lubricants can cause latex to weaken and tear.
- Do *not* use condoms with nonoxynol-9—this spermicide helps prevent pregnancy, but may increase the risk of transmitting HIV and other STDs. Nonoxynol-9 itself may cause genital sores that provide a point of entry for STDs.
- Keep in mind that you can still acquire or transmit some STDs even if you use a condom, because a condom does not cover the surrounding skin areas. But using a condom puts you at significantly less risk than not using one.
- You *cannot* avoid STDs by washing your genital area, urinating, or douching after sex.
- Consider any unusual discharge, sore, or rash, especially in the groin area, as a signal to avoid having sex and see a health-care provider immediately.

HOW TO USE A CONDOM CORRECTLY

A condom is a sheath of latex or other material that fits over an erect penis and protects against STDs by preventing the transfer of body fluids. Condoms can protect you only if you use them correctly. Still, condoms cannot guarantee 100 percent protection. Incorrect use can lead to slipping or breaking of the condom, making it ineffective against STDs. Follow these steps to make sure you are using a condom correctly:

- Use only latex condoms. (Lambskin condoms don't prevent the transmission of STDs including HIV, the virus that causes AIDS.)
- Don't unroll the condom before placing it on the penis.
- Put the condom on after the penis is erect but before the penis touches any part of a partner's body.
- If you have not been circumcised, pull back your foreskin before putting on the condom.
- Holding the rim of the condom, place it over the tip of the penis. While holding the rim in place, unroll the condom over the penis. If the condom is not prelubricated, place a few drops of a water-based lubricant on the outside of the condom. Never use creams, lotions, or petroleum jelly to lubricate a condom because they can cause the condom to break.
- Pinch the tip of the condom to get the air out and to leave a reservoir at the tip to collect semen.
- After ejaculation but before the penis gets soft, hold onto the rim of the condom and carefully and gently withdraw the condom and the penis from your partner. Don't spill any contents onto your partner.
- Remove the condom from the penis, wrap the used condom it in a tissue, and throw it away.
- Wash your hands with soap and water.

LESS RISKY SEXUAL PRACTICES

If you want to make sure you are protected against STDs but want to have an intimate relationship, here are some safe ways to show affection.

- **Kissing**   This can be a safe way to be physically close, as long as both partners are free of cuts and sores in the mouth.
- **Massage**   Caressing and stroking can express affection and give pleasure.
- **Masturbation**   Masturbation with your partner (on unbroken skin), or alone, can provide sexual pleasure safely.
- **Fantasy**   The brain is one of the most powerful sex organs. Use your imagination.

You can never be too careful when it comes to protecting yourself from STDs. Because these infections are so widespread and many people who don't have symptoms are unaware they are infected, you need to take measures to reduce your exposure and risk of infection. Prior planning and good communication with your partner enables you to enjoy the pleasures of a sexual relationship while reducing the risks involved. In addition to always using a condom for any type of sexual activity, here are some more safer-sex guidelines:

- **Know your partner.** Before having sex, establish a committed relationship that fosters trust and open communication. You should be able to discuss both of your past sexual histories, any previous STDs, or intravenous (IV) drug use. You should never feel pressured or forced into having sex.

- **Stay sober.** Being under the influence of alcohol or drugs impairs your judgment and your ability to communicate and makes you more likely to engage in unprotected sex.

- **Be responsible.** If you have an STD, especially an active infection or an STD such as HIV or herpes that is long-lasting, you need to tell any prospective sexual partner. Allow him or her to decide how to proceed. If you mutually agree to engage in sexual activity, use latex condoms and other measures to protect your partner.

- **If you are pregnant, take precautions.** If you have an STD, learn about the risk to your fetus or baby before you become pregnant. HIV-positive women can take medication during pregnancy that significantly reduces the risk that their baby will be born with the infection. Also, HIV-infected women should not breast-feed because the virus can be transmitted to a nursing child in breast milk.

- **Have regular medical checkups.** If you are sexually active, especially if you have more than one sexual partner, be sure to see your doctor regularly for checkups and screening tests for STDs. Many common STDs do not produce symptoms, especially in women, and the only way to know you're infected is with a laboratory test.

6

HEALTH CARE TO KEEP YOU WELL

PREVENTION IS MOST EFFECTIVE when you know the medical conditions for which you're most at risk. This chapter explains how you can learn your personal health risks by compiling a family health history and learning how genes, your environment, and your behavior interact to play a role in the development of health problems. You'll also learn how to choose a trusted doctor for yourself and your family. This chapter includes a section that covers the routine health tests and screenings recommended by doctors to keep you healthy and detect disorders in the early stages. You will learn how each screening test is done and what you should do to prepare for it.

Compiling a personal and family health history

Doctors have long known that common diseases (including heart disease, cancer, and type 2 diabetes) and rare disorders (such as hemophilia, cystic fibrosis, and sickle cell anemia) can run in families. For example, if someone in one generation of a family has high blood pressure, particularly if it occurs at a younger age, the risk for high blood pressure in the next generation is likely to be increased. Tracing the medical conditions that your parents, grandparents, and other blood relatives have had can help your doctor predict the disorders for which you may be at risk. Once you know your family health history, you can take the steps needed to reduce your risk as much as possible. Complete a family health history for every person in your household to make sure everyone in your family stays healthy.

Maybe you already agree that your family history is important to your health. A recent survey found that 96 percent of all Americans believe that knowing their family history is important. However, the same survey found that only one out of three Americans has ever tried to gather the information and write down their family's health history.

Family members share common habits, lifestyles, and environments. They also share inherited traits that are passed on from one generation to the next, which is why family members often resemble one another. The family health history tree reflects all of these shared influences. Lifestyle changes will be especially important to you if your family health history shows an increased risk for specific health problems. For many diseases, people may be able to overcome their inherited risk by knowing their family history and taking steps to minimize their risk for those conditions by leading a healthy lifestyle.

We suggest that you make copies of the health history form on pages 182 to 185 and fill in the information. Once you have completed the form, keep a copy for your records and take a copy with you each time you see your doctor or other health-care professional. The more completely you fill out the form, the better able your doctor will be to determine your health-care needs. Update the form as circumstances change or if you learn more about your family's health history.

If you don't know the health histories of many of your relatives, ask them. If they feel uncomfortable sharing personal information, explain to them that their health information can help improve the future outlook for all family members. Try to get as much specific information as possible. Ask about chronic illnesses such as heart disease and diabetes; pregnancy complications such as miscarriage; and any developmental disabilities. If you need to, create a separate page with detailed information and descriptions about any medical conditions your relatives may have had. Don't forget to include your grandparents, uncles and aunts, nieces and nephews, half-brothers and half-sisters, cousins, great-uncles, and great-aunts.

In addition to your family history, there are many aspects of your personal health and habits that can affect your risk for disease and determine what screening tests you may need. It's a good idea to fill out the Personal Health History form on the following pages, keep it up to date, and take it to all your doctor appointments. The more specific you can be, the more helpful the form will be to you and your doctor. It's also important to be truthful as you fill it out. If there is something you don't want to write down, you should still share it with your doctor verbally.

Evaluating your risk profile

The genes you inherited from your parents and grandparents can affect your personal health risks. Most common diseases result from the interaction of a number of genes with environmental factors, such as smoking, exposure to pollution or radiation, or even not getting enough sleep. These complex interactions are unlikely to be understood fully in the near future. In the meantime, you can use your family health history to get an idea of the genetic, environmental, and behavioral factors that might affect your health.

Ultimately it's up to your doctor to thoroughly evaluate your inherited risks for any health problems. Giving your doctor helpful tools such as your personal health history and your family health history can make your doctor's job easier and may help streamline the diagnosis of a disorder.

HOW GENES INFLUENCE HEALTH RISK

Inside the cells of your body, two sets of chromosomes carry your genetic blueprint written in the genetic alphabet of DNA (deoxyribonucleic acid). One set of chromosomes was passed to you by each of your parents. DNA is present in all living cells and carries all the information required for life. Your genes determine characteristics like eye color or height, and contribute to your chances of developing certain diseases. The influence of genes on some traits, such as intelligence and behavior, is difficult to determine. Each of us has a unique identity that results from the complex interaction of our genes and our environment.

Throughout history, people have observed that diseases run in families. But it was only after the genetic discoveries of the 20th century that doctors began to understand how specific genes affect disease and health. They

Family Health History Tree

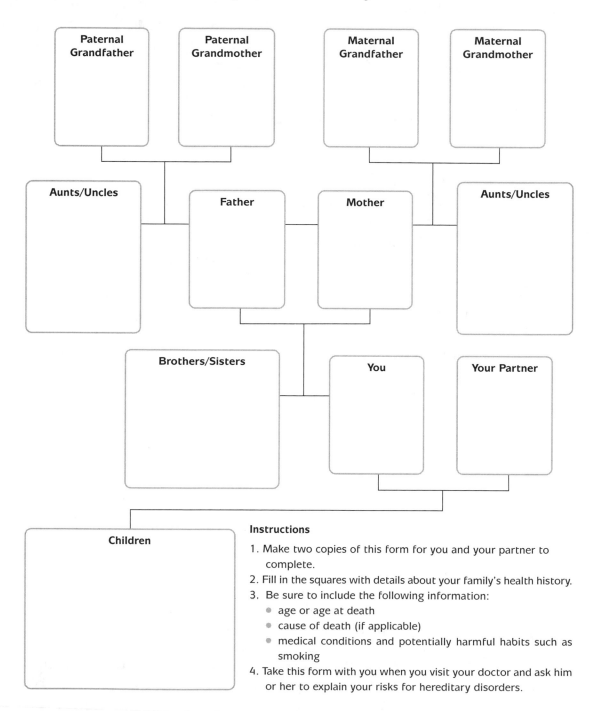

Instructions

1. Make two copies of this form for you and your partner to complete.
2. Fill in the squares with details about your family's health history.
3. Be sure to include the following information:
   - age or age at death
   - cause of death (if applicable)
   - medical conditions and potentially harmful habits such as smoking
4. Take this form with you when you visit your doctor and ask him or her to explain your risks for hereditary disorders.

Personal Health History

Name _____

Sex _____ Birth date _____ Age _____

Place of birth _____ Ethnicity _____

MEDICAL HISTORY _____

Current Conditions   Year Diagnosed

_____   _____

_____   _____

_____   _____

_____

Previous Operations   Year   Hospital

_____   _____   _____

_____   _____   _____

_____   _____   _____

_____   _____   _____

Previous Injuries/Medical Conditions   Year

_____   _____

_____   _____

_____   _____

Mental Illnesses   Year Diagnosed

_____   _____

_____   _____

CURRENT PRESCRIPTION MEDICATIONS _____

Medication   *Dose*   *How Long You*
                                              Have Taken It

_____   _____   _____

_____   _____   _____

_____   _____   _____

_____   _____   _____

_____   _____   _____

_____   _____   _____

_____   _____   _____

CURRENT NONPRESCRIPTION MEDICATIONS

Medication	Dose	How Long You Have Taken It
_____	_____	_____
_____	_____	_____
_____	_____	_____
_____	_____	_____

Drug Allergies

Medication	Reaction
_____	_____
_____	_____

SOCIAL HISTORY

Marital status: Married or single   No. of children _____

Sexual history:
   No. of sex partners in your lifetime _____
   Sex of sex partners: Male, female, or both
   Practice safer sex? Yes or No

LIFESTYLE

Tobacco   Have you ever used tobacco products? Yes or No
               No. of cigarettes smoked per day (on average) _____
               No. of cigars smoked per day _____
               No. of years you smoked _____
               Amount of chewing tobacco or snuff used per day _____
               No. of years you used chewing tobacco or snuff _____
               Have you ever quit? Yes or No

Alcohol   No. of drinks per week (on average) _____
               Have you ever quit? Yes or No
               Have you abused alcohol? Yes or No

Illegal drugs Have you ever used illicit drugs? Yes or No
               Which drug(s) have you used? _____
               When was your last use? _____

Exercise   Do you regularly exercise? Yes or No
               If yes, what type of exercise? _____
               How often do you exercise per week (on average)? _____
               Length of exercise sessions (on average) _____

VACCINATIONS

Vaccination	Year of Last Vaccination	Vaccination	Year of Last Vaccination
Influenza	_____	Hepatitis A	_____
Measles, mumps, rubella	_____	Hepatitis B	_____
Pneumococcal (pneumonia)	_____	Human papillomavirus (HPV)	_____
Polio	_____	Meningococcal (meningitis)	_____
Tetanus, diphtheria	_____	Varicella (chicken pox)	_____

FAMILY HEALTH HISTORY

Relative	Living (yes/no)	Age at Death	Medical Conditions and/or Cause of Death
Father	_____	_____	_____
Mother	_____	_____	_____
Partner	_____	_____	_____
Brothers	_____	_____	_____
	_____	_____	_____
Sisters	_____	_____	_____
	_____	_____	_____
Grandparents			
Paternal grandfather	_____	_____	_____
Paternal grandmother	_____	_____	_____
Maternal grandfather	_____	_____	_____
Maternal grandmother	_____	_____	_____
Uncles and aunts	_____	_____	_____

DOCTORS

	Current Doctor(s)— Medical Specialty	Address	Phone No.
Primary doctor	_____	_____	_____
	_____	_____	_____

	Past Doctor(s)— Medical Specialty	Address	Phone No.
Primary doctor	_____	_____	_____
	_____	_____	_____

HEALTH INSURANCE

Health insurance provider _____

Your identification no. _____

Phone no. of insurance company _____

found that some diseases, including cystic fibrosis, muscular dystrophy, and sickle cell disease, are caused by changes (mutations) in a single gene. And they found that it takes multiple genes, acting together, to increase the risk for other, more complex diseases, including heart disease, high blood pressure, and type 2 diabetes; mental disorders such as schizophrenia and depression; and alcohol and drug dependence.

Still, it is apparent that genes alone are not the whole story. For example, it has been shown that when identical twins (who have the same genetic makeup) are raised in different families, they sometimes develop different diseases. This type of finding suggests that lifestyle and environment are also important contributors to health and disease.

The mapping of the entire human genome is providing researchers with powerful tools to identify genetic influences on health and disease. However, there is still a long way to go to understand why one person develops a disease and another does not. Doctors know that genes alone, even in combination, don't cause heart disease, diabetes, cancer, depression, or addictions. Instead, genes influence a person's risk of developing health problems. Whether or not that risk actually leads to disease depends on a lifetime of complex interactions between a person's genes and environment. Some environments or experiences that are known to increase the chances of physical or mental health problems are especially risky for people who have a genetic susceptibility to those problems.

For example, research on gene-environment interactions shows that children in highly stressful environments are more likely to develop depression as adults if they also have a certain version of a gene that affects the level of the brain chemical serotonin. People who experience high levels of stress as children but lack this genetic variation aren't as likely to develop depression. More and more studies are showing that gene-environment interactions during early development can have long-lasting effects on health that often don't appear until adulthood.

As medical researchers identify people with a high risk for disease based on a combination of inherited factors and exposure to unhealthy influences in their environment, they will be better able to recommend the medical tests, screenings, treatments, and preventive strategies necessary to keep them healthy. A person's environment, diet, age, lifestyle, and overall state of health can also have an influence on his or her response to medications. Understanding a person's genetic makeup may be the key to creating personalized drugs that are both safe and effective.

LIFESTYLE VS. GENES

If you, like most of us, have inherited genes that make you susceptible to developing a particular disease or disorder, it does not mean that you are destined to develop the disease. In fact, many doctors think that a healthy lifestyle can overcome most of a person's genetic susceptibilities. For example, if you inherited a tendency toward heart disease, your first step is to find out what lifestyle factors can promote heart disease and then take action to avoid them while adopting the lifestyle measures that can reduce your risk for heart disease. The principle lifestyle risk factors for heart disease include the following:

- Smoking
- A diet high in saturated and trans fats and low in unsaturated fat (such as fish oil and olive oil)
- Getting little exercise
- Being overweight or obese

If you have a high risk for heart disease based on your family history, you should make the effort to stop smoking, eat a healthy diet, get regular exercise, and keep your weight within the normal range. Successfully controlling your lifestyle risk factors can help prevent your inherited susceptibilities from becoming a reality.

Routine screenings and exams

One of the most important steps you can take to prevent health problems is to have all the medical checkups and screening tests your doctor recommends. Some tests (such as a colonoscopy) are recommended for everyone after reaching a certain age (such as 50). Others are recommended only for men or only for women, or only for people who have a high risk for a specific disorder.

A screening test is a test that is performed to identify a problem or condition before it produces symptoms. Sometimes people think, "I feel fine; I don't need that test," but that is the point—screening tests try to find problems before they make you sick. Some screening tests can actually prevent disease; others identify a disease at an early stage, making treatment more effective. The specific screening tests recommended by your doctor depend on your age, gender, ethnicity, and risk factors for a specific disease.

This section discusses the routine screening tests recommended by most doctors.

Screening tests for cancer

Cancer screening tests are tests or exams that test for specific cancers in people who have no symptoms of cancer. Some tests, such as a colonoscopy or a skin cancer check, are recommended for everyone. Other tests, such as the Pap test for women or the PSA test for men, are recommended for specific groups of people. Screening tests enable doctors to diagnose cancer at an early stage or, ideally, before abnormal cells have become cancerous. When diagnosed at an early stage, most cancers are easier to treat and have better survival rates.

PELVIC EXAM AND PAP TEST

A pelvic exam and Pap test are important parts of a woman's routine health care because they can detect infection, inflammation, cancer, or abnormalities that may lead to cancer of the cervix (the lower part of the uterus). A pelvic exam is a physical examination in which the doctor feels for lumps or changes in the shape of a woman's reproductive organs, including the vagina, cervix, uterus, fallopian tubes, and ovaries. During a pelvic exam, you lie on your back on an examining table with your feet in stirrups and your legs apart. The doctor uses a device called a speculum to open your vagina so he or she can look at the cervix and take samples for a Pap test or to detect infections.

The Pap test, also called a Pap smear, is a way to examine cells collected from the cervix. The main purpose of the Pap test is to detect cancerous cells or abnormal cells that could become cancerous. Most types of cervical cancer can be prevented if women have Pap tests on a regular basis. And—as with many types of cancer—cancer of the cervix is more likely to be treated successfully when it is detected early. The test can also detect some noncancerous conditions such as infection and inflammation.

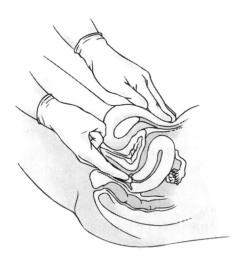

Pelvic examination

During a pelvic exam, a doctor examines a woman's reproductive organs to detect any abnormalities.

A Pap test is simple, quick, and usually painless. It can be done in a doctor's office, a clinic, or a hospital. The doctor takes a sample of cells from the cervix with a wooden scraper or a small cervical brush. The specimen (or smear) is placed either on a glass slide or directly into a jar filled with preservative. It is then sent to a laboratory for examination under a microscope.

How often should you have a Pap test? That depends on a number of factors, including your age and sexual activity. You should talk with your doctor about when and how often you need to have a Pap test. Current general guidelines recommend that women have a Pap test at least once every three years, beginning about three years after they first have sexual intercourse, but no later than age 21. Doctors recommend waiting about three years after the start of sexual activity to avoid unnecessary treatment for common, but usually temporary, abnormal changes that often occur when a woman first starts having sex. It's safe to wait three years, because cervical cancer usually develops slowly and because cervical cancer is extremely rare in women under age 25.

Women between the ages of 65 and 70 who have had at least three normal Pap tests and no abnormal Pap tests in the previous 10 years may decide, after talking with their doctor, to stop having Pap tests. Women who have had a hysterectomy (surgery to remove the uterus and cervix no longer need to have Pap tests, unless the surgery was done to treat a precancerous condition or cancer.

It is best not to have a Pap test when you are menstruating, but it can be done if necessary. Ideally, you should avoid using vaginal medicines or spermicidal foams, creams, or jellies (except as directed by your doctor) for two or three days before your Pap test because they can wash away or hide abnormal cells. Also, avoid having sexual intercourse for one or two days before a Pap test, to reduce the likelihood of inconclusive results.

To report Pap test results, most laboratories in the United States use a standard set of terms called the Bethesda System. In the Bethesda System, Pap test samples that have no cell abnormalities are reported as "negative." About 55 million Pap tests are performed each year in the United States. Of these, roughly 3.5 million (6 percent) are abnormal and require medical follow-up.

The following terms are used to describe the results of Pap tests:

- **Negative or normal** The cervical cells have been found to be healthy and normal.

- **Abnormal cells** Referred to as atypical squamous cells, they are clearly not normal, but are not abnormal enough to be classified as precancerous. These abnormal cells often result from HPV infection (see box), but can also result from other infections, inflammation, or injury. They usually clear on their own, but should be monitored by repeat Pap tests.

- **Mild changes** Classified as low-grade SIL, mild dysplasia, or CIN 1, these are cells that are mildly abnormal, do not invade healthy tissue, and often clear on their own with time.

- **High-grade changes** Classified as high-grade SIL, moderate or severe dysplasia, CIN 2, CIN 3, or carcinoma-in-situ, these are more advanced precancerous changes that involve more cell layers in the cervix, may invade nearby healthy tissue, and require treatment so they do not progress to cancer.

- **Squamous cell carcinoma** This is cervical cancer, and requires treatment.

After an abnormal Pap test result, ask your doctor to explain the specific type of abnormality and what it means. It's important to remember that abnormal cells don't always become cancerous, and some conditions are more likely to lead to cancer than others. If the Pap test shows an unclear result or minor abnormality, your doctor may repeat the test to determine if further follow-up is needed. In many cases, cell changes in the cervix return to normal without treatment.

Following an abnormal Pap test, your doctor may perform another test called a colposcopy, using an instrument similar to a microscope to examine your vagina and cervix. If the colposcopy finds abnormal tissue, the doctor may take a biopsy (removal of cells or tissues from the abnormal area for examination under a microscope). If the biopsy shows abnormal cells that have a high chance of becoming cancerous, further treatment is needed. Without treatment, these cells could turn into invasive cancer. Treatment usually involves removing the abnormal tissue surgically, or freezing it.

HPV TESTING

It is now possible to test directly with a Pap test for the human papillomavirus (HPV), the virus that causes most cervical cancers. Your doctor may recommend that you have this test, or he or she may test for it automatically if your Pap smear returns abnormal. Knowing if you have the HPV virus helps determine your risk of developing cervical cancer and how often you need to have a repeat exam.

SCREENING FOR CHLAMYDIA

Chlamydia (see page 166) is a common sexually transmitted disease (STD) that, without treatment, can damage a woman's reproductive organs and lead to irreversible problems including infertility. Many women who are infected with chlamydia do not know it because it usually does not cause symptoms in women, or only mild symptoms that go unnoticed. Because of the serious complications resulting from chlamydia and because the infection is curable with antibiotics, routine screening is recommended for women who have had a new sex partner, unprotected sex, or risk factors for STDs since their last pelvic exam. If you have any of these risk factors, talk to your doctor about being tested for chlamydia. Doctors often do the chlamydia test at the same time as the Pap smear.

MAMMOGRAMS

A screening mammogram is an X-ray of the breasts used to detect breast changes in women who have no signs or symptoms of breast cancer. Mammograms make it possible for doctors to detect tumors that cannot be felt. Mammograms can also detect microcalcifications, tiny deposits of calcium in the breast that sometimes indicate the presence of breast cancer. A screening mammogram is different from a diagnostic mammogram, which doctors use to check for breast cancer after a lump or other possible signs of breast cancer have been found. A diagnostic mammogram usually includes two X-rays of each breast.

The benefits of having regular mammograms every one to two years are clear for women over age 50. Breast cancer screening with mammograms reduces the number of deaths from breast cancer for women ages 50 to 69. But experts continue to debate whether screening mammography should be recommended for women younger than 50. In women under 50, some experts argue, the possible risks—such as false positive results, with invasive follow-up tests (such as a biopsy) that may not be needed, excess cost, and exposure to radiation—may outweigh the benefits. If you're a woman between ages 40 and 49, the best advice is to discuss the benefits and risks of mammography with your doctor. Only your doctor knows your personal health history and family health history. He or she can fully explain the pros and cons of having a mammogram so you can make an informed decision.

To date, studies have not shown a benefit from regular screening mammograms, or from a baseline screening mammogram (a first mammogram used for comparison in subsequent years), in women under age 40.

You can obtain a high-quality mammogram in a breast clinic, hospital radiology department, mobile van, private radiology office, or doctor's office. The Mammography Quality Standards Act (MQSA) is a federal law to ensure that mammograms are safe and reliable. Through the MQSA, all mammography facilities in the United States must meet stringent quality standards, be accredited by the U.S. Food and Drug Administration (FDA), and be inspected annually. The FDA ensures that mammography facilities across the country meet MQSA standards. These standards apply to all of the employees at a mammography facility including the technologist who takes the mammogram, the radiologist who interprets the mammogram, and the medical physicist who tests the mammography equipment.

Before making an appointment for your mammogram, ask your doctor or the staff at the mammography clinic about their FDA certification. All mammography facilities have to display their FDA certificate. Look for the MQSA certificate at the clinic and check its expiration date. MQSA regulations also require mammography facilities to give patients an easy-to-read report on the results of their mammogram.

Having a mammogram

Before having a mammogram, you will be asked to remove your clothing above the waist and put on a hospital gown. (Consider wearing a two-piece outfit the day of your test.) For a mammogram, the technician will position each breast, one at a time, between two plates that compress the breast, and take a low-intensity X-ray. Usually, you are standing up, and the technician will have you place your arms in certain positions during the test.

The technician will take images of your breasts from a number of different positions to enable the radiologist who interprets the X-rays to see all of the breast tissue. The exam takes about 20 minutes. After looking at the X-rays, the radiologist might ask the technician to take additional images or do a breast ultrasound to obtain a more precise reading.

When a radiologist reads a mammogram, discrepancies sometimes occur, resulting in what are called false negatives or false positives. False negatives describe mammograms that appear normal even though breast cancer is present. Overall, mammograms miss up to 20 percent of breast cancers that are present at the time of screening. False negatives occur more often in younger women than in older women because younger women tend to have denser breasts, which make breast cancers more difficult to detect on a mammogram. As women age, their breasts usually become more fatty and less dense, making breast cancers more noticeable and easier to detect with screening mammograms.

False positives occur when a radiologist interprets a mammogram as abnormal but no cancer is present. All abnormal mammograms need to be followed up with additional testing—usually a diagnostic mammogram, an ultrasound, or a biopsy—to verify if cancer is present. False positives are more common in younger women, women who have had previous breast biopsies, women with a family history of breast cancer, and those who are taking estrogen in hormone replacement therapy (see page 520).

Digital mammography has been available since the year 2000. Both digital and conventional mammography use X-rays to produce images of the breast, but conventional mammography produces an image on film, while digital mammography takes an electronic image of the breast and stores it directly in a computer. This ability allows the radiologist reading the mammogram to enhance, magnify, or manipulate the image during his or her evaluation. The difference between conventional mammography and digital mammography is like the difference between a traditional film camera and a digital camera. Conventional mammograms use a low dose of radiation, and digital mammograms expose you to even less radiation. Both are equally effective screening tools.

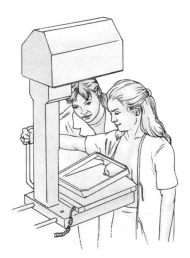

Having a mammogram

During a mammogram, you may feel some discomfort or pain when your breasts are being compressed between the plates, but the discomfort will last for just the brief time it takes to get the image. If the discomfort is too great, tell the technician. Scheduling the appointment 7 to 10 days after the beginning of your period, when your breasts are less likely to be tender, may help minimize the discomfort.

Having breast implants is no reason to refrain from having a mammogram. Be sure to tell the mammography clinic staff about your breast implants when scheduling a mammogram so they can provide a technician and radiologist who are experienced in screening patients with breast implants. Implants can hide some breast tissue, making it more difficult for the radiologist to detect an abnormality on the mammogram. If the technologist performing the procedure knows that you have breast implants, he or she can take steps to make sure that as much breast tissue as possible can be seen on the X-ray.

FECAL OCCULT BLOOD TEST

Doctors recommend that every adult have a fecal occult blood test every year or every other year starting at age 50. People who have risk factors for colon cancer, such as a family history of the disease, should begin having the test at age 40. A fecal occult blood test checks for blood in the stool because blood may be a sign of colon or rectal cancer (see page 263).

You can perform the test at home. You are instructed to place small samples of stool from three different bowel movements on a special card and send it to your doctor or to a laboratory for testing. The samples will be tested for the presence of "occult" (unseen) blood.

You can also buy a test called a flushable reagent stool blood test from a drug store over the counter. To use this test, you place a chemically treated tissue in the toilet after having a bowel movement. Look for a change in the color of the tissue, note your findings on a card, and mail the results to your doctor.

Before either test, you should avoid taking aspirin or vitamin C for several days because they can cause bleeding that could invalidate the test. You should also refrain from eating certain raw vegetables. (The list of foods to avoid will be in the instructions to the test you are taking.) Don't use either test if you are menstruating or if you have bleeding hemorrhoids.

COLONOSCOPY

A colonoscopy allows a doctor to look inside the large intestine (colon) to make an accurate diagnosis of or treat colon abnormalities without the need for major surgery. The colon, about 5 feet long, is the lower part of the intestinal tract that ends at the rectum and anus. The colon's main functions are to absorb water and minerals and form and eliminate waste from the body in the form of stool.

A screening colonoscopy is done in order to find and remove polyps or precancerous changes before they produce any symptoms. In this way, colon cancer can actually be prevented. Everyone should have their first colonoscopy after they turn 50. If no abnormal results show up on the first test, another test is not needed for ten years, unless recommended by your doctor. If you have a family history of colon cancer or have had a polyp removed during a prior colonoscopy, you should have the procedure every three to five years, or as recommended by your doctor.

Before scheduling the procedure, your doctor will ask about any medical conditions you have or medications you take on a regular basis, including aspirin, arthritis medications, blood thinners, diabetes medication, or vitamins that contain iron. The doctor will also want to know if you have heart disease, lung disease, or any other serious medical condition. You must arrange for someone to take you home after the procedure because you will be groggy from the sedative.

Preparing for a colonoscopy

Before having a colonoscopy, you will get instructions from the doctor's office that will explain what you need to do to prepare for the test. Your colon must be completely empty and cleaned out for the colonoscopy. You will be asked to follow a clear liquid diet for one or two days beforehand. The list of foods you are allowed to consume before having a colonoscopy includes water, fat-free bouillon or broth, plain coffee, plain tea, clear soda such as ginger ale, and gelatin.

Starting on the day or evening before your colonoscopy, you probably will be asked to drink a gallon of electrolyte lavage solution. The solution is a laxative designed to cleanse the colon by inducing diarrhea. At the same time, the solution replaces electrolytes (substances responsible for moving nutrients into cells and removing wastes out of cells) that may be lost with the diarrhea. You need to follow the package directions exactly when taking the solution. If you don't understand the instructions, ask your doctor or pharmacist to explain them to you.

Your doctor will tell you when to start drinking the solution and to drink the recommended amount of solution every 10 minutes until your stool becomes watery and clear. Although fruit-flavored, this solution is notoriously bad-tasting, but you have to drink it all so that the colon is cleansed and any abnormalities are more clearly visible to the doctor. Be sure to tell the doctor performing the colonoscopy if you could not consume all of the solution. Incomplete cleansing of the colon could affect the outcome of the procedure, or require a repeat test. If you take a blood-thinning medication—including aspirin, warfarin, or clopidogrel—check with the doctor who prescribed it before discontinuing it prior to your colonoscopy (or any other procedure). You should also find out when to resume taking the medication if you do stop taking it for the procedure.

Having a colonoscopy

During the colonoscopy, you will lie on your side on the examining table. You will be given pain medication and a mild sedative through an intravenous line to keep you comfortable and help you relax during the examination. The doctor and a nurse will monitor your vital signs, look for any signs of discomfort, and make adjustments as needed.

The doctor inserts a long, flexible, lighted tube called a colonoscope into the rectum and slowly guides it into the colon. The scope transmits an image of the inside of the colon onto a video screen to enable the doctor to carefully examine the lining of the colon. The scope bends so the doctor can move it into and around the curves of the colon. Many people fall asleep during the test and don't remember it afterward.

During a colonoscopy, a doctor can remove any polyps (growths in the lining of the colon) he or she sees, using tiny instruments passed through the scope. Most polyps are not cancerous, but some have the potential to become cancerous. Any polyps that are removed are sent to a laboratory for testing. By identifying and removing polyps, a colonoscopy can prevent most colon cancers from forming.

A colonoscopy usually takes 30 to 60 minutes. The sedative and pain medication should keep you from feeling much discomfort during the exam. You may feel some cramping or the sensation of having gas after the procedure is completed, but these sensations usually stop within an hour or so. You will need to stay at the medical office or clinic for one or two hours to allow the sedative to wear off. You won't be able to drive for the rest of the day, but you can resume your normal activities the next day.

FLEXIBLE SIGMOIDOSCOPY

Flexible sigmoidoscopy enables a doctor to look at the inside of the lowest part of the large intestine (colon), from the rectum. This section of the colon is called the sigmoid or descending colon. Doctors use sigmoidoscopy to look for early signs of cancer in the descending colon and rectum. They also use the test to find the cause of diarrhea, abdominal pain, or constipation. Using flexible sigmoidoscopy, the doctor can see any bleeding, inflammation, abnormal growths, and ulcers in the descending colon and rectum. Flexible sigmoidoscopy cannot be used to detect polyps or cancer in the ascending or transverse colon (the other two-thirds of the colon).

Preparing for a sigmoidoscopy

Your colon and rectum must be completely empty before the doctor can perform a flexible sigmoidoscopy thoroughly and safely. You will probably be asked to drink only clear liquids—including fat-free bouillon or broth, gelatin, water, plain coffee, plain tea, or clear soda, such as ginger ale—for 12 to 24 hours before the procedure. You may also be asked to drink an electrolyte lavage solution or give yourself an enema to clean out your intestines. Your doctor may give you other special instructions.

Having a sigmoidoscopy

During a sigmoidoscopy, you lie on your side on an examining table. The doctor will insert a short, flexible, lighted tube called a sigmoidoscope into your rectum and carefully guide it up into the sigmoid colon. The scope transmits an image of the inside of the rectum and sigmoid colon, to enable the doctor to thoroughly examine their linings. The scope also injects air into these organs, inflating them to allow the doctor to see them better.

If anything unusual shows up in the rectum or sigmoid colon, such as a polyp or inflamed tissue, the doctor can remove a piece of it using instruments inserted into the scope. The doctor then sends the tissue to a laboratory for testing.

Flexible sigmoidoscopy takes about 10 to 20 minutes. During the procedure, you might feel pressure and slight cramping in your lower abdomen, but you will feel better as soon as you pass gas.

DIGITAL RECTAL EXAM

To check for abnormalities in the rectum or lower abdomen, doctors often perform a digital rectal examination. To perform the exam, the doctor inserts a lubricated, gloved finger into the rectum and inspects the area through touch for any abnormalities. The digital rectal exam is often part of a routine physical examination in men (to examine the prostate gland for enlargement or cancer) and a routine pelvic examination (see page 188) in women. The test can also be used to find the cause of symptoms such as pelvic pain or rectal bleeding.

PSA TEST

As men age, prostate conditions, both noncancerous (benign) and cancerous (malignant), tend to become more common. The most common benign prostate conditions (see page 502) are prostatitis (inflammation of the prostate) and benign prostatic hyperplasia (enlargement of the prostate). There is no evidence that prostatitis or an enlarged prostate leads to cancer, but it is possible for a man to have one or both of these conditions and to also develop prostate cancer (see page 291).

Prostate-specific antigen (PSA) is a protein produced by the cells of the prostate gland. The PSA test measures the level of PSA in the blood. It is normal for men to have low levels of PSA in their blood, but prostate cancer often produces higher levels. For this reason, PSA can be used as a screening test for prostate cancer. For a PSA test, a blood sample is taken and sent to a laboratory, which measures the amount of PSA in the blood. Because PSA is produced by the body and can be used to detect disease, doctors call it a disease marker or tumor marker.

However, there are other, noncancerous prostate conditions that can raise the PSA level. For this reason, PSA levels alone do not give a doctor enough information to distinguish between benign prostate conditions and prostate cancer. Doctors take the results of PSA tests into account when deciding whether to recommend further testing. Many doctors use the PSA test along with a digital rectal examination (see previous page) to help detect prostate cancer in men ages 50 and older. Together, these tests can be effective screening tests for detecting prostate cancer in men who have no symptoms.

Who should have a PSA screening test? The recommendations from the American Cancer Society, the American Urological Society, and the U.S. Preventive Services Task Force vary widely. Some encourage yearly screening for men over age 50; others recommend that men who are at an increased risk for prostate cancer begin yearly screening at age 40 or 45. (Men who are at increased risk include those with a family history of prostate cancer and blacks, who are at higher risk for the cancer than whites.) Still other guidelines do not recommend routine screening; they caution against routine PSA screening, or counsel men about the risks and benefits on an individual basis, encouraging them to make their own decisions about testing. Medicare provides coverage for an annual PSA test for all men ages 50 and older.

PSA TESTING: PROS AND CONS

Detection of prostate cancer does not necessarily mean saving lives. The PSA test sometimes detects a small cancer that will never become life-threatening, putting men at risk for complications from unnecessary follow-up diagnostic tests and treatments such as surgery or radiation. Also, PSA testing may not help if it detects a fast-growing or aggressive cancer that has already spread to other parts of the body.

The PSA test can produce false positive or false negative results. A false positive occurs when the PSA level is elevated but no cancer is present. False positives may lead to unnecessary medical procedures that carry potential risks and cause needless worry. False negative test results occur when the PSA level is in the normal range but prostate cancer is present. Most prostate cancers are slow-growing and can exist for decades before they are large enough to cause symptoms. Your best bet is to discuss the pros and cons of PSA testing with your doctor, who can recommend what's best for you.

What your PSA numbers mean

PSA test results are usually reported as nanograms of PSA per milliliter (ng/ml) of blood. In the past, most doctors considered PSA values below 4.0 to be normal but recent research has found prostate cancer in men with PSA levels below 4.0. Many doctors use the following ranges established by the National Cancer Institute to evaluate the likelihood of prostate cancer; the higher a man's PSA level, the more likely that cancer is present.

- 0 to 2.5 is low risk
- 2.6 to 10 is slightly to moderately elevated risk
- 10 to 19.9 is moderately elevated risk
- 20 or higher is significantly elevated risk

However, keep in mind that several factors can cause PSA levels to fluctuate, so one abnormal PSA test does not necessarily indicate a need for other tests or treatment. Many factors—including prostate cancer, benign prostate enlargement, inflammation, age, and race—could explain an elevated PSA level. Smoking can also increase the PSA level. Most men with an elevated PSA test turn out *not* to have prostate cancer. In fact, only 25 to 30 percent of men who have a biopsy after an elevated PSA level on a test actually have prostate cancer.

If you don't have any symptoms that suggest cancer, your doctor may recommend having the PSA test and digital rectal exam regularly to watch for any changes. But if your PSA level continues to rise over time or the doctor feels a suspicious lump, he or she may recommend other tests to determine if you have prostate cancer or another prostate problem.

Blood screening tests

Some screening tests can analyze a sample of blood to determine a person's risk for diseases such as heart disease (by testing blood fats such as cholesterol) or diabetes (by testing the level of the sugar glucose in the blood). The HIV screening test can detect the presence in the blood of antibodies (specific proteins the body produces to fight the AIDS virus).

CHOLESTEROL SCREENING

To test your blood cholesterol levels, a sample of blood is taken from your arm and sent to a laboratory for evaluation. The test is usually done after a

10- to 12-hour fast and gives information about the following components of your cholesterol profile:

- Total cholesterol
- LDL (bad) cholesterol, the main source of the buildup of fatty deposits in arteries
- HDL (good) cholesterol, which helps clear the arteries of harmful LDL cholesterol
- Triglycerides, fats that store energy and are gradually released between meals to meet the body's requirement for fuel; in excess, they can be harmful

If you are 20 years of age or older, it is recommended that you have your cholesterol measured at least once every five years, and more often (every two years) if you have a family history of heart disease or high cholesterol or if you have diabetes.

What your cholesterol numbers mean

Total cholesterol

Less than 200	Desirable
200–239	Borderline high
240 and above	High

LDL (bad) cholesterol (lower is better)

Less than 100	Optimal
100–129	Near optimal
130–159	Borderline high
160–189	High
190 and above	Very high

HDL (good) cholesterol (higher is better)

60 and above	High
40–59	Average
39 or less	Low

Triglycerides (lower is better)

Less than 150	Normal
151–199	Borderline high
200–499	High
500 and above	Very high

DIABETES TESTS

To diagnose type 2 diabetes, doctors use blood tests to measure the level of glucose (sugar) in the blood. Several factors, such as your activity level and the type of medication you are taking, can affect blood sugar levels, so your doctor will probably perform more than one type of blood test before reaching a diagnosis. Some tests may have to be repeated to make sure the diagnosis is correct. The following are the two most common tests used for diagnosing type 2 diabetes.

Fasting plasma glucose test

A fasting plasma (blood) glucose test measures the level of sugar in the blood. It is a test that is used to screen for diabetes and is recommended for everyone starting at age 20. The test should be repeated every five years if you have no risk factors for diabetes, or every two years if you do.

The test measures your blood sugar after you have fasted (have not had anything to drink except water overnight or for at least eight hours). The fasting plasma glucose test is a fairly reliable and convenient way to diagnose diabetes. It's most reliable when performed in the morning. A test result of 60 to 99 is a normal reading. If your fasting blood sugar level is 100 to 125, you have a form of prediabetes called impaired fasting glucose and you are at high risk of developing diabetes. Levels of 126 and above suggest a diagnosis of diabetes; the doctor will repeat the test to confirm the diagnosis.

Oral glucose tolerance test

An oral glucose tolerance test measures the body's ability to use glucose. To prepare for the test, you will be asked to eat foods rich in carbohydrates, such as whole grains, cooked dried beans, and vegetables, for two or three days and then to fast overnight or for at least eight hours. The oral glucose tolerance test is more sensitive than the fasting plasma glucose test, but requires more effort. The amount of glucose in your blood is measured just before you drink a liquid containing glucose dissolved in water and again every half hour for two hours after drinking it. If your blood sugar levels are between 140 and 199 two hours after drinking the liquid, you don't yet have type 2 diabetes, but you are likely to develop it. Levels of 200 or above, confirmed by a repeat test, indicate that you have diabetes.

HIV SCREENING

Doctors recommend screening for the human immunodeficiency virus (HIV) for all adolescents and adults between ages 13 and 64. This recommendation calls for routine but voluntary HIV screening as a normal part of health care, similar to the screening tests for other health conditions. If your doctor doesn't recommend the test during a regular appointment or checkup, you should feel free to request it.

HIV screening is recommended because HIV infection is a serious health problem that can be detected by reliable, noninvasive screening tests and diagnosed early, before symptoms appear. People who are infected with HIV can gain years of life when treatment is started early. Also, the costs of screening are reasonable when weighed against the potential benefits. For pregnant women, routine screening has proven much more effective for detecting unsuspected HIV infection and preventing transmission to the fetus than testing based on individual risk factors.

The HIV test is usually done on blood taken from a vein or fingerstick sample. Another way the test may be done is by taking a sample from a person's gums with a swab. Do not rely on home HIV tests because some home kits can give false information about a person's HIV status. The federal government tested HIV kits advertised and sold on the Internet for home use and, in every case, the kits showed a negative result when used on a known HIV-positive sample (when they should have shown a positive result). Using one of these kits could give the false impression that you are not infected with HIV when you are.

Self-examinations

Self-examinations are exams that you can do at home to check for any abnormal changes in your body. The most commonly recommended self-exams include the breast self-exam for women, the testicular self-exam for men, and the skin cancer self-exam and fecal occult blood test (see page 194), which are recommended for all adults.

BREAST SELF-EXAM

A breast self-exam is an at-home self-check used to detect breast lumps, changes in the size or shape of a breast, or any other changes in the breasts or underarm area. Regular breast self-exams help you to become familiar with how your breasts normally look and feel, so you'll be able to easily notice any changes. When you notice something different, you should see your doctor. Most breast changes or lumps are not cancerous, but only a doctor can tell for sure. If it does turn out to be breast cancer, finding it early gives you more treatment options and a better chance for a cure.

Regular breast self-exams can help detect breast cancer early, but they should not take the place of having regular mammograms (see page 191). The combination of regular self-exams and annual mammograms remains the most effective way to find breast cancer early and to improve a woman's chances for survival.

While examining your breasts, look for a lump or other feature that is noticeably different from the rest of your breast tissue. If you find a lump or other change in your breast, either during a breast self-exam or by chance, carefully examine the other breast. If both breasts feel the same, the lumpiness is probably normal. As you get to know your breasts better by doing breast self-exams, you should be able to tell the difference between your normal lumpiness and something different. Besides a lump or swelling, other changes in your breasts to look for include the following:

- Any changes in the shape or feel of the breasts
- Hard or soft lumps
- Changes in skin texture such as scaling
- Changes in color such as redness
- Puckering or depression (such as dimpling) in part of the breast
- A newly inverted nipple
- Discharge of any kind from a nipple

If you notice any of these changes, see your doctor right away. Doctors recommend that all women, especially those at increased risk for breast cancer and those over age 30, do a breast self-exam every month throughout life. If you are menstruating, the best time to perform the exam is right after your period ends, when the breasts tend to be less tender or swollen. It's easiest to examine your breasts when you are lying down so the breast tissue can distribute evenly across your chest wall. This way, you'll be better able to feel all of your breast tissue and more likely to notice anything unusual. Another option is while you are standing in the shower; raise your arm over your head to help spread the breast tissue.

How to examine your breasts

There are several effective ways to examine your breasts. Ask your doctor to teach you how to do a breast self-exam to make sure you're doing it correctly and thoroughly. Here's one method accepted by most doctors:

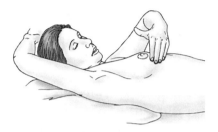

Lie down with a folded towel or pillow under the shoulder of the breast you're examining.

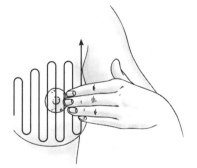

Examine each breast in an up-and-down pattern to make sure you don't miss any of your breast tissue.

- Lie down and put a folded towel or pillow under your right shoulder. Bring your right arm up and put it behind your head.

- Use the three middle fingers of your left hand to press on the tissue in your right breast in round, dime-sized motions. Feel for any lumps or other changes in the breast tissue.

- Press on each part of your breast in three ways. First, press lightly, to examine the tissue just under your skin. Then, press a little harder to probe a bit deeper. Finally, press firmly to inspect the tissue closest to your chest. A firm ridge underneath each breast is normal. Use all three types of pressure on each area of breast tissue, then move on to the next area.

- Examine your breast in an up-and-down pattern, starting at the underarm and moving down and then up to the collarbone, then down again, across the breast to the middle of your breastbone. (The up-and-down pattern seems to be the most effective pattern for covering the entire breast without missing any breast tissue.) Then, circle each nipple with your fingers to look for any changes.

- Cover each breast systematically, so you don't miss any part of your breast tissue.

- Move the towel under your left shoulder and duplicate the exam on your left breast, using the three middle fingers of your right hand.

- If you are large-breasted, examine your breasts in two stages. First, lie down and examine the outside of your breast. Then, lie on your side and check the inside of the breast.

- Check your underarms. Sit or stand up and raise your arm slightly, and press in a circular motion in the armpit. (Don't raise your arm

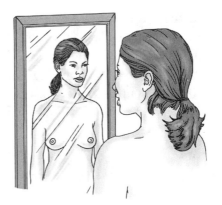

Use a mirror to examine your breasts.

straight up because the muscle and tissue will become too tight to feel anything.)

- For a visual examination of your breasts, stand in front of a mirror with your hands pressing firmly down on your hips and look at your breasts to check for any change in size, shape, or outline. See if there is any dimpling, pulling, redness, or scaling on the skin or nipples. Relax your arms down at your sides and see if you notice any changes. Then, put your arms above your head, press your palms together, and look for changes. Squeeze each nipple between your thumb and index finger and check for discharge.

TESTICLE SELF-EXAM

All males who have reached puberty or are over age 15 should examine their testicles at least once a month to check for any changes that could signal testicular cancer (see page 292). Testicular cancer affects mostly young men between the ages of 20 and 39. It is also more common in men who have had abnormal testicle development, have had an undescended testicle, or have a family history of the cancer.

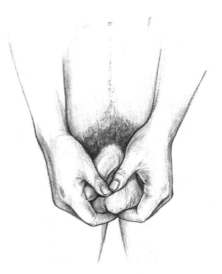

Roll each testicle between your fingers and thumbs.

The best time to do the test is during or after a shower, when the skin on your scrotum is warm and relaxed. Always do the test while standing up. Here's the process:

1. Carefully feel your scrotum to find a testicle.

2. Roll the testicle between the thumb and fingers of both hands to check the entire surface of the testicle. You may notice along the back side of the testicle that there is a structure that feels like a bag of worms. This is the epididymis, a normal structure.

3. Repeat the process with the other testicle.

Your testicles should feel firm, but not rock hard. One testicle usually hangs lower and may be a bit larger than the other. Testicles contain blood vessels and other tissues that can feel like something abnormal. That's why it's important to do the exam at least every month; you can become familiar with how your testicles normally feel and you will more easily notice any changes. Always contact your doctor if you find anything suspicious, such as a hard lump (like a pea) or an enlarged testicle. It could just be an infection, but it could also be the first sign of testicular cancer. Some cases of testicular cancer don't produce symptoms until they reach an advanced stage. Other signs of testicular cancer include the following:

- A testicle that seems smaller than before
- A heavy feeling in the scrotum
- A dull ache in the lower abdomen or groin
- An unexpected collection of fluid in the scrotum
- Pain or discomfort in a testicle or in the scrotum
- Enlarged or tender breasts

You should also talk to your doctor about any of the following situations, which are treatable and not life-threatening:

- You can't find one or both testicles. (A testicle may not have descended properly into the scrotum.)
- You feel a soft collection of thin tubes above the testicle. (It could be a collection of dilated veins.)
- You feel pain or swelling in the scrotum. (You could have an infection or a fluid-filled sac called a hydrocele causing obstructed blood flow to the area; both can be treated.)

SKIN CANCER CHECK

If you're over age 20, you should be examining the skin on your entire body every month for any changes. This advice is especially important if you've ever had frequent or prolonged exposure to the sun or bad sunburns earlier in life. Checking your skin routinely will help you become familiar with your freckles, moles, birthmarks, and other skin discolorations so you can recognize a change or something new when you see it. What you are primarily looking for are changes that could be a sign of skin cancer (see page 260), especially melanoma, the most dangerous kind. A new mole or suspicious patch of skin, or changes in an existing mole may be a sign of skin cancer.

The best time to do a skin check is after a shower or bath. You should check your skin in a room with plenty of light. Use both a full-length mirror and a hand-held mirror. Check for anything new, including the following:

- Moles that look different from your other moles
- Red or dark-colored flaky patches that may be a little raised
- Flesh-colored firm bumps
- Changes in the size, shape, color, or feel of a mole
- Sores that don't heal

Check yourself from head to toe.

- Look at your face, neck, ears, and scalp. You may want to use a comb or a hair dryer to move your hair so that you can see your scalp better. You could also ask a relative or friend to check your scalp because it can be hard to do it yourself.
- Look at the front and back of your body in the mirror. Then, raise your arms and look at your left and right sides.
- Bend your elbows. Look carefully at your fingernails, palms, forearms (including the undersides), and upper arms.
- Examine the back, front, and sides of your legs, and look at the skin around your genital area and between your buttocks.
- Sit and closely examine your feet, including your toenails, your soles, and the spaces between your toes.

It may be helpful to record the dates of your skin exams and to write notes about the way your skin looks. Or take pictures of certain areas you question to help your doctor see whether something has changed over time. If you ever find anything unusual, see your doctor. Many skin cancers can be cured when detected and treated early.

Bone density testing

A bone density test is the best way to evaluate the health and strength of your bones. Bone density tests can diagnose the bone-thinning disorder osteoporosis (see page 325), determine the risk for fractures, and evaluate the effectiveness of osteoporosis treatment. Fractures—especially of the hip—are the leading cause of loss of independence in older people.

The most widely recognized bone density test is dual-energy X-ray absorptiometry (DEXA). DEXA assesses a person's bone density and compares it to an established standard (the bone density of a healthy 30-year-old). Although no bone density test is completely accurate in determining a person's risk for fractures, DEXA is the most reliable predictor of the likelihood of having a future fracture. Talk to your doctor about your risk for osteoporosis and ask if you should have a bone density test. The information provided by a bone density test can help your doctor determine which prevention or treatment options are right for you. Treatment and lifestyle changes can reduce your risk for fractures and other effects of osteoporosis.

HAVING A BONE DENSITY TEST

For a bone density test, you lie on a table as a scanner measures the concentration of bone in your lower spine, wrist, forearm, and hip. You will not have to remove your clothing. The entire test usually takes only a few minutes. Bone scanners use very small doses of radiation and, like any X-ray, the procedure is painless.

All women age 65 and older should be screened regularly for osteoporosis. For women who are at increased risk for fractures from osteoporosis, routine screening should begin at age 60. People who are younger than 65 and don't have any risk factors for osteoporosis may not need a bone density test yet. If you are 45 or older and have one or more risk factors for

DEXA: WHAT THE NUMBERS MEAN

After the DEXA test, the results are scored. A score of 0 indicates that your bone mineral density equals the norm for a healthy young adult. Differences between your bone density and that of the norm are measured in units called standard deviations, indicated as negative or positive numbers. The lower your score is below 0, the lower your bone density and the higher your risk of having a fracture.

- A score between $+1$ and -1 is considered normal and healthy.
- A score between -1 and -2.5 indicates low bone density (referred to as osteopenia), but not low enough to be diagnosed as osteoporosis.
- A score of -2.5 or lower indicates osteoporosis. The lower the negative number, the more severe the osteoporosis.

osteoporosis, you may want to consider having the test. If you are a woman past menopause and you have fractured a bone, you may want to have a bone density test to determine if you have osteoporosis and determine what treatment will be most effective. Your doctor is the best person to recommend when you should begin having routine bone density tests.

Routine eye exams

Sight is precious, so you owe it to yourself to have regular eye examinations, especially if you notice changes in your vision. People 45 and older tend to have more vision problems than younger people. By age 65, you should have eye exams every six months to a year, depending on your risk factors for eye disorders such as glaucoma (see page 410) and age-related macular degeneration (see page 413).

A routine eye test is called a refraction and can be performed by either an ophthalmologist, a medical doctor (M.D.) who specializes in disorders of the eye, or an optometrist, a doctor of optometry (O.D.) who diagnoses, manages, and treats vision disorders. During a refraction test, you sit in a chair with a special device called a phoroptor. The doctor will ask you to look through the phoroptor at an eye chart that is about 20 feet away. The phoroptor holds lenses of varying strengths that the doctor can move into your field of vision so you can see which lens, if any, improves your vision. The doctor will ask you if the chart looks clearer or blurrier with each lens in position, information that will help determine if you have normal vision or are nearsighted or farsighted. He or she can also tell if you have astigmatism (a distortion of the image on the retina caused by an asymmetrical cornea) or presbyopia (the inability to focus on nearby objects). Most people start to develop presbyopia in their 40s. The refraction test helps the doctor determine the right prescription for corrective eyeglasses or contact lenses.

Often, a routine eye exam includes a test for glaucoma called an air puff test, which measures eye pressure. However, this test by itself cannot accurately diagnose glaucoma. Doctors usually find evidence of glaucoma during a test that dilates the pupils; drops are put into the eyes to enlarge the pupils and enable the doctor to see the insides of the eyes, to check for signs of glaucoma such as subtle changes to the optic nerve, which can appear before noticeable symptoms develop.

If the doctor sees signs that could indicate glaucoma or age-related macular degeneration (a disorder in which central vision is lost), he or she will conduct a more comprehensive eye examination that may include the following tests:

- **Visual acuity test** An eye-chart test that measures how well you see at various distances.

- **Vision field test** An exam that measures side (peripheral) vision. It helps determine if a person has lost peripheral vision, which is a sign of glaucoma.

- **Dilated eye exam** An exam in which drops are placed into the eyes to widen (dilate) the pupils, allowing the doctor to examine the retina at the back of the eye and the optic nerve for signs of damage. After this exam, near vision can be blurry for a few hours.

- **Tonometry** An examination that measures the pressure inside the eye. During the test, which is painless and takes only a few seconds, you will see a bright blue circle of light move toward your eye.

- **Pachymetry** An exam that uses an ultrasonic wave instrument to measure the thickness of the cornea (the transparent covering over the front of the eye). This test is used for accurately measuring pressure in the eye to diagnose glaucoma and is performed before a person has a vision-correcting procedure such as LASIK (laser-assisted in situ keratomileusis), which removes tissue from the cornea.

- **Amsler grid** This test is used to help diagnose age-related macular degeneration. The pattern of the grid resembles a checkerboard. You cover one eye and stare at a black dot in the center of the grid. While staring at the dot, if you notice that the straight lines in the pattern appear wavy or that some of the lines are missing, you could have age-related macular degeneration. Further testing will need to be performed to make a definite diagnosis.

Routine dental exams

Going to the dentist may not seem like such a big deal, but getting regular dental exams and cleanings is an important part of prevention. Gum disease is a serious bacterial infection that destroys the gum fibers and bone that hold the teeth in the mouth. No one is immune to gum disease, but there are many things you can do to avoid it as part of your routine dental hygiene. Do your gums bleed when you brush your teeth? If they do, you could have the first stage of gum disease, called gingivitis. The best way to prevent gum disease is to brush your teeth twice a day, floss your teeth every day, and see the dentist for a checkup and cleaning every six months.

THE DENTAL CHECKUP

During a routine dental exam, the dentist will conduct a thorough examination of the soft tissue in your mouth and throat, to look for any signs of precancerous conditions or oral cancer (see page 274). This exam will include a visual inspection and a finger exploration of your tongue, the floor of your mouth (under the tongue), the palate (roof of the mouth), salivary glands, insides of the cheeks, and the back of the throat. The dentist will also examine your face, head, and neck to check for enlarged lymph nodes. He or she may also check the joint that connects the jaw to the skull for misalignment.

Next, the dentist or dental hygienist will use a metal probe to measure how deep the band of gum tissue extends (pocket depth) around each tooth. This technique helps the dentist identify gum disease in its early stages, when treatment is most effective. Depths greater than 3 millimeters signal that the tooth has become less attached to the surrounding bone, which is a characteristic of gum disease.

The dentist or hygienist will note any cavities, existing fillings and crowns, and the general condition of each tooth. This information is written down in your dental record. The dentist will periodically order X-rays of your teeth to detect any small areas of decay, bone loss, or abscesses that can't be seen from a visual inspection. You may not need to have X-rays every year.

BREAKING NEWS **Saliva tests may detect oral cancer**

Researchers are developing simple, inexpensive diagnostic tests that can detect oral cancer and other disorders by analyzing a person's saliva. Saliva contains proteins and DNA molecules that have characteristic sequences, or "alphabets," that can be decoded. Each code indicates the presence of a particular disorder. Oral cancer can be recognized in saliva by testing for five proteins and four types of genetic material that form a distinctive pattern in 9 out of 10 cases.

If you don't need to have any cavities filled or other restorative work, the hygienist will then clean your teeth with an instrument called a scaler or curette, which removes plaque from the surface of the teeth. He or she will then polish your teeth. The purpose of polishing is to make the teeth smoother, so plaque can't build up as easily. Polishing also removes surface stains from the teeth.

You should see your dentist for a checkup and cleaning every six months. More frequent visits may be needed if you are pregnant, smoke, use chewing tobacco, drink alcohol excessively, or have gum disease or certain medical conditions such as type 2 diabetes or HIV infection. Your dentist will tell you how often you should have your teeth cleaned.

Your child should have his or her first dental checkup within six months of the eruption of the first tooth and no later than 12 months of age. During this first exam, the dentist can teach you how to properly clean your child's teeth and tell you about the normal schedule of tooth development in children. Unless your child has frequent dental problems, he or she should not need to see the dentist more than once a year, until about the age of 10. Then visits should be every six months.

Genetic testing and counseling

Genetic testing covers a wide range of techniques used to analyze the human genetic material DNA and RNA. Doctors use genetic tests to detect variations in genes that might signal a susceptibility to a specific disease or medical condition. Genetic counseling refers to the education and guidance provided to help people make informed decisions based on their genetic risk profile. Genetic counselors can help a person decide whether to have a genetic test, and what to do with the information found by the test.

GENETIC TESTING

Doctors sometimes order genetic tests on blood and other tissues to detect genetic disorders or inherited risks for disease. There are more than 1,000 genetic tests available, and the number is rapidly increasing. Doctors may order genetic tests for several reasons, including the following:

- To find possible genetic diseases in fetuses during pregnancy
- To find out if people carry a gene for a disease they might pass on to their children

At-home genetic tests

Be wary of the benefits that at-home genetic tests claim to offer. Some companies declare that at-home genetic tests can measure the risk of developing a particular chronic disease such as heart disease, type 2 diabetes, cancer, or Alzheimer's disease. But the FDA (Federal Drug Administration) and CDC (Centers for Disease Control and Prevention) say there are no valid studies showing that these tests give accurate results or that they can reliably predict risk for disease. Also, having a particular gene doesn't necessarily mean that a disease will develop, and not having a particular gene doesn't necessarily mean that you won't get the disease. Depending on your environment and lifestyle, specific genes or groups of genes may or may not become "switched on."

Some companies also claim that a person can protect against a serious disease by choosing special foods and nutritional supplements. The results of their at-home tests often include dietary advice and sales offers for "customized" dietary supplements. However, no valid scientific studies have shown that genetic tests can determine a person's nutritional needs. If you have a genetic predisposition to a disease that may be affected by nutrition or lifestyle, you might want to see a dietitian, who can teach you how to make smart dietary choices.

You should also be skeptical of claims that genetic tests can evaluate your ability to withstand the effects of certain environmental exposures such as pollution or cigarette smoke. No existing genetic tests can predict whether a person's genetic makeup can enable him or her to withstand specific environmental exposures. Additionally, the results of genetic tests are not always black and white, making interpretations and explanations difficult. In most cases, diseases occur as a result of the interaction between genes and environment—factors such as a person's diet, level of physical activity, smoking, and exposure to sunlight. The interaction between environmental factors and genes can be very complicated and science does not yet fully understand these issues.

For these reasons, genetic testing should be used only in settings in which a person has been given adequate counseling before the test is done (to make sure he or she understands the test and wants to be tested) and adequate counseling when the results are received. To make sure that any genetic information you get is accurate and correctly interpreted, you need to discuss it with your doctor and a genetic counselor.

- To screen embryos for disease (called preimplantation screening)
- To test for specific genetic diseases in adults with a family history before they have symptoms
- To confirm a diagnosis in a person who has symptoms of a particular disease

People have many different reasons for having a genetic test or choosing not to be tested. For example, if a disease gene is found by a test, it would be important to know whether the disease can be prevented or treated. For diseases for which there is no treatment, a person may not want to know the results of the test. On the other hand, test results might help a person make important life decisions, such as career choice, family planning, or the type of health insurance to get. A genetic counselor can give you information to help you evaluate the pros and cons of genetic testing in your situation.

GENETIC COUNSELING

If you've been diagnosed with a genetic disease or have been recommended for genetic testing, your doctor will probably refer you to a genetic counselor or medical geneticist. Genetic counselors are health professionals with specialized graduate degrees and experience in the areas of medical genetics and counseling. They often come from backgrounds such as biology, genetics, nursing, psychology, public health, and social work. Genetic counselors work with doctors to provide information, answer questions, and offer support to people with genetic disorders, those who are undergoing genetic testing, those who may be at risk for inheriting genetic disorders, or people who could have children with a genetic disorder. The genetic counselor conducts one-on-one counseling to help people understand genetic disorders and their testing and treatment options.

Genetic counselors generally work with a health-care team, providing information and support to people with birth defects or genetic disorders and to families who may be at risk for an inherited condition. They identify families at risk, interpret information about the disorder, analyze inheritance patterns and risks of recurrence, and review available options with the family. They also provide supportive counseling to families, serve as patient advocates, and refer people and their families to community or state support services. They serve as educators and resource people for other health-care professionals and for the general public.

PART TWO

Preventing
Health Problems

7

PREVENTING HEART ATTACKS AND STROKES

THE CARDIOVASCULAR SYSTEM, or circulatory system, consists of the heart and blood vessels (arteries and veins). The heart is a muscular pump about the size and shape of a fist. As the heart beats, it moves blood continuously around the body through the blood vessels. On average, the heart pumps more than a gallon of blood through the entire circulatory system every minute.

The arteries carry oxygen-rich blood from the left side of the heart to the rest of the body, including vital organs such as the brain, kidneys, and liver, as well as all of the other tissues. Veins carry oxygen-depleted blood back to the right side of the heart, which pumps it to the lungs. In the lungs, blood releases carbon dioxide to be exhaled, and picks up a fresh supply of oxygen. From the lungs, veins carry the blood back to the left side of the heart, where the cycle of circulation begins again.

Heart disease

If you're like most people, especially if you are a woman, you may think that you're not at risk for heart disease. But you very well could be. Heart disease is the No. 1 killer of both men and women in the United States. Nearly 700,000 Americans die of heart disease each year—about 29 percent of all U.S. deaths. When you add in stroke and other forms of vascular (blood vessel) disease, which all have common underlying risk factors, nearly 40 percent of all deaths occur as a result of all forms of cardiovascular disease. Even if you have no family history of heart disease, you could be at risk, especially if you are overweight, eat a diet high in saturated and trans fats, and are not physically active.

The good news is that heart disease is highly preventable, as long as you're willing to make some lifestyle changes—including following a heart-healthy diet, getting regular exercise, quitting smoking if you smoke, losing weight if you need to, and handling stress in a positive way. "Heart disease" is a term that includes several more specific heart and blood vessel conditions, including angina and heart attack. "Cardiovascular disease" is a term that encompasses heart disease, stroke, and peripheral artery disease.

Atherosclerosis

Atherosclerosis, one of the major causes of cardiovascular disease, is a process in which arteries become hardened and narrowed from the buildup of fatty deposits called plaque inside artery walls. Plaque is made up of cholesterol, fibrous tissue, calcium, and inflammatory cells. There are two types of plaque: hard and stable, and soft and unstable. Hard plaque causes artery walls to thicken and harden. Soft plaque is more likely to cause ruptures or splits in the inner lining of the artery walls, which can cause a blood clot to form abruptly, cutting off the blood supply to tissues downstream. When bloodflow to the heart muscle is reduced by hard or soft plaque, a person may feel chest pain called angina (see page 221). When an artery leading to the heart or brain is completely blocked, a heart attack or stroke can occur.

Atherosclerosis is a slow and complex disease that sometimes starts as early as childhood. In some people, atherosclerosis develops faster as they grow older. Scientists think that the buildup of plaque usually begins when the lining of an artery is damaged or injured. Injury can result from a number of factors, such as chemicals in cigarette smoke, high blood pressure, elevated levels of cholesterol or other blood lipids, diabetes, inflammation, or turbulence in a blood vessel at a point where it branches. LDL cholesterol (the "bad" cholesterol) can then gain entry into the wall of the damaged

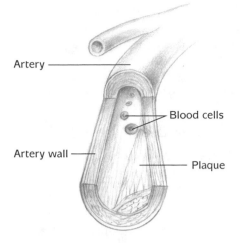

Atherosclerosis

Atherosclerosis is the buildup of fatty deposits called plaque inside artery walls. A buildup of plaque can reduce or block the flow of blood to tissues supplied by an artery.

Artery

Blood cells

Artery wall

Plaque

artery and trigger a cascade of processes that promote the development of plaque.

Inflammation appears to play an important role in altering cholesterol and promoting the process of atherosclerosis. Over time, atherosclerosis can damage and weaken the heart muscle by interfering with its blood supply, which can lead to heart failure (see page 230), a serious problem in which the heart is too weak to pump blood adequately. Atherosclerosis also contributes to poor circulation in the legs, stroke, and heart rhythm disorders.

Complications resulting from atherosclerosis are the leading cause of illness, disability, and death in the United States. Researchers estimate that at least half of adult men and 40 percent of women will have some form of atherosclerotic cardiovascular event during their lifetime. As plaque builds up, it can cause serious diseases and complications affecting the arteries leading to different parts of the body, including the following:

- Brain, causing a stroke
- Heart, causing a heart attack
- Kidneys, causing renovascular hypertension (high blood pressure caused by a narrowing of the arteries that supply blood to the kidneys) or kidney failure
- Arms and legs, causing peripheral artery disease (which restricts blood flow to the limbs, fingers, and toes)

RISK FACTORS

Scientists have identified a number of factors that are responsible for atherosclerosis, and hundreds of others that are clearly associated with an increased risk for atherosclerosis. Your chances of having atherosclerosis rise with the number of risk factors you have. You can control some of these risk factors, but not all of them. These are the risk factors you cannot control:

- **Age** As you get older, your heart disease risk increases.
  - In men, risk increases especially after age 45.
  - In women, risk increases especially after age 55.

- **Family history of early heart disease**   Your risk for atherosclerosis is greater if:
  - Your father or brother was diagnosed with heart disease before age 55.
  - Your mother or sister was diagnosed with heart disease before age 65.

Following are the risk factors you can do something about:

- **Unfavorable cholesterol profile**   An unfavorable cholesterol profile (see page 199), especially a level of LDL (bad) cholesterol over 100, promotes the buildup of fatty deposits, including cholesterol, in arteries. Low levels of HDL (good) cholesterol may also be an important indicator of risk, especially in people with a family history of early heart disease.
- **High blood pressure**   Uncontrolled high blood pressure (see page 235) promotes atherosclerosis by damaging artery walls and causing the arteries to "harden" more quickly. (Normal blood pressure is lower than 120/80.)
- **Smoking**   Smoking (including exposure to secondhand smoke) raises blood pressure, damages artery walls, and increases the risk for blood-clot formation.
- **Diabetes**   Diabetes (see chapter 8), or elevated blood sugar, appears to directly affect artery walls, and also promotes atherosclerosis by altering cholesterol levels.
- **Obesity**   Being overweight (see chapter 3) increases the risk for unfavorable cholesterol levels, high blood pressure, and type 2 diabetes—all of which promote atherosclerosis. Overweight and obesity also appear to promote inflammation in arteries.
- **Lack of physical activity**   Being physically inactive can increase the risk for weight gain and unfavorable cholesterol and blood pressure levels.
- **Excess alcohol**   Drinking excessively can lead to high blood pressure and can raise blood levels of triglycerides (a potentially harmful type of fat in the blood that can promote atherosclerosis).

PREVENTION

Preventing atherosclerosis and its potential consequences—including heart attack, stroke, and peripheral artery disease—starts by knowing your risk factors and taking action to lower the risk factors you can control. It is most important to prevent the development of risk factors in the first place, so atherosclerosis does not get a start in your arteries. But even if you already have one or more risk factors, it is never too late to try to improve them. With lifestyle changes and, perhaps, medication, you can prevent or significantly slow the progression of atherosclerosis.

Knowing your family history (see page 179) of the disorder is key. If you or someone in your family has heart disease, be sure to tell your doctor. Make sure everyone in your family is physically active (see chapter 2) and maintains a healthy body weight (see chapter 3). If you have any other medical conditions, carefully follow your doctor's recommendations for treating them. By staying as healthy as possible, you can lower your risk for atherosclerosis and heart disease, and prevent serious complications such as a heart attack.

Angina

Angina is chest discomfort or pain that occurs when the heart muscle is not getting enough blood. Symptoms of angina usually occur during exertion, because the blood supply may be insufficient to meet the extra demand placed on the heart to increase its pumping during exertion. Angina does not typically occur if the heart arteries are normal or only mildly narrowed.

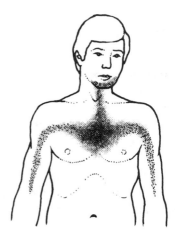

Location of angina pain

The pain or pressure of angina can be moderate to severe. It usually starts in the center of the chest and sometimes radiates to the left or right shoulder and then down the arm. Angina can also radiate to the throat, jaw, and lower teeth. Symptoms that accompany angina can include difficulty breathing, sweating, nausea, and dizziness.

Angina is a symptom of heart disease, which develops when fatty deposits called plaque build up in the walls of arteries leading to the heart, in a process called atherosclerosis (see page 218). Plaque buildup can cause angina in the following two ways: by rupturing and forming blood clots that partially or totally block an artery, or by narrowing an artery to the point at which blood flow to the heart is greatly reduced. More than 6 million people in the United States have angina.

Some people experience angina as the usual symptom of heavy pressure in the center or upper part of the chest. Others experience shoulder or arm discomfort, or just shortness of breath. Within the same person, episodes of angina tend to be similar. After a person has had several episodes of angina, he or she learns to recognize the pattern and signs. The symptom usually goes away in a few minutes (five minutes or less) after rest or after taking angina medication. Angina is not a heart attack, but makes it more likely that a heart attack will occur in the future. Angina symptoms that last longer than 10 or 20 minutes could be a sign of a heart attack, and are a reason to seek immediate medical attention.

Physical exertion is a common trigger of pain and discomfort from angina. Severely narrowed arteries may allow enough blood to reach the heart when the demand for oxygen is low (such as when you're sitting). But when you do something strenuous, like walking up a hill or climbing stairs, the heart works harder and needs more oxygen. Other factors that can trigger angina include the following:

- Emotional stress
- Exposure to very hot or cold temperatures
- A heavy meal
- Smoking

RISK FACTORS

The more of the following risk factors you have, the greater your chances of developing angina. These are the same risk factors that increase your risk for atherosclerosis and heart disease.

- Diabetes
- Family history of heart disease at a young age
- High blood pressure
- High LDL (bad) cholesterol and/or low HDL (good) cholesterol
- Being physically inactive
- Being overweight or obese
- Smoking

PREVENTION

The following preventive measures for angina are the same as those for heart disease in general:

- Stop smoking if you smoke.
- Lose weight if you're overweight.
- Control your blood pressure, blood sugar levels, and cholesterol levels.
- Consume a heart-healthy diet (see page 27).
- Get regular exercise.
- Eat oily fish (such as salmon or mackerel) at least twice a week, or ask your doctor if you should take fish oil supplements.
- If you already have angina, your doctor may tell you to take a nitroglycerin tablet a few minutes before any planned activity that might trigger angina pain.
- Remember to get a fresh batch of nitroglycerin at least every six months so it is fresh and will work when you need it.

WARNING

Chest pain

Chest pain that lasts longer than a few minutes and cannot be relieved by rest or by taking angina medication may indicate that you are having, or are about to have, a heart attack. If you have this kind of chest pain, sit down and call 911 or your local emergency medical number right away. Leave your phone off the hook so medical personnel can locate your address if you should become unconscious. If you have nitroglycerin tablets, take up to three pills one at a time every five minutes. If you have aspirin and are not allergic to it, chew and swallow a full-strength (325-milligram) tablet, or four baby-strength (81-milligram) tablets.

- Work with your doctor to make sure you are on appropriate doses of medications to prevent heart attack (such as aspirin and cholesterol-lowering medications), to control cholesterol and blood pressure, and to prevent angina and the underlying problem of blood supply to your heart (such as beta blocker medications or longer-acting forms of nitroglycerin).

Heart attack

Heart attack is the single leading killer of both men and women in the United States. Each year, more than 1.2 million Americans have a heart attack, and about a third of them die as a direct result. Even more people die as a result of the long-term consequences of heart attacks, such as heart failure and heart rhythm disorders. Most people could limit the damage and recover from a heart attack if they got treatment more quickly. Of people who die from a heart attack, about half die within an hour of the first symptoms and before they reach the hospital.

Heart attacks occur most often when a fatty substance called plaque builds up over many years in the walls of the arteries that supply blood and oxygen to the heart (atherosclerosis; see page 218). Eventually, an area of plaque can rupture, or split open the inner lining of the artery, causing a blood clot to form on the surface of the plaque. If the clot becomes large enough, it can completely block the flow of oxygen-rich blood to the part of the heart muscle fed by the artery. During a heart attack, if the blockage in the coronary artery is not treated quickly, the heart muscle will begin to die. Dead heart muscle will ultimately be replaced by scar tissue, which diminishes the pumping ability of the heart. This heart damage may not always be obvious, but it weakens the heart. In other cases, it can cause severe or long-lasting problems, including heart failure (see page 230) and life-threatening abnormal heart rhythms (see page 241).

A medical problem called microvascular disease can also cause a heart attack or angina. Microvascular disease affects the smallest arteries and often occurs in people

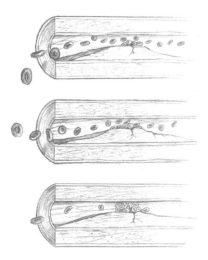

From plaque to blood clots

A buildup of plaque in an artery can cause blood clots to form. Cracks develop in the roughened surface of plaque (top). The body reacts as though the cracks are an injury and forms blood clots to seal them and promote healing (center). If a clot grows large enough (bottom), it can block blood flow in an artery to the heart (causing a heart attack) or an artery to the brain (causing a stroke).

who have had diabetes for a long time. Uncontrolled diabetes can damage the small arteries, including those leading to the heart. Microvascular disease, which appears to be a more common form of heart disease in women, can be difficult to diagnose but can have significantly harmful long-term consequences for the heart.

Another, less common cause of heart attack is a severe spasm (tightening) of an artery that cuts off blood flow to the heart. These spasms can occur even in arteries that don't have obvious plaque buildup. It's not fully clear what triggers a coronary artery spasm, but some possible factors include the following:

- Use of certain stimulant drugs such as cocaine
- Emotional stress or pain
- Exposure to extreme cold
- Cigarette smoking
- Undetected plaque

CPR AND AEDS CAN SAVE LIVES

Cardiopulmonary resuscitation (CPR) is a lifesaving technique that is performed to maintain a person's circulaton and breathing after they have stopped. The procedure involves keeping the person's airway open, doing chest compressions to pump blood through the heart, and giving rescue breaths. But newer guidelines suggest that a simpler technique may be just as effective. The chances of surviving cardiac arrest outside a hospital setting have been found to be twice as high if bystanders, even if they have not been trained, perform resuscitation with continual chest compressions without mouth-to-mouth breathing. The continual forceful compressions to the center of the chest, at a rate of 100 per minute, can keep the person's blood circulating until rescue personnel arrive. Ask your doctor, local hospital, or fire department about CPR classes in your community, or contact the local chapter of the American Red Cross or the American Heart Association. CPR training can mean the difference between life and death.

Many places where people gather (including airports, airplanes, shopping malls, theaters, and other public places) now have automated external defibrillators (AEDs). These machines can save the life of someone whose heart stops beating by delivering a jolt of electricity to the heart to restart it. The more quickly this jolt is delivered to a person in cardiac arrest, the more successful it is likely to be, and the more likely it is that the person will survive. If you take a CPR class and get certified, you will learn how to operate an AED. If you or a family member has significant heart disease or a history of prior cardiac arrest, you should talk with your doctor about the possibility of getting an AED for your home.

Save a life: Recognize the symptoms of a heart attack

Not all heart attacks begin with the kind of sudden, crushing pain you often hear about. The warning signs and symptoms of a heart attack are not the same for everyone. Some people don't have symptoms at all (this is called a silent heart attack). Sometimes the signs and symptoms of a heart attack occur suddenly, but warning signs and symptoms can develop hours, days, and even weeks before a heart attack occurs. If you have already had a heart attack, your symptoms may not be the same during another one, but they often are. The more signs and symptoms you have, the more likely it is that you are having a heart attack.

Know the warning signs of a heart attack so you can act quickly to get treatment for yourself or someone else. The sooner treatment is given, the less damage to the heart. Treatment is most effective when started within one hour of the onset of symptoms, so acting fast at the first sign of a heart attack can save a life and limit damage to the heart. Following are the most common heart attack signs and symptoms:

- Chest discomfort or pain—uncomfortable pressure, squeezing, fullness, tightness, or pain in the center of the chest that can be mild or strong. The discomfort or pain lasts more than a few minutes or goes away and comes back. Heart attack pain can sometimes feel like indigestion or heartburn.

- Angina pain that doesn't go away with medication or rest or that changes from its usual pattern (occurs more frequently or occurs at rest). Unusual angina can be a sign of the beginning of a heart attack and requires emergency medical evaluation and, if necessary, immediate treatment.

- Upper body discomfort in one or both arms, the back, the neck, the jaw, or the stomach.

- Shortness of breath during or before chest pain or discomfort.

- Nausea, vomiting, lightheadedness or fainting, or breaking out in a cold sweat.

RISK FACTORS

Some risk factors for heart attack can be controlled, while others cannot. Major controllable risk factors for heart attack include the following:

- Smoking
- High blood pressure
- Unfavorable blood cholesterol (including high LDL cholesterol and triglyceride levels, and low HDL cholesterol levels)
- Being overweight or obese
- Eating a lot of saturated and trans fats
- Being physically inactive
- Having diabetes
- Having uncontrolled stress

HAVE A HEART ATTACK EMERGENCY ACTION PLAN

Make sure that you have an emergency action plan in case you or someone you are with has a heart attack, especially if you are at high risk or have already had a heart attack. It is critical to get treatment immediately; even a short delay can mean the difference between life and death. Make the following steps part of your plan so you can act fast if you think you or someone else is having a heart attack:

- Call 911 or your local emergency number to get medical help immediately. Don't wait more than five minutes to call for help.
- Chew and swallow an aspirin tablet (after calling 911). Aspirin helps dissolve blood clots and prevent new clots from forming.
- Sit down and take a nitroglycerin pill if your doctor has prescribed this type of medication.

If you are with a person who is having a heart attack and he or she loses consciousness, use a portable defibrillator (see previous page), if one is available, to restart the person's heart. Or perform cardiopulmonary resuscitation (CPR) if you have been trained in the lifesaving technique. These techniques can prevent brain damage or death if the heart stops beating before emergency medical help arrives.

If your symptoms stop completely in less than five minutes, you should still call your doctor to report the episode and ask for further instructions.

Risk factors that cannot be controlled include the following:

- **Age** Risk increases for men especially after age 45 and for women especially after age 55 (or after menopause).

- **Family history of early heart attack** Your risk is increased if your father or a brother had a first heart attack before age 55, or if your mother or a sister had a first heart attack before age 65. For unknown reasons, the risk may be higher if your mother has had a heart attack at an early age than if your father has.

In early to middle adulthood—ages 21 to 55 years—women, especially white women, seem to be more protected from heart disease than men the same age, but this difference narrows

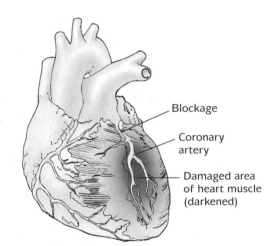

Blockage

Coronary artery

Damaged area of heart muscle (darkened)

Heart attack

A heart attack occurs when an artery leading to the heart becomes blocked by accumulated plaque or a blood clot, depriving part of the heart muscle of blood. Once an artery has been blocked, damage to the heart occurs quickly and can become permanent within minutes. The longer the blockage lasts, the more extensive the damage to the heart muscle is likely to be.

in later years. Significant numbers of men begin to have—and die from—heart attacks at an average age of about 45, while women begin about 10 years later. Of course, people with a family history of heart disease or who have diabetes or very elevated cholesterol levels may have heart attacks at much younger ages (even in their 20s), especially if they also smoke.

Researchers have discovered that approximately 90 percent of people who have a heart attack had at least one unfavorable or notably elevated risk factor that was identifiable prior to their heart attack. This illustrates the importance of seeing your doctor and being screened regularly for risk factors. However, the well-known risk factors don't explain all heart attacks. Talk with your doctor about whether it might be appropriate to consider measuring some newly discovered risk indicators for heart attack.

PREVENTION

Preventing, lowering, or eliminating your controllable risk factors for heart disease can help you prevent a heart attack. Even if you already have heart disease, you can take steps to lower your risk of having a heart attack by making healthy lifestyle choices. You may also need to have treatment for medical conditions that raise your heart attack risk. Adopting the following heart-healthy lifestyle habits can help you avoid a heart attack by reducing plaque buildup in the arteries, lowering blood pressure, improving blood cholesterol levels, and controlling blood sugar levels. The bottom line for lifestyle: Eat less, eat smart, and move more every day.

- **Consume a heart-healthy diet.** Follow a diet that is low in saturated and trans fats and salt, and rich in fruits, vegetables, whole grains, good fats (such as olive oil and fish oil), and fiber (see page 27).

- **Lose weight if you are overweight.** Being overweight increases your chances of having an unfavorable cholesterol profile, high blood pressure, and type 2 diabetes, all of which raise heart attack risk. At a minimum, don't gain any more weight. Try to focus especially on decreasing portion sizes and lowering the amount of calories you consume every day.

- **Quit smoking.** Smoking, and exposure to secondhand smoke, raise blood pressure, damage artery walls, and promote blood clot formation.

- **Get regular exercise.** Physical activity improves heart fitness and endurance. Ask your doctor how much and what kinds of physical activity would be most beneficial for you. Do something active every day—ideally for at least one hour.

- **Eat fatty fish twice a week.** The omega-3 fatty acids in fatty fish such as salmon and mackerel can reduce the risk for heart attack and blood vessel disease and lower the risk for death from heart disease. Ask your doctor about taking fish oil supplements if you don't eat fish regularly.

- **Manage your stress.** The amount of stress your body can take without health consequences is, in part, genetically influenced. But you can change your response to stressful situations by learning new ways to cope, such as relaxation techniques (see page 122) like yoga, breathing exercises, biofeedback, and meditation; and by being more physically active.

- **Take an aspirin every day.** If your doctor recommends it, taking a daily aspirin tablet can help lower your risk of having a heart attack by helping to prevent the formation of blood clots. Aspirin also fights inflammation, which may contribute to heart disease. However, because aspirin's blood-thinning effects can also elevate the risk for hemorrhagic stroke (bleeding inside the brain) and peptic ulcers (see page 341), do not start taking aspirin without talking to your doctor about it first.

- **Avoid taking hormone replacement therapy.** Hormone replacement therapy (HRT; see page 520) relieves the symptoms of menopause, but it also may slightly increase a woman's risk for heart disease and breast cancer. If you are having severe symptoms from menopause, you may want to consider HRT, but you should not use it to reduce your risk for heart disease.

In addition to making lifestyle changes, you can reduce your risk of having a heart attack by treating medical conditions that can make a heart attack more likely, including the following:

- **High blood cholesterol levels**   You may need to take a cholesterol-lowering medication such as a statin to improve your cholesterol profile (see page 200) if you have not been able to improve it with diet, exercise, and weight loss.

- **High triglyceride levels**   Like cholesterol, triglycerides (another fatty substance in the blood) also raise heart disease risk, especially in women. You can reduce them with a diet low in saturated and trans fats and carbohydrates, and by limiting alcohol.

- **High blood pressure** Know your blood pressure level (see page 235). If you need medication to control it, make sure you take it. Limit your salt intake and lose weight if you are overweight.

- **Diabetes** If you have diabetes, carefully control your blood sugar levels through diet and physical activity, as your doctor recommends. Also, if you have diabetes it is very important to control your blood pressure and cholesterol. If you need medication, take it exactly as prescribed.

Heart failure

Heart failure, also known as congestive heart failure, is a common but serious condition in which the heart is too weak to pump sufficient blood through the body. About 5 million people in the United States have heart failure, and the number is growing. Each year, about 550,000 people are diagnosed with heart failure for the first time. The condition contributes to or causes about 300,000 deaths each year. The lifetime risk of developing heart failure is at least one in five for adult men and women.

Despite how it sounds, heart failure does not mean that the heart has stopped or is about to stop working. It means that it cannot pump blood the way it should: it cannot properly fill with enough blood or pump with enough force, or both. Heart failure develops over time as the pumping action of the heart grows weaker. It can affect the left side, the right side, or both sides of the heart. Most cases affect the left side, making the heart unable to pump enough oxygen-rich blood to the rest of the body. In a person with right-sided heart failure, the heart cannot effectively pump blood to the lungs (which nourish the blood with oxygen). This weakening of the heart's pumping ability may result in any or all of the following problems:

- Blood and fluid back up into the lungs.
- Fluid builds up in the feet, ankles, and legs.
- The person becomes tired and short of breath.

Heart failure is always caused by other diseases or conditions that damage or overwork the heart muscle over a period of time. High blood pressure (see page 235) and coronary artery atherosclerosis (plaque buildup in arteries that can lead to heart attack; see page 218) are the most common underlying causes of heart failure. People who have had a heart attack are at especially high risk of developing heart failure. Other conditions that can lead to heart failure include the following:

- Cardiomyopathy (a disease in which the heart muscle becomes enlarged or abnormally thick or rigid). In rare cases, the muscle tissue in the heart is replaced with scar tissue.
- Diseases of the heart valves (leaky or tight valves)
- Influenza or other severe infections
- Abnormal heartbeats or arrhythmias
- Congenital heart defects (developmental heart defects that are present at birth)
- Treatments for cancer (such as radiation and some chemotherapy drugs)
- Thyroid disorders (having either too much or too little thyroid hormone in the body)
- Alcohol abuse
- Having HIV/AIDS
- Use of stimulant drugs such as cocaine

Most forms of heart failure cannot be cured, and people with heart failure usually need to take medication for the rest of their life. The symptoms may get worse over time and a person may not be able to do many of the things he or she did before having heart failure. Still, heart failure is treatable with a low-salt, heart-healthy diet (such as the DASH eating plan; see page 27) and appropriate medications.

RISK FACTORS

Anyone can develop heart failure, but it is more common in people 65 years of age and older and in African Americans. Men have a higher rate of heart failure than women, but in actual numbers, more women have heart failure because many more women live into their 70s and 80s, when heart failure is most common. Children with congenital (present at birth) heart defects are at increased risk for heart failure because some of these problems can weaken the heart muscle.

PREVENTION

The major underlying causes of heart failure are heart disease, high blood pressure, and diabetes. Getting treatment for these conditions can greatly reduce the risk for heart failure. Other steps you can take to reduce your risk are the following:

- Eat a heart healthy diet that's low in salt, saturated fat, and cholesterol.
- Quit smoking if you smoke.
- Lose weight if you're overweight.
- Control your diabetes.

Peripheral artery disease

Peripheral artery disease (PAD) occurs when a hardened fatty buildup called plaque accumulates on the inside walls of the arteries that carry blood from the heart to the limbs, most commonly the legs. The buildup of plaque in artery walls is called atherosclerosis (see page 218), which can cause the arteries to narrow or become blocked by a blood clot. Reduced blood flow can cause pain and numbness in the arms or legs, increase the risk for infections in the limbs, and make it difficult for the body to fight the infections. A severe blockage can prevent the legs and feet from getting sufficient oxygen and nutrition for cell growth and repair, causing painful leg or foot sores. In the advanced stages, blood flow to one or both legs can be completely blocked, causing the tissue to die (gangrene). In this case, the foot or leg may need to be amputated. PAD is the leading cause of amputation.

PAD is common. The disorder affects 8 to 12 million people in the United States—an estimated 5 percent of Americans over age 50. Men are more likely to have symptoms of PAD, but both men and women can develop the disorder. PAD can affect general health and limit a person's ability to walk. A person with PAD has a six to seven times greater-than-normal risk of having a heart attack, stroke, or transient ischemic attack (TIA; see page 241). If a person already has heart disease, he or she has a one in three chance of having narrowed or blocked arteries in the legs.

Early diagnosis and treatment of PAD are essential for preventing disability and saving lives. PAD can be successfully treated. The buildup of plaque in the arteries can often be stopped or reversed by quitting smoking, making dietary changes, being more physically active, losing weight, and improving blood cholesterol and blood pressure levels. In some people, blood flow in the vessels in the limbs can be improved with medication or surgery.

RISK FACTORS

Major risk factors for developing PAD include the following:

- **Smoking**   Smoking is more closely linked to the development of PAD than any other risk factor, raising the risk three to five times. Smoking harms the blood vessels in a number of ways. The nicotine and carbon monoxide in tobacco smoke make the heart work harder, increase heart rate, raise blood pressure, and narrow blood vessels. Smoking damages cells in the walls of blood vessels, making it easier for harmful fats and other blood components to build up in the arteries. Long-term smoking also boosts total blood cholesterol and lowers good HDL cholesterol. On average, smokers who develop PAD experience symptoms 10 years earlier than nonsmokers who develop the disorder. Quitting smoking slows the progression of PAD. Smoking as few as one or two cigarettes a day can interfere with treatment for the condition. Smokers have a high risk for complications from the disorder, including gangrene (tissue death) in the leg, caused by decreased blood flow.

- **Diabetes**   One in three people over the age of 50 who have diabetes is likely to have PAD. If you are over 50 and have diabetes, ask your doctor about being tested for PAD. Like smokers, people with diabetes have a high risk for complications from the disorder, including gangrene (tissue death) in the leg, caused by decreased blood flow.

- **Age**   Men over age 50 and women over age 55 are at increased risk for PAD.

- **Other conditions**   Several other underlying conditions or disorders that affect the blood vessels, including the following, can also increase the risk for PAD.
  - Kidney disease
  - High blood pressure or a family history of hypertension

○ Unfavorable cholesterol profile or a family history of abnormal cholesterol levels

○ Heart disease or a family history of heart disease

○ Stroke or a family history of stroke

PREVENTION

You can prevent PAD by taking the following steps:

- **Quit smoking.** If you smoke, this is the most important step you can take.

- **Control your blood pressure, cholesterol, and blood sugar levels.** This includes eating right and exercising regularly. Talk with your doctor about beginning a supervised exercise therapy program, and whether you need medication.

WHAT IS AN ANEURYSM?

An aneurysm is an abnormal bulge or ballooning in the wall of an artery (a blood vessel that carries oxygen-rich blood from the heart to other parts of the body). An aneurysm that grows large enough can burst, causing dangerous, often fatal, bleeding inside the body.

Most aneurysms develop in the aorta, the main artery from the heart to the rest of the body. An aneurysm that occurs in the aorta in the abdomen is called an abdominal aortic aneurysm. But aneurysms can also occur in arteries in the brain, heart, intestines, neck, spleen, back of the knees and thighs, and other parts of the body. If an aneurysm in the brain bursts, it causes a stroke.

About 15,000 Americans die each year from a ruptured aortic aneurysm. It is the 10th leading cause of death in men over age 50 in the United States. Many cases of ruptured aneurysms could be prevented with early diagnosis and timely treatment. Because

aneurysms can develop and grow large before they cause any symptoms, it is important to look for them in people who are at risk. Experts recommend that men ages 65 to 75 who have ever smoked (at least 100 cigarettes in their lifetime) should be checked for abdominal aortic aneurysms with a simple ultrasound test.

The best way to prevent an aneurysm is to avoid the risk factors that increase your chances of developing one. Take these steps:

- Quit smoking if you smoke.

- Eat a heart-healthy diet to reduce the buildup of plaque in the arteries.

- Control your blood pressure (eating a low-salt diet helps; see pages 27 and 36).

- Get treatment for unfavorable cholesterol levels.

- Be physically active every day—for at least 30 minutes to an hour.

PREVENTING BACTERIAL ENDOCARDITIS

Bacterial endocarditis is an infection that affects the inner lining of the heart or the heart valves. The infection, which can severely damage the heart valves, develops when bacteria in the bloodstream settle on malformed heart valves or other heart tissue that has become damaged. The disorder most often occurs in people who have had bacterial endocarditis before, who have a congenital (present at birth) heart defect, who have had a heart valve replaced, or who have had a heart transplant and developed heart-valve abnormalities. Although bacterial endocarditis is more likely to occur after exposure to bacteria during routine daily activities, it can, in rare cases, result after dental procedures. For this reason, dentists have routinely recommended that people who are at increased risk for endocarditis take antibiotics preventively before having some dental procedures. If you have any of the heart conditions mentioned previously, you probably will need to take antibiotics prior to having any dental work, including routine cleanings.

However, people with other types of heart conditions (such as mitral valve prolapse) do not appear to benefit from routine antibiotics prior to dental work, and they are no longer recommended for them. The recommendation changed when leading experts in heart medicine and infectious diseases, after reviewing numerous published studies about bacterial endocarditis, concluded that no convincing evidence exists to prove that dental procedures actually cause endocarditis.

If you have any heart damage from rheumatic fever or any other condition, you should still tell your dentist about it before you have any dental procedures, including routine cleanings. Your dentist will determine whether you need preventive antibiotics before these procedures.

- **Maintain a healthy weight.** If you are overweight, work with your doctor to develop a sensible weight-loss plan.
- **Eat a heart-healthy diet.** Consume foods that are low in saturated and trans fats and cholesterol. Reduce your intake of salt. Eat more plant foods: fruits, vegetables, beans, nuts, and whole grains.

High blood pressure

Blood pressure is the force of the blood pushing against the walls of the arteries. Each time the heart beats (about 60 to 90 times a minute at rest), it pumps blood out into the arteries. Blood pressure is at its highest when the heart beats; this is called systolic pressure. When the heart is at rest, between beats, blood pressure falls; this is called diastolic pressure. A

✓ **Control your blood pressure**

If you have been diagnosed with high blood pressure, it's essential to get your blood pressure down to a healthy level and keep it there to avoid the life-threatening complications of uncontrolled high blood pressure. Most people who are prescribed medication for high blood pressure will need to take it for the rest of their life, and most people require more than one medication to control it. Make sure you take any blood pressure medication exactly as prescribed, and every day. Doing so could save your life.

blood pressure reading is given as two numbers—the systolic and diastolic pressures—such as 120/80 (120 over 80). Systolic pressure is the first number; diastolic pressure is the second number.

Blood pressure changes during the day. It is lowest when you sleep and highest shortly after you wake up. It can also increase when you become excited, nervous, or active. But for most of the time you are awake, your blood pressure stays pretty much the same whether you're sitting or standing still. Normal blood pressure is lower than 120/80. In general, lower is better, but very low blood pressure can sometimes be a cause for concern and should be checked by a doctor.

When blood pressure stays high—140/90 or higher in either the top or bottom number—you have high blood pressure. High blood pressure makes the heart work harder and can damage the blood vessels and other tissues, increasing the risk for stroke, heart attack, and kidney problems. About 65 million American adults—nearly one in three—have high blood pressure. Many people do not know they have it because it does not cause symptoms, even as it is damaging tissues. Once high blood pressure develops, it usually lasts a lifetime. The good news is that it can be treated and controlled.

BLOOD PRESSURE CLASSIFICATIONS FOR PEOPLE 18 AND OLDER

A diagnosis of high blood pressure, or hypertension, is based on two or more blood pressure readings taken at separate visits to the doctor or a clinic. If your systolic pressure (the first number) falls into one category and your diastolic pressure (the second number) falls into another, the higher reading is used to classify your blood pressure. Doctors classify blood pressure in the following way:

Category	Systolic pressure	Diastolic pressure
Normal blood pressure	Lower than 120	Lower than 80
Prehypertension	120 to 139	80 to 89
Stage 1 hypertension	140 to 159	90 to 99
Stage 2 hypertension	160 or higher	100 or higher

In most people with high blood pressure, a single specific cause is never found; this is called essential or primary high blood pressure. Researchers are trying to find the causes of essential high blood pressure. In some people, high blood pressure results from an underlying medical problem or a medication a person is taking. When the cause of high blood pressure is known, doctors call it secondary high blood pressure.

RISK FACTORS

Although the cause of high blood pressure is usually unknown, the following factors can increase your risk or worsen existing high blood pressure:

- Family history of high blood pressure (especially in a parent or sibling)
- Being African American (Blacks tend to develop high blood pressure earlier in life than whites and usually have more severe high blood pressure.)
- Being older (More than half of all Americans age 60 and older have high blood pressure.)
- Being overweight
- Having prehypertension (blood pressure in the 120–139/80–89 range)

The following lifestyle issues can also raise blood pressure:

- Smoking (smoking can also cause a temporary rise in blood pressure)
- Eating too much salt
- Drinking more than two alcoholic drinks per day
- Not getting enough of the mineral potassium in the diet
- Not being physically active
- Having long-term stress

PREVENTION

You can significantly reduce your risk for high blood pressure by doing the following:

- Maintain a healthy weight (see chapter 3).
- Become more physically active (see chapter 2).
- Follow a healthy eating plan such as the DASH diet (see page 27), which emphasizes fruits, vegetables, and low-fat dairy foods, and minimizes salt.

- Choose and prepare foods with less salt and sodium. (Read package labels for sodium content.)
- Quit smoking if you smoke (see page 125).
- Drink alcohol only in moderation if you drink at all (fewer than two drinks a day for men and one drink a day for women).

Stroke

A stroke occurs when the blood supply to part of the brain is suddenly interrupted or when a blood vessel in the brain bursts, spilling blood into the spaces between brain cells. Brain cells die when they no longer receive oxygen and nutrients from the blood or when sudden bleeding occurs in the brain. Stroke is the third leading cause of death in the United States and is a major cause of serious, long-term disability in adults. About 600,000 strokes are reported in the United States each year. Strokes often recur—one in four people who recovers from a first stroke will have another stroke within five years.

There are two major kinds of stroke. The first, called an ischemic stroke, is caused by a blood clot that blocks a blood vessel or artery in the brain, cutting off the supply of blood to an area of the brain. About 80 percent of all strokes are ischemic strokes. The second type, called hemorrhagic stroke, is caused by a blood vessel in the brain that breaks and bleeds into the brain. About 20 percent of strokes are hemorrhagic strokes.

The good news is that treatments are available that can greatly reduce the damage caused by a stroke. The window of opportunity to minimize damage from a stroke through treatment is within three hours of the onset of symptoms. However, because it takes time for emergency personnel to evaluate a stroke and begin treatment, you need to get to the hospital within 60 minutes of the first signs of a stroke for treatment to be most effective. For these reasons, it is crucial to be able to recognize the symptoms of a stroke and get to a hospital quickly.

RISK FACTORS

High blood pressure (see page 235) is the single most important risk factor for stroke. High blood pressure is sometimes called the silent killer because it usually has no noticeable symptoms until other serious problems, such as a stroke, occur. Many people are not aware that they have high blood

Know the symptoms of a stroke

Prompt treatment for a stroke can be lifesaving and can significantly reduce the paralysis and loss of function that often result from a stroke and improve the chances of recovery. The earlier that treatment is given, the better the outcome. Consider a mild stroke a warning signal of more serious strokes to come. Become familiar with the following symptoms of a stroke so you can get immediate help for yourself or a loved one. These symptoms, when caused by a stroke, occur suddenly and may be accompanied by drowsiness or nausea and vomiting (especially if there is bleeding in the brain). If you recognize these symptoms, call 911 or your local emergency number immediately:

- Sudden numbness or weakness on one side of the body—especially in the face or in an arm or a leg
- Sudden severe headache (probably the worst you have ever had)
- Sudden confusion or trouble speaking or understanding speech
- Sudden vision problems such as dimness or blurred vision in one or both eyes
- Abrupt difficulty walking, dizziness, or loss of balance or coordination

Here's an easy test to help you quickly determine if someone is having a stroke. If the person cannot do the following things appropriately, call 911 or your local emergency number immediately.

1. Ask the person to smile.
   - Normal response: Both sides of the face move equally.
   - Possible sign of a stroke: One side of the face does not move (looks like it is drooping).

2. Ask the person to close his or her eyes and hold both arms out straight for 10 seconds.
   - Normal response: Both arms move equally or are held in a steady position.
   - Possible sign of a stroke: One arm cannot move or drifts down, or the person loses his or her balance.

3. Ask the person to say a common phrase like "Dogs are our friends."
   - Normal response: The person says the correct words with no slurring.
   - Possible sign of a stroke: The person slurs the words, says the wrong words, or cannot speak at all.

Note: Even if the person has normal responses to all of these, he or she could still be having a stroke. Call 911 or your doctor immediately if you are concerned.

pressure. Have your blood pressure checked at least once a year. If your blood pressure is high, it can be controlled with diet, exercise, and medication. The most important treatable conditions linked to stroke are the following:

- **High blood pressure** Eat a low-salt, heart-healthy diet (see the DASH eating plan, page 27); maintain a healthy weight; and exercise to reduce blood pressure. Your doctor may have to prescribe medication if lifestyle changes don't bring your blood pressure down into the normal range.

- **Cigarette smoking** Quit now if you smoke (see page 135). Talk to your doctor about a smoking-cessation program.

- **Heart disease** If you have heart disease, your doctor will treat it and may prescribe medication to help prevent the formation of blood clots, which could obstruct an artery leading to the brain and cause a stroke. An abnormal heart rhythm called atrial fibrillation is also a major risk factor for stroke. If you're over 50, your doctor may recommend taking an aspirin tablet daily.

- **Diabetes** Keeping your blood sugar levels in the normal range can prevent complications that increase the risk for stroke.

- **Transient ischemic attacks** Usually referred to as TIAs (see box on next page), these are small strokes that last for only seconds or a few minutes. They should never be ignored and can be a warning that a stroke is likely to occur.

PREVENTION

Prevention is the best course when it comes to stroke. Have your blood pressure checked regularly. If you already have high blood pressure, follow your doctor's instructions for bringing it down into the normal range. If you have heart disease, diabetes, or unfavorable cholesterol levels, get them under control—and keep them under control—

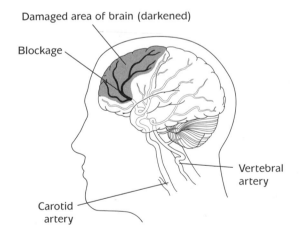

Damaged area of brain (darkened)

Blockage

Vertebral artery

Carotid artery

How a stroke occurs

A stroke occurs when a blood vessel in the brain becomes obstructed, cutting off the blood supply to that part of the brain. Blockage of blood flow to one side of the brain usually produces symptoms, such as numbness or paralysis, on the opposite side of the body.

A transient ischemic attack (TIA) involves a short-lived symptoms of a stroke, often called a mini-stroke, which lasts only a few minutes (usually from 2 to 15 minutes). TIAs occur when the blood supply to part of the brain is briefly interrupted. TIA symptoms occur suddenly and are similar to those of a stroke but don't last as long. Most symptoms of TIAs disappear within an hour, although they may persist for up to 24 hours. TIA symptoms can include the following:

- Numbness or weakness in the face, arm, or leg, especially on one side of the body
- Confusion or difficulty talking or understanding speech
- Difficulty seeing in one or both eyes
- Trouble walking, dizziness, or loss of balance and coordination

If the symptoms last longer than 24 hours, it is considered a stroke. People can have recurring TIAs, and the symptoms may be the same or different, depending on which area of the brain is affected. However, because there is no way to tell whether your symptoms are from a TIA or a full-fledged stroke, you should assume that any stroke-like symptoms signal a medical emergency. Don't wait to see if the symptoms go away. TIAs are warning signs of a risk for a more serious and debilitating stroke.

About one third of people who have a TIA will have a stroke at some time, usually within five years. Many strokes can be prevented by recognizing the warning signs of TIAs and getting a prompt evaluation (performed within 60 minutes of the initial symptoms) and treatment. The most important treatable factors linked to TIAs and stroke are high blood pressure, cigarette smoking, heart disease, atherosclerosis, diabetes, and heavy drinking. You can take steps to eliminate these risk factors. Lifestyle changes such as eating a low-salt diet that's also low in saturated and trans fats, maintaining a healthy weight, exercising, and enrolling in a smoking-cessation program or alcohol-abuse program help reduce your risk for TIAs or stroke.

and you will greatly reduce your chances of having a stroke. If you smoke, quit now.

Heart rhythm disorders

Arrhythmia is a problem with the speed or rhythm of the heartbeat. During an arrhythmia, the heart can beat too fast, too slow, or with an irregular rhythm. A heartbeat that is too fast is called tachycardia. A heartbeat that is too slow is called bradycardia.

The heart has an internal electrical system that controls the speed and rhythm of the heartbeat. With each heartbeat, an electrical signal spreads from the top of the heart to the bottom. As it travels, the electrical signal causes the heart to contract and pump blood. The process repeats with each heartbeat. An arrhythmia occurs when the normal electrical signals that control the heartbeat are delayed or blocked, or overridden by abnormal signals. This can occur when the special nerve cells that produce the heart's electrical signal don't work properly or when the electrical signal doesn't travel normally through the heart. An arrhythmia can also develop when another part of the heart starts to produce electrical signals, adding to the normal signals and disrupting the normal heartbeat.

Most arrhythmias are harmless, but some can be serious or even life-threatening. When the heart rate is too slow, too fast, or irregular, the heart may not be able to pump enough blood to the body. Lack of blood flow can damage the brain, heart, and other organs. One of the most common arrhythmias is atrial fibrillation, characterized by rapid and random heartbeats. This disorganized beating can lead to stagnation of blood in the upper chambers of the heart (atria), formation of blood clots, and strokes or other emergencies (if the blood clots break off and travel to other tissues).

Millions of Americans have arrhythmias. They are especially common in adults over age 60 because older adults are more likely to have heart disease and other health problems that can lead to arrhythmias. Older people also tend to be more sensitive to the side effects of medications, some of which can cause arrhythmias. In fact, even some medications that are used to treat arrhythmias can cause them as a side effect.

Smoking, heavy alcohol use, severe stress, vigorous exercise, use of some stimulant drugs (such as cocaine or amphetamines), use of some prescription or over-the-counter medications, consuming lots of caffeine, or smoking can trigger arrhythmias in some people. A heart attack or any condition that damages the heart's electrical system—including high blood pressure, heart failure, an overactive or underactive thyroid gland (that produces too much or too little thyroid hormone), and rheumatic heart disease—can also cause arrhythmias. For some arrhythmias, such as Wolff-Parkinson-White syndrome, the underlying heart defect that causes the arrhythmia is present at birth (congenital). Sometimes the cause of arrhythmias cannot be found.

RISK FACTORS

Arrhythmias are more common in people who have a disorder or condition that weakens the heart, such as the following:

- Heart attack

- Heart failure or cardiomyopathy (which weakens the heart and changes the way electrical signals move around it)
- Heart tissue that is too thick or stiff, or that hasn't formed normally
- Leaking or narrowed heart valves (which make the heart work too hard and can lead to heart failure)
- Congenital problems with the heart's structure or function

Other conditions, including the following, also can increase the chances of having an arrhythmia:

- High blood pressure
- Infections that damage the heart muscle or the sac around the heart
- Diabetes (which increases the risk for high blood pressure and heart disease)
- Sleep apnea (when breathing becomes too shallow or stops during sleep; see page 110), which can stress the heart
- An overactive or underactive thyroid gland (producing too much or too little thyroid hormone in the body)
- Anxiety

These other risk factors also can increase a person's chances of having an arrhythmia:

- Having heart surgery
- Taking some stimulant drugs (such as cocaine or amphetamines)
- Having an imbalance of chemicals or other substances (such as potassium) in the bloodstream
- Consuming excessive amounts of coffee or other caffeine-containing foods or drinks

PREVENTION

To prevent arrhythmias, follow these guidelines:

- Limit your consumption of coffee and other caffeine-containing foods and drinks.
- Avoid stimulants (such as amphetamines or cocaine).
- Avoid alcohol, especially binge drinking (having more than five drinks in a row).

- Keep your medical appointments. It's a good idea to bring all your medications with you in a plastic bag to your doctor visits to ensure that all of your doctors know exactly what medications you are taking, which can help prevent medication errors.
- Follow your doctor's instructions for taking medications. And check with your doctor before taking any over-the-counter medications, nutritional supplements, or cold and allergy medications.
- Tell your doctor right away if you are having side effects from any medications. These side effects can often be treated.
- Tell your doctor if your arrhythmia symptoms are getting worse or if you have any new symptoms.
- Let your doctor monitor you regularly if you are taking a blood-thinning medication.

Many arrhythmias are caused by underlying heart disease. Keep your heart healthy by consuming a healthy diet, getting regular physical activity, quitting smoking, maintaining a healthy weight, and keeping your blood cholesterol and blood pressure at healthy levels. Your doctor may recommend avoiding certain things that could make your heart beat too fast, including alcohol, caffeinated coffee, and some cold and cough medications.

You might ask your doctor about learning how to do vagal maneuvers, which are exercises that people with some arrhythmias perform to help stop an episode of rapid heartbeat. Talk with your doctor about what pulse rate is normal for you, and learn how to take your pulse. Keep a record of changes in your pulse rate and share this information with your doctor.

8

AVOIDING TYPE 2 DIABETES

TYPE 2 DIABETES has become an epidemic in many parts of the world. Once known as adult-onset diabetes, type 2 diabetes previously occurred almost exclusively in people over age 40 who were overweight. But now, doctors are seeing more people develop type 2 diabetes at younger ages because of the increasing prevalence of obesity, which often begins in childhood. More than 19 million people in the United States have type 2 diabetes; and an additional 13 million people have prediabetes, a condition that puts them at high risk of developing type 2 diabetes.

Type 2 diabetes is different from type 1 diabetes, which was previously known as juvenile onset diabetes. In type 1 diabetes, the pancreas loses its ability to produce the hormone insulin because the body's immune system has mistakenly attacked and destroyed the specialized pancreas cells that produce insulin. People with type 1 diabetes require insulin replacement to stay alive. People with type 2 diabetes often have very elevated levels of insulin, but their muscle and fat cells become less sensitive to its effects.

In many cases, type 2 diabetes can be prevented, mainly by eating a healthy diet, getting regular physical activity, and maintaining a healthy weight. For people who are overweight, losing just 5 to 7 percent of their weight and keeping it off can cut their diabetes risk in half.

When uncontrolled, diabetes can cause serious long-term complications such as heart disease, nerve damage, kidney failure, blindness, and limb amputation. Many people with type 2 diabetes can control their blood sugar and avoid complications with diet, exercise, and weight loss, but some need to take glucose-lowering medications or insulin injections.

RISK FACTORS

Some risk factors, such as an inherited susceptibility to type 2 diabetes, cannot be changed. If you have a close relative (parent or sibling) with type 2 diabetes, you are at substantially increased risk for type 2 diabetes. It is especially important for you to control the risk factors for diabetes that are modifiable, usually through healthy lifestyle habits. The following factors can put you at risk for type 2 diabetes:

- Being overweight
- Being older than 45
- Having a close relative (parent, brother, or sister) with type 2 diabetes
- Being of Native American, African American, Hispanic, Asian, Pacific Islander, or Native Alaskan descent
- Eating an unhealthy diet (including too many fast foods, saturated and trans fats, added sugars, and salt)
- Being physically inactive
- Smoking (which reduces the body's ability to use insulin)
- Excess stress (which may affect levels of blood glucose and insulin)
- Lack of sleep (which may promote weight gain and interfere with the way the body uses glucose)
- Having impaired fasting glucose or impaired glucose tolerance (characterized by glucose levels that are above normal but below the level required for a diagnosis of type 2 diabetes)
- Having gestational diabetes during a pregnancy
- Having polycystic ovarian syndrome (a disorder in females characterized by increased levels of male hormones and insulin)

WHAT CAUSES TYPE 2 DIABETES?

Being overweight is a major cause of type 2 diabetes. The prevalence of type 2 diabetes in the United States has soared with the national increase in the numbers of people who are overweight. Fewer than half of American adults are at a healthy weight, about one third are obese, and another third are overweight and at risk of becoming obese. Alarmingly, nearly one in five children and teens ages 6 to 19 is also overweight.

Diabetes affects the way the body uses food for growth and energy. When you eat a dinner roll or a banana, your body breaks down the carbohydrates (starches and sugars) into glucose, a simple sugar that is the body's main source of fuel. The glucose gets absorbed into the bloodstream, which carries it to muscle and fat cells. The cells respond to signals from the hormone insulin, which acts like a key that unlocks the doors of the cells to allow glucose to enter and be used for energy or stored for later. In people with type 2 diabetes, the cells become less sensitive to the effects of insulin. Over time, the pancreas can no longer produce enough insulin to overcome the cells' lack of response to insulin, and glucose cannot get into the cells. As a result, glucose begins to build up in the blood—elevated blood sugar levels are the hallmark of diabetes.

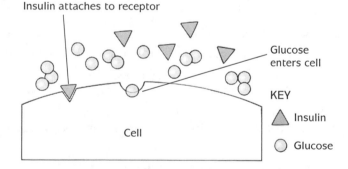

Cells unresponsive to insulin

Insulin is a hormone that enables muscle and fat cells to absorb glucose (sugar) from the bloodstream. Each cell has insulin receptors that act like keys that open the cell to allow glucose to enter. In a person with type 2 diabetes, the cells have become less responsive to insulin. Even though insulin attaches to the receptors, glucose has trouble getting into the cells, and the glucose accumulates in the bloodstream.

Many people who are at risk for type 2 diabetes can prevent or delay the disorder by eating a healthy and balanced diet, being physically active, and losing a little weight. For people who are overweight, even modest lifestyle changes that produce a 5 to 7 percent weight loss can cut their diabetes risk in half. (A 5 to 7 percent weight loss for a person who weighs 200 pounds would be 10 to 14 pounds. So you can see that it doesn't take much!)

Keep your weight down

Being overweight is a major risk factor for type 2 diabetes. Maintaining a healthy weight is one of the most important things you can do to reduce your risk. When you eat too much, the excess calories that are not immediately used get stored as fat. When you regularly overeat, the stored fat keeps accumulating.

These fat stores—especially those that accumulate in the abdominal area—reduce the ability of the cells to respond to the hormone insulin. Losing weight (reducing your fat stores) can significantly lower a person's risk of developing type 2 diabetes. If you already have diabetes, losing weight can reduce its severity by making your cells more sensitive to insulin. How do you know if your weight puts you at risk for type 2 diabetes? Consider these factors: your body mass index (BMI), the distribution of fat on your body, and your waist size.

To check the status of your weight, use the BMI chart on page 85. Body mass index is a mathematical formula that provides an indicator of what weight is appropriate for your height. A BMI of 25 or higher signals an increased risk for diabetes; a BMI of 30 or more indicates obesity and poses an even higher risk. In the United States, 85 to 90 percent of people with type 2 diabetes are obese. In some groups, such as Asians, diabetes risk starts to increase at even lower BMI levels.

People who carry more weight in their abdominal area than on their hips or thighs have a higher risk of developing diabetes, because fat stored in the abdomen has a greater influence on insulin sensitivity than fat stored elsewhere on the body. (Abdominal fat also increases the risk for high blood pressure, heart disease, and stroke.) Waist size is another indicator of unhealthy weight. In general, women with a waist size larger than 35 inches and men with a waist size larger than 40 inches are at increased risk for diabetes because they carry a lot of fat in the abdomen. However, for people of Asian descent, the risk for diabetes appears to increase at even smaller waist sizes.

Consume a healthy diet

Eating a healthy and balanced diet is one of the principal ways to avoid type 2 diabetes. Try to eat 5 to 9 servings of fruits and vegetables every day. It sounds like a lot, but you can do it if you have some fruit at every meal, eat plenty of salads, have cut-up vegetables for snacks, and eat at least 2 servings of vegetables at dinner. Swap breads and pastas made from white flour for those made from whole grains. Work with your doctor or a dietitian to develop a meal plan that includes these important recommendations:

- Consume at least 5 servings of fruits and vegetables each day.
- Limit your intake of saturated fats and cholesterol, and avoid trans fats (see page 11).
- Limit your consumption of added sugars and salt.
- Eat a variety of whole grains every day.
- Equalize the calories you take in with those you burn through regular exercise.
- Boost your intake of fiber.

Getting enough fiber in your diet is especially important in preventing type 2 diabetes, because fiber helps make cells more sensitive to insulin, which regulates blood sugar levels. A high-fiber diet can also help reduce the level of artery-clogging LDL cholesterol in the blood, lowering the risk for heart disease. To achieve these benefits from fiber, you need to consume 14 grams of fiber for every 1,000 calories you take in. That translates into 28 grams of fiber daily for a typical 2,000-calorie daily diet. Twenty-eight grams sounds like a lot, but you can easily reach this goal by following these tips:

- Eat only high-fiber breakfast cereals. Check the label on the cereal box and buy only those that contain 5 grams of fiber or more per serving. (Avoid instant oatmeal because it provides little or no fiber or other nutrients.)
- Eat whole fruits instead of fruit juices. Have fruit for snacks and dessert.
- Eat more raw and cooked vegetables at lunch and dinner.
- Replace white bread, pasta, and rice with the whole-grain versions.
- Make several meals meatless every week by, for example, replacing meat-based main dishes with bean-based entrées.

- Toss some beans, peas, or lentils into salads, soups, casseroles, and egg dishes.

If you have not been eating many high-fiber foods, increase your intake gradually to prevent gas and bloating. Drink six to eight glasses of water every day, because eating a lot of fiber without taking in enough fluids can cause constipation.

Be more active

Even if you have a high risk for type 2 diabetes, you can sharply lower your chances of developing the disorder by becoming more physically active. Exercise, combined with a healthy diet, is a safe and effective way to prevent diabetes. It also helps you manage your weight by using excess calories that your body would otherwise store as fat.

Physical activity prevents or delays the development of diabetes in two important ways. First, exercise helps muscle cells use the circulating blood sugar they need for energy production by making the cells more sensitive to insulin. Exercise improves insulin sensitivity even if you don't lose any weight. If you lose a few pounds, your insulin sensitivity will improve even more. Second, physical activity helps muscle cells absorb glucose more efficiently. Following are the ways in which exercise reduces your risk for type 2 diabetes as well as high blood pressure, heart attack, and stroke:

- Lowers blood sugar levels
- Reduces blood pressure
- Lowers bad LDL cholesterol and raises good HDL cholesterol in the blood
- Strengthens the heart muscle
- Decreases body fat

Any amount of exercise is better than none, but doctors recommend at least 30 minutes of moderate-intensity physical activity on most—preferably all—days of the week. Moderately paced exercises, such as walking, can greatly reduce your risk of developing type 2 diabetes. If you have been physically inactive for a while, start slowly and work up to 30 minutes a day at a pace that is comfortable for you. If you can't sustain physical activity for 30 minutes, or feel that you're just too busy to set aside that much time for exercise, accumulate activity over the course of the day in

10- or 15-minute intervals. The exercise will add up and so will the health benefits.

Excess weight places extra stress on the muscles and joints, especially the hips, knees, and ankles. If you're overweight, you may have discomfort or pain when you exercise. Injuries such as strains and sprains are also a risk. For this reason, start out slowly when beginning an exercise program. Make sure you wear socks with sturdy, comfortable shoes that are right for the activity you're doing. People with diabetes who have nerve damage or blockages in their arteries need to be especially careful about protecting their feet, because a small injury such as a blister can take a long time to heal and could become infected.

Strength-training exercises (see page 52) are especially good for cutting diabetes risk because they can help control blood sugar levels. Strength training, also known as resistance training, refers to activities that make the muscles work against some form of resistance. Strengthening exercises can be done using free weights or weight machines; or without weights, by doing exercises such as sit-ups and push-ups, which make the muscles work against the weight of the body.

Medical research shows that people who consume a healthy diet and regularly lift weights can reduce their blood sugar levels much more than those who try to control blood sugar through diet alone. Not only does resistance training help cells become more sensitive to insulin, it also enables muscles to absorb sugar from the blood more efficiently. Just as important, weight training is good for the heart, a key factor for people at risk for type 2 diabetes, because having diabetes increases the risk for heart disease about fourfold. An extra bonus: strength training helps offset the muscle loss that comes with aging. The goal of resistance training should not be to bulk up too much, but just to improve tone and get good exercise. Be sure not to lift weights that cause you to strain or bear down, since this can lead to injury and may be harmful to your heart.

PREVENTING DIABETES COMPLICATIONS

Having diabetes puts you at two to five times the normal risk for heart disease and stroke, and even prediabetes puts you at twice the risk. People with diabetes also tend to develop heart disease or have strokes at an earlier age than other people. Over time, people with diabetes sometimes sustain damage to the nerves (neuropathy). Neuropathies can lead to numbness and sometimes pain and weakness in the hands, arms, feet, and legs. Nerve damage can also affect every organ system, including the digestive tract, lungs, heart, and sex organs. People with diabetes can develop nerve problems at any time, but the longer someone has diabetes, the greater his or her risk.

If you already have type 2 diabetes, you can lower your risk for complications by keeping your blood sugar levels (see page 201), blood pressure (see page 236), and blood cholesterol (see page 200) below the recommended target levels. Reaching these targets also can help prevent the narrowing or blockage of the blood vessels in the legs, a condition called peripheral artery disease (see page 232). You can reach the target numbers by choosing foods wisely, being physically active, and taking medication if needed. The following measures will also help reduce your risk for complications:

- **Blood sugar monitoring**   Regular blood sugar testing at home helps you find out how well your food intake, exercise, and medication regimen are controlling your blood sugar levels. The closer to normal your blood sugar is, the better you will feel and the less likely you are to develop dangerous complications. Your doctor will recommend how frequently you should test your blood sugar, and what your target level should be. You should test more often when you change diabetes medications, or when you are sick or under more stress than usual.

  A continuous glucose-monitoring system records blood sugar levels at 10-second intervals to identify patterns in the fluctuation of sugar levels over time—patterns that would otherwise go unnoticed using just a fingerstick test. Continuous monitoring of blood sugar can give your doctor information that can help him or her fine-tune your therapy, but it is not intended to replace standard fingerstick testing. You still need to check your blood sugar at regular intervals using your glucose monitor. Controlling blood sugar appears to be especially important for preventing diabetes-related complications of the eyes, kidneys, and nerves, but it is also important for preventing heart disease and stroke.

- **Eye screening**   Damage to the retina of the eye from diabetes is called diabetic retinopathy (see page 416). Without treatment, diabetic retinopathy almost always leads to blindness. Diabetes also plays a role in the development of glaucoma (see page 410) and cataracts (see page

408). If you have type 2 diabetes, you should see an ophthalmologist (a doctor who specializes in diseases of the eye) at least once a year for a dilated eye exam. If you already have diabetic retinopathy, you will probably need to have your eyes examined more frequently. An ophthalmologist can check for diabetic retinopathy and glaucoma using screening tests.

- **Kidney monitoring** Keeping your blood sugar levels under control will help prevent kidney disease. Diabetes can damage the tiny blood vessels in the kidneys in the same way that it harms the blood vessels in other parts of the body. High levels of blood sugar cause the kidneys to filter too much blood. Over years of being overworked, the kidneys can start to leak protein, and their function declines. Waste products accumulate in the blood, and valuable substances, such as protein and red blood cells (which normally stay in the blood), end up being eliminated in urine. Eventually the kidneys can no longer remove the waste products, and the kidneys begin to fail.

  It's also important to control blood pressure (see below) because a small rise in blood pressure can rapidly worsen kidney disease. To maintain the health of your kidneys, your doctor will probably recommend regular kidney function tests.

- **Monitoring of blood pressure and cholesterol** High blood pressure and unhealthy blood cholesterol levels—major risk factors for heart disease—often accompany diabetes. In fact, for people with diabetes, controlling blood pressure and cholesterol levels is probably even more important in preventing heart disease than controlling blood sugar levels. Blood pressure control is especially important. People with diabetes have lower target blood pressure levels than people without diabetes.

  Make sure you have your blood pressure measured at every doctor visit, and at least twice a year. Cholesterol levels should be monitored at least every one to two years. It is important to know your numbers, and to discuss with your doctor what your goal levels are, and what you need to do to achieve them. Diet and physical activity are essential for helping to control blood pressure and cholesterol. Even so, many people with diabetes will require medications to control blood pressure and cholesterol. It is important to understand what the benefits of these medications are, and what your doctor expects to achieve with them.

- **Foot checks** High blood sugar levels from diabetes cause two problems that can harm the feet: nerve damage and poor blood flow. Having damaged nerves makes you less likely to feel pain in your legs and feet. You may not realize that you have a sore or a cut on your foot. The wound could become infected and eventually result in serious foot ulcers. In severe cases, infected foot ulcers don't heal, and the skin and tissue around the sore begin to die (a condition called gangrene). To keep gangrene from spreading up the leg, amputation may be necessary. Examples of common foot problems that can lead to infection in a person with diabetes include corns, calluses, ingrown toenails, blisters, bunions, plantar warts, hammertoes, athlete's foot, and dry, cracked skin. If you notice any of these conditions, you should bring them to your doctor's attention right away.

  The most important thing you can do to take care of your feet is to check them for anything unusual every day. Set a time to do it so you won't forget. Here are some other tips to help you keep your feet healthy:

  - Wash your feet in warm water every day. Test the water temperature with your elbow or a thermometer. Dry your feet thoroughly, especially between your toes.

  - If your skin is dry, rub lotion on your feet after you wash and dry them.

  - File corns and calluses gently with an emery board or pumice stone after you bathe.

  - Cut your toenails once a week. Cut them when they are soft, after washing. Cut them to the shape of your toe, but not too short. File the edges with an emery board.

  - Always wear shoes or slippers to protect your feet.

  - Wear socks or stockings to prevent blisters. Don't wear knee-high nylon stockings, because they may be too tight below your knee and could limit blood flow to the feet.

  - Make sure your shoes fit properly. Shop for shoes at the end of the day when your feet are bigger. Break in new shoes slowly—wearing them only one or two hours a day for the first couple of weeks.

- Before you put on your shoes, check to make sure nothing sharp has fallen inside them.
- Keep the blood flowing to your feet. Put your feet up, wiggle your toes, and move your feet up and down from the ankle. This is especially important if you are spending a lot of time sitting, such as during travel.
- Ask your doctor to examine your feet at least once a year.

9

PREVENTING CANCER

CANCER IS THE SECOND LEADING cause of death in the United States, after heart disease. More than half a million Americans die each year of cancer. One out of two men and one out of three women develop some kind of cancer at some time in their life, most often after age 55. Early detection of cancer increases the chances for a cure, so perform all the routine self-examinations (see page 202), have all the recommended screening tests (see page 187), and tell your doctor about any suspicious symptoms.

All cancers result from mutations, or changes, in genes that control cell growth and behavior. These genes normally curb cell proliferation and tell cells to mend DNA damage when necessary, or to self-destruct when DNA damage can no longer be repaired. Sometimes DNA damage can cause cells to bypass normal controls, mutate, and become cancerous; they divide constantly and pass on the mutation to their offspring.

Some people seem to be more vulnerable than others to factors that can cause cancer, but doctors often cannot explain why one person develops cancer and another doesn't. But scientists have studied general patterns of cancer to learn what factors in the environment and what things people do

CANCEROUS VERSUS NONCANCEROUS

Cancer cells, unlike normal cells, divide uncontrollably, ignoring the usual signals to stop dividing. Cancer can spread through the body in two ways: invasion or metastasis. Invasion is the spread of cancer cells into neighboring tissues. Metastasis occurs when cancer cells penetrate blood vessels or lymphatic vessels, circulate through the bloodstream or lymphatic system, and invade healthy tissue in another part of the body.

When cancer spreads from its original place to another part of the body, the new tumor has the same kind of abnormal cells and the same name as the original tumor. For example, if colon cancer spreads to the liver, the cancer cells in the liver are actually colon cancer cells, and the disease is termed metastatic colon cancer, not liver cancer.

Characteristics of noncancerous growths

- They are usually not life-threatening.
- They can usually be removed and tend not to grow back.
- They do not invade surrounding tissues.
- Their cells do not spread to other parts of the body.

Characteristics of cancerous growths

- They are more serious than noncancerous growths.
- They can often be removed but can grow back.
- They can invade and damage nearby tissues and organs.
- Their cells can break away and spread to other parts of the body.

How cancer spreads

If cancer cells enter blood vessels, they can be carried through the bloodstream to another part of the body and invade tissues and organs there. The spread of cancer from one area of the body to another is called metastasis. Another way in which cancer can spread is by invading nearby tissue as a tumor grows.

Blood vessel

1 Cancer cells break through blood vessel wall

2 Cancer cells travel through bloodstream

3 Cancer cells invade new site

during their lives, might boost their risk of developing cancer. You can avoid some of the risk factors for cancer, but you can't avoid them all. For example, although you can choose to quit smoking, you cannot choose your family history. Both smoking and inheriting specific genes could be considered risk factors for certain kinds of cancer, but only smoking can be avoided. Prevention means reducing the risk factors you can control and amplifying the protective factors that can lower your cancer risk.

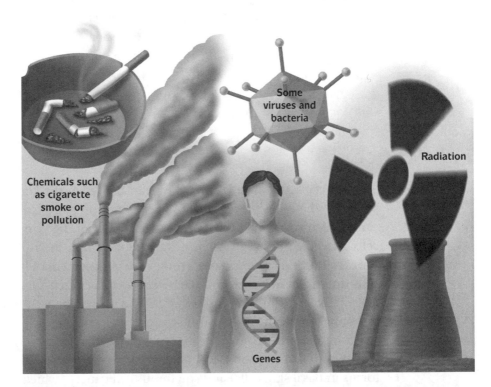

What causes cancer?

Many factors can combine to cause cancer. Gene mutations (changes) that increase susceptibility to a particular cancer can be inherited or, most often, occur after exposure to substances that can cause genetic damage. For example, exposure to cigarette smoke can cause lung cancer, excessive sun exposure can cause skin cancer, and the human papillomavirus (HPV) causes most cases of cervical cancer. No one gene mutation is responsible for cancer; multiple genetic changes in specific genes are necessary to change normal cells into cancerous cells that grow out of control.

TEN TOP CANCERS

Although more people have breast cancer or prostate cancer than lung cancer or colon cancer, lung cancer and colon cancer kill more Americans each year.

Most common cancers	Major killers
1. Skin	1. Lung
2. Breast	2. Colon and rectum
3. Prostate	3. Breast
4. Lung	4. Prostate
5. Colon and rectum	5. Pancreas
6. Bladder	6. Non-Hodgkin's lymphoma
7. Non-Hodgkin's lymphoma	7. Leukemias
8. Melanoma	8. Ovarian
9. Uterine (endometrial)	9. Stomach
10. Leukemias	10. Brain and nervous system

Skin cancer

Skin cancer is the most common type of cancer in the United States, and probably the most preventable. About 1 million Americans develop skin cancer each year. Skin cancer begins in the cells of the skin. Normally, skin cells grow old and die every day, and new cells take their place. But sometimes this orderly process goes wrong: new replacement cells form when the skin doesn't need them, and old cells don't die when they should. These extra cells can form a mass of tissue called a growth or a tumor. Tumors can be benign (noncancerous) or malignant (cancerous).

Skin cancers are named for the type of cells that have become cancerous. The two most common types of skin cancer are basal cell cancer (which forms in basal skin cells) and squamous cell cancer (which forms in squamous cells). Basal cell cancer rarely spreads to other parts of the body, while squamous cell cancer sometimes spreads to the lymph nodes and to internal organs. Both basal cell and squamous cell cancers usually form on the head, face, neck, hands, or arms—areas that are most often exposed to the sun. However, skin cancer can occur anywhere on the body. If your skin tans poorly or burns easily after sun exposure, if you have red or blond hair and fair skin that freckles easily, or if you have blue eyes, you are especially susceptible to developing skin cancer.

A third type of skin cancer, melanoma, is much rarer than basal cell and squamous cell cancers, but can be much more serious. Melanoma develops in cells called melanocytes, which lie in the deepest layer of the skin. Melanoma usually begins in a mole. People whose skin tans poorly or who have a large number of abnormal moles may also have an increased risk of developing melanoma. The incidence of melanoma among whites is twenty times higher than it is among blacks and about four times higher than it is among Hispanics.

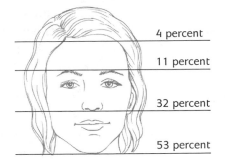

Squamous cell cancer on the face
Squamous cell cancers that develop on the face usually appear on the lower part of the face, especially between the bottom of the nose and the chin.

RISK FACTORS

People with certain risk factors are more likely than others to develop skin cancer. Risk factors vary for different types of skin cancer, but some general risk factors include the following:

- Light skin color
- Family history of skin cancer
- Personal history of skin cancer
- Excessive exposure to the sun (either through work or leisure activities)
- History of sunburns early in life
- Skin that burns, freckles, reddens easily, or becomes painful in the sun
- Blue or green eyes
- Blond or red hair
- Certain types of moles or a large number of moles

PREVENTION

The best way to prevent skin cancer is to protect yourself from exposure to the sun. Because skin cancer has been linked to sunburns in childhood or adolescence, it is also important to protect children from the sun starting at an early age. Doctors suggest that people of all ages limit their time in the sun and avoid other sources of ultraviolet (UV) radiation, such as tanning beds. UV radiation is the stream of invisible high-energy rays coming from the sun. Follow these guidelines to reduce your chances of developing skin cancer:

- Stay out of the midday sun—from 10 a.m. until 4 p.m.—whenever you can.

- Protect yourself from UV radiation reflected by sand, water, snow, and ice. UV radiation can easily pass through light clothing, windshields, windows, and clouds.

- Wear long sleeves and long pants of tightly woven fabrics, a hat with a wide brim, and sunglasses that absorb both types of UV radiation— UVA and UVB.

- Use sunscreen lotions. Sunscreen may help prevent skin cancer, especially broad-spectrum sunscreen (that filters both UVA and UVB rays) with a sun protection factor (SPF) of at least 15. But you still need to avoid the sun and wear clothing to protect your skin.

- Reapply sunscreen every two hours, more often when swimming or sweating.

- When possible, stay in the shade.

- Avoid using sunlamps and tanning booths.

The regular use of sunscreen has been shown to reduce the risk for basal cell and squamous cell skin cancers. However, doctors are concerned that

ABCDs of melanoma

See your doctor right away if you notice any of the following signs of possible melanoma in a mole, or if a mole seems to be growing:

- **Asymmetry** If you draw an imaginary line down the middle of the mole, each side is a different size or shape.
- **Border** The mole has an irregular or blurred border.
- **Color** The mole has more than one shade or color, such as black, brown, blue, red, and white.
- **Diameter** The mole is larger than ¼ inch across (about the size of a pencil eraser).

people who use only sunscreen (without other protection) could actually increase their risk for skin cancer if using sunscreen gives them a false sense of security and they end up spending more time in the sun than they might if they didn't use sunscreen. For extra protection when you're going to be in the sun for a long time, wear a hat and a long-sleeved shirt and long pants.

As for the effectiveness of sunscreen against melanoma, the evidence is mixed. Although melanoma incidence is higher in regions near the equator, where ultraviolet exposure is most intense, melanoma often occurs in areas of the body that are not exposed to the sun.

Regularly checking your skin for new growths or other skin changes is a good idea, especially if you have several moles. Report any changes in your skin or moles to your doctor right away.

Colon cancer

Colon cancer is a disease in which cancerous cells form in the tissues of the colon (large intestine) or rectum. It is also referred to as colorectal cancer. Colon cancer is the second leading cancer killer in the United States, after lung cancer. Over the past decade, both the incidence and the death rates for colon cancer have modestly decreased. Until age 50, men and women have similar risks for colon cancer, but after age 50, men are more vulnerable. There are striking differences in incidence and death rates among racial and ethnic groups. Death rates from colon cancer for Hispanics, Asians, and Native Americans are lower than those for whites and African Americans.

Colon cancer has a strong genetic component. Most cases are caused by the interaction of multiple genes and environmental factors such as eating a diet high in animal fat (especially from red meat) and being obese. Because colon cancer occurs more frequently in people who are obese than in those who are at a healthy weight, researchers theorize that high levels of insulin in obese people may promote tumor development in the colon. Fat that accumulates in the abdominal area may be more important in colon cancer risk than fat carried on other parts of the body. Having an inflammatory condition in the intestine called ulcerative colitis for longer than 10 years or having intestinal polyps called adenomatous polyps that are not detected and removed from the colon can also increase colon cancer risk.

RISK FACTORS

The list of factors that can raise your risk of colon or rectal cancer is long. Some factors are controllable and some are not, but regular screening with a colonoscopy (see page 194) helps to detect adenomatous polyps in the colon and remove them before they can become cancerous. As with most cancers, early detection leads to better long-term outcomes. The most common risk factors for colon cancer are the following:

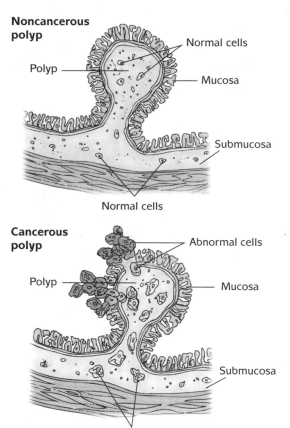

Noncancerous polyp

Normal cells

Polyp

Mucosa

Submucosa

Normal cells

Cancerous polyp

Abnormal cells

Polyp

Mucosa

Submucosa

Abnormal cells

Colon polyps

Intestinal polyps are mushroom-like growths in the inner lining of the wall of the colon. They are usually made up of normal cells. When a polyp becomes cancerous, its cells grow and multiply abnormally. The abnormal cells can grow into the adjacent layers of the colon wall and, if the cells keep multiplying unchecked, they can invade blood vessels and spread throughout the body.

- **Age**   The risk for colon cancer starts to go up after age 40 and continues to increase with age. More than 90 percent of people with colon cancer are diagnosed after age 50. The average age at diagnosis is 72.

- **Family history**   Close relatives (parents, siblings, or children) of a person with colon cancer are somewhat more likely to develop the disorder, especially if the relative developed the cancer at a young age. If many close relatives have had colon cancer, the risk is greater. If you have close relatives who have had colon cancer, you should have regular colonoscopies.

- **Polyps**   Polyps are growths on the inner wall of the colon or rectum. They are common in people over age 50. Most polyps are not cancerous, but some, called adenomatous polyps, can become cancerous. Finding and removing polyps can help prevent colon or rectal cancer.

- **Genetic changes**   Changes (mutations) in specific genes can cause two distinct medical conditions that increase the risk for colon cancer: hereditary nonpolyposis colon cancer and familial adenomatous polyposis. Hereditary nonpolyposis colon cancer is the most common type of inherited colon cancer, accounting for about 2 percent of all cases; the average age at diagnosis is 44. Familial adenomatous polyposis is a rare inherited condition in which hundreds of polyps form in the colon and rectum.

- **Personal history of cancer**   If you have already had colon or rectal cancer, you are at increased risk of developing it a second time. Women with a history of cancer of the ovary, uterus (endometrium), or breast have a somewhat higher risk of developing colon cancer than women who don't have a history of these cancers.

- **Ulcerative colitis or Crohn's disease**   People who have, over many years, had a condition such as ulcerative colitis or Crohn's disease (both of which cause inflammation in the colon), have a heightened risk of developing colon cancer.

- **Obesity and lack of exercise**   Obesity and a lack of physical activity are linked to an increased risk for colon cancer. Obesity and physical inactivity may account for as much as 25 to 30 percent of the increased risk for several major cancers—including cancer of the colon.

- **Smoking**   Studies have found that smoking cigarettes raises the risk of developing noncancerous polyps in the colon as well as colon cancer. In cigarette smokers who have had surgery to remove noncancerous intestinal polyps, recurrence of the polyps is more likely than in nonsmokers.

- **Alcohol**   Heavy drinking, especially drinking hard liquor, can increase the risk for colon cancer. Having nine or more drinks made with liquor every week for 10 years or more can triple the risk for colon cancer.

- **Diet**   Studies seem to show that a diet high in fat (especially animal fat) and low in calcium, the B vitamin folic acid, and fiber may raise the risk for colorectal cancer. However, the evidence is weak for fiber (although there are plenty of other good reasons to increase your intake of fiber). Some studies suggest that people who eat few fruits and vegetables may also have an increased risk for colon cancer, but the results from diet studies are often contradictory and inconclusive.

PREVENTION

Having a colonoscopy to detect polyps in the colon and remove them is the single most effective way to prevent and reduce the risk for colon cancer. Most polyps in the colon and rectum are adenomatous polyps, which can eventually develop into cancer. Doctors routinely remove polyps during a colonoscopy. If you have no personal or family history of colon cancer, you should have your first colonoscopy at age 50. People who are at higher-than-average risk for colon cancer should talk with their doctor about whether to have a colonoscopy before age 50.

People who have colon cancer can develop the disorder a second time, so it's important to have regular checkups. Talk to your doctor about how often to have a colonoscopy. The general rule for people who have already had colon cancer is every three to five years, depending on the type of cancer found. If you have colon cancer, you might also be concerned that your family members could develop the cancer. Encourage your family members to see their doctor, who can plan an appropriate schedule for screening exams and checkups. Depending on a person's preferences and situation, in place of a colonoscopy a doctor may recommend a flexible sigmoidoscopy (see page 196), which examines just the lower part of the colon (sigmoid), and a fecal occult blood test (see page 194), which checks for hidden blood in the stool (which can be a sign of colon cancer).

The following have shown promise in preventing colon cancer in some studies, but their true effect on colon cancer risk is not yet known:

- **Nonsteroidal anti-inflammatory drugs** Nonsteroidal anti-inflammatories (NSAIDs) such as aspirin, ibuprofen, and naproxen may lower the risk of developing noncancerous polyps in the colon. However, it is not clear if taking NSAIDs results in a lower risk for cancerous polyps. The use of some NSAIDs can increase the risk for heart attack and stroke, and some can cause bleeding in the stomach and intestines, so don't take NSAIDS without talking to your doctor first.

- **Hormone replacement therapy** Hormone replacement therapy (HRT; see page 520) that includes both estrogen and progestin may lower the risk for colon cancer in women after menopause. HRT with estrogen alone does not appear to lower the risk. However, hormone use may increase the risk for breast cancer, heart disease, and blood clots in some women.

- **Vitamins and minerals** Calcium and vitamin D, especially when taken in supplements up to the recommended daily dose, may reduce the risk for colon cancer. The recommended daily dose is 1,200 milligrams of calcium and 800 international units (IUs) of vitamin D.

- **Statins**   Studies have found that taking statins (cholesterol-lowering drugs) may affect the risk for colon cancer by helping cells control the development, growth, and spread of tumors. However, this research is ongoing, and no doctors recommend taking statins for cancer prevention.

- **Diet**   It's not yet known whether a diet low in fat and high in fiber, fruits, and vegetables lowers the risk for colon cancer. Some studies have shown that a diet high in fat, protein, calories, and red meat raises colon cancer risk, but other studies have not found the same increase in risk.

Lung cancer

Lung cancer is the leading cancer killer of both men and women in the United States. More people die from lung cancer each year than from any other type of cancer. In the early 2000s, lung cancer accounted for more deaths than breast cancer, prostate cancer, and colon cancer combined. More than 100,000 men and 84,000 women are diagnosed with lung cancer each year in the United States, and nearly 90,000 men and 70,000 women die from it each year. Nearly all of these deaths could have been prevented, because cigarette smoking causes nearly 90 percent of all cases of lung cancer.

It takes years for lung cancer to develop, but adverse changes in lung tissue can start soon after you start smoking. Every time you light up, the normal cells in your lungs get exposed to the cancer-causing chemicals in tobacco. Cells in the lungs can eventually become cancerous, multiply out of control, and travel to other parts of your body before you ever have any symptoms. Women seem to be especially susceptible to developing lung cancer from smoking. Women develop lung cancer earlier in life after fewer years of smoking and are more likely than men to have slow-growing tumors that seldom show symptoms in the initial stages.

RISK FACTORS

Lung cancer has been linked to the following risk factors:

- **Smoking**   Smoking is the No. 1 cause of lung cancer. People who stop smoking for good lower their risk of developing lung cancer or of having lung cancer return. The earlier you quit, the lower your risk.

- **Secondhand smoke** Smoke that comes from a burning cigarette, cigar, or pipe or that is exhaled by smokers also causes lung cancer. People who inhale secondhand smoke are exposed to the same cancer-causing agents as smokers, although in lesser amounts. Inhaling secondhand smoke is called involuntary or passive smoking. There is no safe level of secondhand smoke for nonsmokers. About 3,000 lung cancer deaths occur each year from secondhand smoke.

- **Family history** Doctors suspect that one or more defective genes can be passed down in families to increase a person's risk for lung cancer. For example, someone who has a close relative (a parent or sibling) with lung cancer has twice the risk for lung cancer as someone who does not have a relative with lung cancer. However, it is difficult to pinpoint a lung cancer gene because of the major role of smoking in lung cancer. In addition, family members of smokers are often exposed to cigarette smoke, which increases their risk for lung cancer.

- **Radon exposure** Radon, a radioactive gas that is found in soil and rock in all parts of the United States, is the second leading cause of lung cancer after smoking. Radon, which is formed by the decay of uranium, may be found in all types of homes and buildings in the United States. If radon gas is in the ground, it can seep into a building. Inhaling indoor air containing radon over many years can increase the risk for lung cancer.

- **Workplace exposure** Some substances found in the workplace—such as asbestos, arsenic, chromium, nickel, tar, and soot—can cause lung cancer in people who have never smoked and, in smokers, can further increase lung cancer risk. However, the effects of these substances on lung cancer rates is small compared with cigarette smoking.

- **Air pollution** Lung cancer rates are higher in cities with higher levels of air pollution.

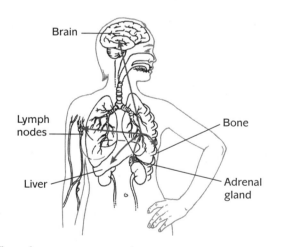

Where lung cancer spreads

Lung cancer can spread to the lymph nodes or other tissues in the chest, including the other lung. In many cases, lung cancer also spreads to other organs of the body, such as the bones, adrenal glands (which sit on top of the kidneys), liver, or brain. The symptoms vary, depending on which organs are affected. For example, a tumor in the brain can cause paralysis.

The most important step you can take to prevent lung cancer is to stop smoking if you smoke (see page 135). Even if you have smoked for many years, quitting can lower your risk for lung cancer. Take the following measures:

- **Don't smoke.** Smoking is the single most preventable cause of death in the United States.
- **Stay away from secondhand smoke.** Inhaling someone else's smoke can be almost as damaging to your lungs as smoking.
- **Check for radon.** Get the radon levels in your home tested, especially if you live in a location where radon is known to exist.
- **Avoid cancer-causing chemicals.** Protect yourself from toxic chemicals such as vinyl chloride, nickel. and coal products. If you are exposed to such chemicals at work and you smoke, your risk is multiplied.
- **Avoid excessive amounts of alcohol.** Heavy drinking may slightly increase your risk for lung cancer.

Liver cancer

Primary liver cancer, or hepatocellular carcinoma, is cancer that originates in the tissues of the liver. In the United States, primary liver cancer is not common, and is related to some lifestyle factors and medical conditions that can be prevented. For example, hepatitis (inflammation of the liver), especially hepatitis B (an infection caused by a virus that attacks the liver), can cause lifelong infection and lead to cirrhosis (scarring) of the liver and liver cancer. In cirrhosis, scar tissue replaces normal, healthy tissue, blocking the flow of blood through the liver and preventing it from working as it should. Cirrhosis has many causes. In the United States, the most common causes are long-term alcohol abuse and hepatitis C infection.

The following are the major risk factors for primary liver cancer. The more risk factors you have, the higher your risk. But keep in mind that many people with known risk factors for liver cancer may never develop the disease.

- **Chronic liver infection** The most important risk factor for liver cancer is chronic, long-term infection with the hepatitis B or hepatitis C virus. These viruses can be passed from person to person through blood (such as by sharing needles); hepatitis B can be also be spread through sexual contact or from a pregnant woman to her baby during a vaginal delivery. These infections may not cause symptoms, but blood tests can show whether either virus is present. Hepatitis B vaccine can prevent chronic hepatitis B infection and can protect against liver cancer in people who have not been infected with hepatitis B. Researchers are still working on a vaccine to prevent hepatitis C infection.

- **Cirrhosis**   Cirrhosis is a disease that develops when liver cells are damaged and replaced with scar tissue. Cirrhosis can be caused by alcohol abuse, taking certain drugs and other chemicals, and exposure to certain viruses or parasites. About 5 percent of people with cirrhosis develop liver cancer.

- **Being male**   For unknown reasons, men are twice as likely as women to develop liver cancer.

- **Family history**   People who have family members with liver cancer may be more likely to develop it.

- **Age**   In the United States, liver cancer occurs most often after age 60.

- **Aflatoxin**   Liver cancer can result from consumption of a substance made by certain types of mold, called aflatoxin. Aflatoxin can form on peanuts, corn, and other nuts and grains. In Asia and Africa, aflatoxin contamination is a problem, but the U.S. government does not allow the sale of foods that have high levels of aflatoxin.

PREVENTION

The following steps can help you reduce your risk of developing primary liver cancer:

- **Limit your consumption of alcohol.** In the United States, alcohol abuse is a chief cause of the cirrhosis, or scarring, that can proceed to liver cancer. Men should drink no more than two drinks a day and women should have no more than one drink daily.

- **Consider having the hepatitis B vaccination.** If you are a health-care worker, have multiple sex partners, travel internationally, or are otherwise considered at high risk for hepatitis, you should have the hepatitis B vaccination. The vaccination is recommended for all American children.

There is no vaccination for hepatitis C, so you should avoid situations in which it is spread—including sharing needles (during intravenous drug use), having unsanitary tattooings or body piercings, or, less commonly, during sex. The virus used to be spread primarily through blood products (before 1987) or blood transfusions (before 1992) but now all donor blood and blood products are screened for the virus.

Esophageal cancer

The esophagus is the muscular tube that connects the throat and stomach. Cancer can form in the tissues that line the esophagus. The two main types of esophageal cancer are squamous cell carcinoma (cancer that begins in flat cells lining the esophagus) and adenocarcinoma (cancer that begins in cells that make and release mucus and other fluids).

Doctors do not know all the causes of esophageal cancer, but they recognize several factors that can damage the esophagus and possibly set the stage for cancer to develop. Cigarette smoking and heavy drinking are the two major causes of esophageal cancer, especially when combined. Severe, long-term untreated or recurring gastroesophageal reflux disease (GERD; see page 338) can cause chronic inflammation in the esophagus from the backflow of stomach acid. This chronic inflammation can damage the lining of the esophagus and cause bleeding or ulcers (esophagitis). Some people develop a condition called Barrett's esophagus, in which cells in the esophagus lining take on an abnormal shape and color. Over time, the cells can become cancerous. Esophageal cancer is usually fatal but it can be successfully treated if it is diagnosed at an early stage.

RISK FACTORS

The two most important risk factors for esophageal cancer are cigarette smoking and heavy drinking, especially when combined. Smoking and drinking, and many of the other risk factors listed here cause irritation and inflammation in the esophagus, which can damage the cells in the lining of the esophagus. These damaged cells can eventually become cancerous:

- Smoking
- Heavy drinking
- Chronic GERD (heartburn)
- Being over age 55

- Being male
- Being obese
- Being infected with the Helicobacter pylori (H. pylori) bacterium (which causes inflammation and ulcers in the stomach lining)
- Having long-term exposure to silica dust (which can affect quarry workers, miners, construction workers, and others who work with granite, sandstone, brick, concrete, and tile)
- Having had radiation therapy to the chest

PREVENTION

You can reduce your chances of developing esophageal cancer by adopting the following healthy lifestyle habits:

- Don't smoke. If you smoke, quit.
- If you drink alcohol, drink only moderately.
- Get treatment for GERD.
- Maintain a healthy weight.

Bladder cancer

Most bladder cancers begin in cells that make up the inner lining of the bladder, sometimes as a result of chronic irritation and inflammation. Each year in the United States, about 67,000 new cases of bladder cancer are diagnosed, and the disease causes nearly 14,000 deaths.

No one knows the exact cause of bladder cancer. Cigarette smoking greatly increases the risk for bladder cancer and increases the death rate from bladder cancer. Researchers have looked at a couple of factors that may play a role in the development of bladder cancer—such as chlorine added to drinking water and the artificial sweetener saccharin—but little solid evidence has emerged to link them with the disease.

RISK FACTORS

People who develop bladder cancer are likely to have certain risk factors. Still, most people with known risk factors do not get bladder cancer, and many who do get the cancer have none of the risk factors. If you have any of the following risk factors, discuss your concerns with your doctor. He or she can suggest ways to reduce your risk and can plan a schedule of checkups.

- **Smoking** The use of tobacco is a major risk factor for bladder cancer. Cigarette smokers are two to three times more likely than nonsmokers to develop bladder cancer. Pipe and cigar smokers are also at increased risk. In addition, exposure to secondhand smoke raises the risk.

- **Age** As with most cancers, the chances of developing bladder cancer go up with age. People under 40 rarely have bladder cancer.

- **Occupational exposure** Some workers have an increased risk for bladder cancer because of exposure to cancer-causing chemicals in the workplace. At-risk occupations include working in the rubber, chemical, or leather industries, and being a hair stylist, machinist, metal worker, printer, painter, textile worker, or truck driver.

- **Long-term inflammation of the bladder** Chronic inflammation from recurrent urinary tract infections (see page 359) or kidney stones can boost bladder cancer risk.

- **Treatment with the drugs cyclophosphamide or arsenic** These drugs are used to treat some cancers and other conditions, but they also can increase bladder cancer risk.

- **Race** Whites are twice as likely to develop bladder cancer as blacks and Hispanics. The lowest rates of the cancer are among Asians.

- **Being male** Men are two to three times more likely than women to develop bladder cancer.

- **Family history** People with family members who have bladder cancer are more likely to develop the cancer than those without a family history. Researchers are studying changes in certain genes that may increase the risk for bladder cancer.

- **Personal history of bladder cancer** People who have had bladder cancer previously are at increased risk of having a recurrence of the cancer.

- **Infection** Infection with certain parasites has been linked to an increased risk for bladder cancer, but these parasites are common only in tropical areas, not in the United States.

If you smoke, the most important thing you can do to reduce your risk for bladder cancer is to quit smoking (see page 135).

- **Quit smoking if you smoke.** Cancer-causing chemicals in tobacco can accumulate in the urine and damage the bladder lining, where most bladder cancers start. Breathing in someone else's secondhand smoke can also be dangerous, so quitting can benefit your whole family. Never expose children to secondhand smoke.

- **Stay away from industrial chemicals.** Prolonged and repeated exposure to chemicals used in the manufacturing of dyes, rubber, leather, textiles, and paint can raise your risk of developing bladder cancer years later. At work, always follow the safety instructions for handling chemicals to minimize your exposure.

- **Avoid chronic bladder inflammation.** Long-term or recurring urinary tract infections or inflammation increase the risk for bladder cancer. Although doctors do not believe that infection or inflammation alone causes bladder cancer, it can be a factor in this type of cancer.

- **Drink more fluids.** People who drink plenty of water and other fluids have lower rates of bladder cancer than those who don't drink many fluids. Doctors think this may be because fluids flush out potential carcinogens in the urine, making them less likely to come in contact with the bladder lining.

Oral cancer

Oral cancer is part of a group of cancers called head and neck cancers. Oral cancer can develop in any part of the mouth, throat, or voice box, including the lips, lining of the cheeks, salivary glands, roof of the mouth, back of the mouth, floor of the mouth, gums, tongue, and tonsils. Most oral cancers begin in the tongue and in the floor of the mouth. Almost all oral cancers first form in the flat cells (squamous cells) that cover the surfaces of the mouth, tongue, and lips. Medically, these cancers are called squamous cell carcinomas, and are the same as squamous cell skin cancer (see page 260).

When oral cancer spreads (metastasizes), it usually travels through the lymphatic system (a network of vessels that carries infection-fighting cells throughout the body in a clear, watery fluid called lymph). The spreading cancer cells often first appear in nearby lymph nodes in the neck. Cancer cells can also spread to other parts of the neck, to the lungs, and to other parts of the body

Oral cancer is diagnosed in about 30,000 Americans each year, and causes more than 8,000 deaths—killing one person every hour. Oral cancer is a disease whose survival rate—about 50 percent—has not improved much in the last 20 years. It also has a high rate of second oral tumors; people who survive a first cancer of the oral cavity are up to 20 times more likely to develop a second oral cancer than those who have never had oral cancer. This heightened risk can last 5 to10 years, sometimes longer, after the first cancer.

Oral cancer is usually diagnosed between the ages of 65 and 74, but it tends to occur 10 years earlier in blacks, and blacks have a lower survival rate from the cancer. In fact, black males experience the highest incidence and lowest survival rates of any group.

Doctors can't always explain why one person develops oral cancer and another doesn't, but they do know that it is not contagious. Oral cancers develop out of a multistep process of accumulated changes (mutations) in many genes—changes triggered by a number of factors. Tobacco and alcohol use, diet, exposure to viruses, and a possible genetic susceptibility probably interact to cause oral cancer.

RISK FACTORS

The following factors have been shown to increase the risk for oral cancer. If you have any of these risk factors, talk with your doctor or dentist. Ask how often you should have dental checkups and cleanings, and then be sure to keep every appointment.

- **Tobacco** Tobacco in any form contains numerous cancer-causing chemicals. Tobacco use accounts for most oral cancers. Smoking cigarettes, cigars, or pipes; using chewing tobacco; and dipping snuff are all linked to oral cancer. The use of other tobacco products (such as bidis and kreteks; see page 275) may also increase cancer risk. Long-term heavy smokers are at high risk, but the risk is even higher for tobacco users who also drink alcohol heavily. In fact, three out of four oral cancers occur in people who use alcohol, tobacco, or both alcohol and tobacco.

- **Alcohol** People who drink alcohol are more likely to develop oral cancer than people who don't drink. The risk increases with the amount of alcohol consumed. The risk increases even more if a person both drinks alcohol and uses tobacco. Exposure to alcohol by the mouth and throat might also make it easier for the cancer-causing agents in tobacco to penetrate tissues in the mouth and throat.

- **Sun** Cancer of the lip can be caused by exposure to the sun, and the risk is further increased in smokers.

- **A personal history of head and neck cancer** People who have had head and neck cancer have an increased risk of developing another head and neck cancer. Smoking further increases this risk.

- **Viruses** Viruses are thought to play a part in the development of oral cancers. Researchers are zeroing in on the human papillomavirus (HPV), especially the HPV-16 and HPV-18 strains, and the herpes viruses as possible contributors to some cases of oral cancer. DNA from HPV and certain herpes viruses—including Epstein-Barr, cytomegalovirus, and herpes simplex—has been detected in oral cancer biopsies (samples of tissue that are removed and examined under a microscope for cancer cells).

- **Inherited factors** More and more evidence suggests that genes are implicated in head and neck cancers.

- **Diet** Research hints that a diet lacking in antioxidant-rich fruits and vegetables could contribute to oral cancer. Antioxidants may help prevent genetic mutations that can lead to cancer.

PREVENTION

If you smoke or use tobacco products, quitting can dramatically reduce your risk of developing oral cancer. Quitting also lowers the chance that a person with oral cancer will get a second cancer in the head or neck. People who stop smoking can also reduce their risk for cancer of the lung, larynx, mouth, pancreas, bladder, and esophagus. There are many resources available to help smokers quit (see page 135). Talk to your doctor to find out what kind of help might be appropriate for you.

To reduce your chances of developing oral cancer, take the following steps:

- **Don't use tobacco in any form.** Your doctor and dentist will probably tell you that not using tobacco and limiting your use of alcohol are the most important things you can do to prevent oral cancer.

- **Limit your alcohol intake.** The more alcohol you drink, the higher your odds of developing oral cancer, especially if you smoke.
- **Restrict your time in the sun.** If you spend a lot of time in the sun, use a lip balm that contains sunscreen and wear a hat with a brim to help protect your lips from harmful radiation from the sun.
- **Have regular oral checkups.** Regular dental and medical checkups are a good time for your dentist or doctor to check your entire mouth for signs of cancer. Regular checkups can detect the early stages of oral cancer or conditions that could lead to oral cancer. Ask your doctor or dentist about checking the tissues in your mouth as part of your routine exams.

Women's cancers

For women, a long-term increase in overall cancer incidence leveled out beginning in 1999, after increasing since 1979. Cancers of the female breast and reproductive system remain common, but the incidence of breast cancer began to stabilize in 2001 after increasing since the 1980s. Some types of cancer in women are linked to infection with the human papillomavirus (HPV; see page 170), underscoring the importance of practicing safer sex (see page 165) and having regular Pap tests and pelvic exams (see page 188) to detect HPV and any abnormal changes that might signal a precancerous condition.

Breast cancer

In the United States, breast cancer is the most common cancer after skin cancer, and is the second leading cause of cancer-related deaths in women. (Lung cancer is No. 1.) Breast cancer forms in the tissues of the breast, usually in the ducts (tubes that carry milk to the nipple) and lobules (the glands that make milk). Although the number of breast cancer cases diagnosed has increased, the overall breast cancer death rate has dropped steadily since the early 1990s. There are nearly 180,000 new cases of breast cancer in American women each year, and more than 40,000 deaths from the cancer. About 2,000 men in the United States are diagnosed with breast cancer every year, and about 450 men die from it each year.

The increased incidence of breast cancer among women with a family history of the disorder shows that it has a genetic component. Five to 10 percent of women with breast cancer have a mother or sister with breast cancer. Scientists have identified two inherited gene mutations, called BRCA1 and BRCA2, that significantly increase breast cancer risk.

RISK FACTORS

Medical research has identified several factors that may raise the risk for breast cancer, including the following:

- **Age**   Age is the most important risk factor for breast cancer. The cancer is not common in women under age 35, more common in women over 50, and especially common in women over age 60. The risk of developing breast cancer at age 60 is 26 times greater than it is at 35.

- **History of breast cancer**   If you have had breast cancer in one breast, you are at increased risk of developing it in your other breast.

- **Family history**   The vast majority of women who develop breast cancer have no family history of the disease. However, heredity can play a role. Women who have a close relative (mother, sister, or daughter) with breast cancer (especially if it develops at a young age) are at increased risk of developing the cancer.

- **Estrogen**   The female hormone estrogen helps develop and maintain female sex characteristics. Being exposed to estrogen over a long time may increase a woman's risk for breast cancer. Estrogen levels are highest during the years a woman is menstruating. Early menstruation (starting at age 12 or younger) and late menopause (after age 50) extend the body's exposure to estrogen. The more years a woman menstruates, the longer her breast tissue is exposed to estrogen. Because estrogen levels are lower during pregnancy, breast tissue is exposed to more estrogen in women who become pregnant for the first time after age 35 or who never have a pregnancy.

- **Genes**   Women who have inherited certain mutations in the BRCA1 and BRCA2 genes have an increased risk for breast cancer. If several members of your family have had breast cancer, your doctor may discuss genetic testing (see page 212) to determine if you have a genetic mutation in one of these genes. You may be able to delay or prevent the cancer or at least have it diagnosed at an early stage.

- **Radiation therapy**   Women whose breasts have been exposed to radiation therapy, such as for lymphoma, are at increased risk for breast cancer. Treatment with radiation during childhood or puberty, especially radiation to the chest and neck, seems to increase breast cancer risk more than treatment as an adult. Keep in mind, however, that the low level of radiation used in mammograms (see page 191) does not increase a woman's risk for breast cancer. Any potential risk from mammograms is greatly outweighed by the benefit of getting regular mammograms to detect cancer early, when a cure or effective treatment is more likely.

- **Hormone replacement therapy** Combination hormone replacement therapy (HRT; see page 520) using estrogen and a form of the female hormone progesterone (progestin) is linked to a slightly increased risk for breast cancer. But evidence of a link between estrogen-only therapy and breast cancer is not conclusive.

- **Obesity** After menopause, women who are obese have a higher risk of developing breast cancer and a higher risk of dying from breast cancer than women who are at a healthy weight. The increased risk may result from higher levels of estrogen in obese women because, after menopause, fat cells produce estrogen. The high death rates may be due to the cancer being diagnosed at a later stage in heavier women because breast tumors may be more difficult to detect.

- **Alcohol** Drinking alcohol has been linked to increased breast cancer risk. The more you drink, the higher the risk.

PREVENTION

The following factors may help protect against breast cancer. Some of these factors are more controllable than others:

- **Pregnancy** Estrogen levels are lower during pregnancy. The risk for breast cancer appears to be lower if a woman has her first full-term pregnancy before she is 20 years old. This may be because early pregnancy causes breast cells to mature, which makes them less likely to undergo changes that could lead to cancer.

- **Breastfeeding** Estrogen levels tend to remain lower while a woman is breastfeeding, especially when breast milk is a baby's sole source of nourishment.

- **Late menstruation** Beginning to have menstrual periods at age 14 or older decreases the number of years the breast tissue is exposed to estrogen.

- **Early menopause**   The fewer years a woman menstruates, the shorter the time her breast tissue is exposed to estrogen.

- **Hormone replacement therapy**   Long-term use of hormone-replacement therapy with estrogen and progesterone slightly increases breast cancer risk. If you have difficult menopause symptoms, it is probably all right to take HRT for up to five years. After that, breast cancer risk seems to go up. This may also be true for using HRT after age 60, because breast cancer risk rises with age.

- **Fiber intake**   Boosting fiber consumption to between 20 and 30 grams daily—double the amount most people take in—may lower the amount of estrogen circulating in the bloodstream. Eat more beans, lentils, fresh fruit, vegetables, and whole grains.

- **Alcohol**   No matter what type of alcoholic beverage you prefer—beer, wine or liquor—they all increase breast cancer risk to the same extent. Drinking more than three alcoholic drinks a day boosts breast cancer risk by 30 percent.

- **Healthy weight**   Women who have an inherited risk for breast cancer are 65 percent less likely to develop the disease if they lose weight between the ages of 18 and 30 years.

- **Exercise**   Numerous studies suggest that people who exercise regularly are less likely to get breast cancer. Exercising four or more hours a week may lower estrogen levels and help reduce breast cancer risk.

- **Aspirin**   Taking one aspirin a week may help protect against breast cancer, but don't do this without talking to your doctor first. Over the long term, aspirin can cause stomach inflammation, bleeding, and ulcers. Don't take aspirin if you have ever had ulcers, liver or kidney disease, bleeding disorders, or bleeding in the stomach or intestines.

More extreme preventive measures that should be considered only by women with a very high risk of breast cancer include the following:

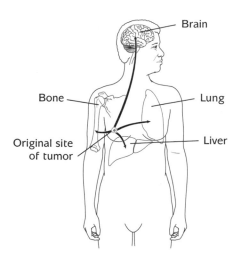

Where breast cancer spreads

Groups of lymph nodes under the arms and in the chest can act as passages for the spread of breast cancer. Breast cancer cells can enter the lymph nodes and be carried in the lymphatic system and bloodstream throughout the body. The sites to which breast cancer most often spreads are the lungs, liver, bones, or brain.

- **Ovary removal**   The amount of estrogen made by the body can be greatly reduced by removing one or both ovaries, which produce estrogen. There is also medication available that lowers the amount of estrogen the ovaries make.

- **Breast removal**   Surgical removal of both breasts (a double mastectomy) greatly lowers a woman's chances of developing breast cancer. However, prophylactic breast removal should be considered only in women who have a strong family history of the disorder or have been found to have the breast cancer genes BRCA1 or BRCA2.

Ovarian cancer

Growths found in the ovaries may be noncancerous fluid-filled growths called cysts or cancerous growths that can spread to other parts of the body. In the United States, ovarian cancer is a major cause of cancer death in women; more women die of ovarian cancer each year than of cervical and endometrial cancers combined. Survival rates for ovarian cancer have not improved much in recent years, and no good screening test is available to detect the cancer at an early stage. The exact cause of ovarian cancer remains unknown, but the disorder has a strong inherited component.

Ovaries, uterus, and cervix

The ovaries and the uterus make up the primary female reproductive organs. The ovaries sit on either side of the uterus, just above the pubic bone. Each ovary contains thousands of eggs, most of which a woman is born with. During each menstrual cycle, one egg (sometimes more) ripens and is released into a fallopian tube. As the egg travels slowly down the tube toward the uterus, it can be fertilized by a sperm. The uterus lies in the pelvis, behind the bladder. The walls of the uterus consist of powerful muscles that contract to push out a baby during delivery. At the lower end of the uterus is a narrow, thick-walled structure called the cervix, which opens into the vagina.

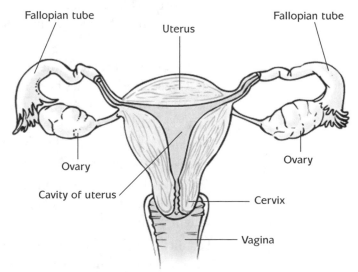

Fallopian tube

Uterus

Fallopian tube

Ovary

Ovary

Cavity of uterus

Cervix

Vagina

RISK FACTORS

Most women with ovarian cancer do not have any known risk factors, and only a small number of women who have risk factors develop ovarian cancer.

- **Age**   The risk of developing ovarian cancer increases after menopause. Half of all cases occur in women over age 63.

- **Reproductive history**   Women who started menstruating at a young age (before age 12), had no children or had their first child after age 30, or went through menopause after age 50 may be at increased risk for ovarian cancer. The increased risk seems to be related to the number of times a woman ovulates during her lifetime, with the risk lower in women who have ovulated less, such as women who have taken birth-control pills or who have had several pregnancies.

- **Family history of ovarian, breast, or colon cancer**   Women with a strong family history of ovarian cancer (in a mother, a sister, or a daughter) are at increased risk of developing the cancer, especially if the cancer occurred at a young age (younger than 55). The younger the age at which the cancer occurred, the higher the risk. About 10 percent of cases develop in women who have inherited the breast cancer gene BRCA1 or BRCA2 or the gene for hereditary nonpolyposis colon cancer, an inherited form of colon cancer.

- **History of breast cancer**   Women who have had breast cancer are at increased risk for ovarian cancer. Some of the inherited risks for breast cancer, such as the BRCA1 and BRCA2 genes, are the same for ovarian cancer.

- **Hormone replacement therapy**   Hormone replacement therapy (HRT; see page 520) has been linked to an increased risk for ovarian cancer in women after menopause, but studies have been contradictory. The risk may go up with longer use of HRT (for 10 or more years), and the risk may be higher with estrogen-only therapy than with estrogen-progestin therapy.

- **Obesity**   Being obese seems to worsen ovarian cancer. Heavier women have a higher risk of dying from ovarian cancer than normal-weight women.

- **Fertility drugs**   Some research has found an increased risk of ovarian cancer in women who have used fertility drugs, especially in those who don't become pregnant. But infertility also increases the risk for ovarian cancer. More research is needed to clarify these relationships.

PREVENTION

The following steps may help you reduce your risk for ovarian cancer even if you have a family history of the disorder:

- **Birth-control pills**   Taking oral contraceptives reduces a woman's risk of developing ovarian cancer. The longer you use oral contraceptives, the lower your risk might be, and the decreased risk may last up to 25 years after you stop taking them. This lower risk occurs both in women who have given birth and in women who have not. Oral contraceptives may even protect against ovarian cancer in women who are at higher risk because they have inherited a BRCA1 or BRCA2 gene. Disadvantages of taking birth-control pills include an increased risk for blood clots that can block blood vessels, especially in smokers over age 35, and a slightly increased short-term risk of breast cancer that decreases over time after a woman stops taking them.

- **Pregnancy and breastfeeding**   Women who have had at least one pregnancy are less likely to develop ovarian cancer than women who have never had children. Breastfeeding also reduces the risk. Both pregnancy and breastfeeding block ovulation, thereby reducing the cell turnover that occurs during ovulation that can increase the chances for abnormal cell changes that can lead to cancer.

- **Tubal ligation or hysterectomy**   Women who have undergone surgical sterilization (tubal ligation) or hysterectomy (surgical removal of the uterus) seem to have a lower risk of developing ovarian cancer.

- **Removal of ovaries**   Women who have a very strong family history of ovarian cancer or who have been found by genetic testing (see page 212) to have inherited the BRCA1 or BRCA2 genes sometimes decide to have prophylactic oophorectomy (removal of both ovaries) and salpingectomy (removal of the fallopian tubes). This greatly reduces their risk for ovarian cancer. After removal of the ovaries, there is still a small chance that ovarian cancer may develop in nearby abdominal and pelvic tissue. Before making this irreversible decision, have a cancer risk assessment and genetic counseling. The disadvantages of having your ovaries removed include the loss of fertility, hot flashes, lowered sexual desire, vaginal dryness, frequent urination, bone loss, and an increased risk for heart disease.

Endometrial cancer

In the United States, endometrial cancer is the most common cancer of the female reproductive system. Also known as uterine cancer, the disease primarily affects women after menopause. In the past few years, the number of new cases of endometrial cancer has been decreasing, as has the number of deaths from the cancer. Endometrial cancer occurs more often in white women than in black women. The cancer is less likely to be fatal than most other female reproductive cancers because it tends to grow very slowly and is relatively easy to diagnose at an early stage.

RISK FACTORS

As with most types of cancer, certain risk factors make it more likely for women to develop endometrial cancer. But keep in mind that many women with one or more of these risk factors never develop endometrial cancer, and some women who have endometrial cancer do not have any of these risk factors. Even after a diagnosis of endometrial cancer, it is impossible to determine which, if any, of the following risk factors is responsible:

- **Estrogen therapy**   Women who have not had their uterus removed and who take hormone replacement therapy (HRT; see page 520) with estrogen alone for five years or more to treat the symptoms of menopause have a 10 times greater risk of developing endometrial cancer than women who don't take estrogen. Adding progesterone (in the form of progestin) to the estrogen in HRT lowers the risk; progestin counteracts the buildup of tissue in the endometrium (lining of the uterus) that is stimulated by estrogen; this buildup of tissue can lead to cancerous changes in cells in the endometrium.

- **Reproductive history**   The more menstrual cycles (ovulation) a woman has during her lifetime, the higher her risk for endometrial cancer. Starting to menstruate at a young age (before age 12) and going through menopause after age 50 increase the risk for endometrial cancer. For the same reason, women who have never been pregnant have a greater risk of developing endometrial cancer than women who have had children (perhaps because progesterone, which reduces endometrial growth, is more prominent than estrogen during pregnancy). Women who breastfeed may also lower their risk because they usually don't ovulate when breast milk is their baby's sole source of nourishment.

- **Being overweight**   Being overweight greatly increases a woman's risk for endometrial cancer. Overweight women have higher levels of circulating estrogen because fat cells can change other hormones into estrogen. Compared with women who are at a healthy weight, endometrial cancer is twice as common in overweight women and more than three times as common in obese women.

- **Being physically inactive**   Being physically inactive can double your risk for endometrial cancer compared with women who exercise every day.

- **Tamoxifen**   Tamoxifen is a selective estrogen receptor modulator (SERM) that is used to treat breast cancer and to prevent breast cancer in high-risk women. Although it acts against estrogen in breast tissue, tamoxifen acts like an estrogen in the uterus, causing the endometrium to grow and slightly increasing a woman's risk for endometrial cancer. Raloxifene, another SERM, has not been shown to increase the risk for endometrial cancer.

- **Ovarian conditions**   An ovarian tumor called a granulose-theca cell tumor can increase a woman's estrogen levels. Women with polycystic ovarian syndrome (a disorder involving the hormones made by the ovaries) have higher-than-normal estrogen levels and lower-than-normal levels of progesterone. Both of these conditions increase the risk for endometrial cancer.

- **Diabetes**   For unknown reasons, women with diabetes have a four-fold higher risk for endometrial cancer than women without diabetes.

- **Hereditary conditions**   In a small number of women, endometrial cancer is caused by genes that also put them at risk for breast cancer or ovarian cancer (the BRCA1 or BRCA2 genes), or colon cancer (the genes for hereditary nonpolyposis colon cancer).

- **Radiation therapy to the pelvis**   Women who have had radiation therapy to treat a previous cancer in the pelvic area may be at increased risk of developing a second cancer in the area, such as endometrial cancer. Radiation can damage the DNA of cells and cause changes that could lead to cancer.

Although most cases of endometrial cancer cannot be prevented, the following measures may help you lower your risk:

- **Take birth-control pills.** The use of combination estrogen-progestin oral contraceptives by women before menopause has been shown to lower the risk for endometrial cancer, ranging from a 50 percent decrease after 4 years of use to a 72 percent decrease after 12 or more years of use. However, because birth-control pills can increase the risk for blood clots in some women (especially in women over age 35 who smoke), talk to your doctor about the benefits and risks for you.

- **Avoid estrogen-only hormone therapy.** Taking hormone replacement therapy (HRT) with estrogen alone greatly elevates endometrial cancer risk. Taking progesterone (progestin) along with the estrogen in HRT counteracts the effects of estrogen on the buildup of endometrial tissue.

- **Have symptoms checked out by your doctor.** Abnormal vaginal bleeding is the most common sign of endometrial precancers (such as endometrial hyperplasia) or endometrial cancer. If you notice any unusual vaginal bleeding or spotting, see your doctor right away. To prevent endometrial hyperplasia from possibly becoming cancerous, it can be treated by taking progestins (to block cell growth in the endometrium); by a dilation and curettage (D&C), which scrapes away the abnormal endometrial tissue; or by a hysterectomy (surgical removal of the uterus).

- **Keep your weight down.** Because being overweight increases endometrial cancer risk, keeping your weight in a healthy range may help reduce your risk.

- **Exercise regularly.** Women who exercise every day are half as likely to develop endometrial cancer as women who are not physically active.

- **If you have diabetes, carefully control it.** Because women with diabetes are at increased risk for endometrial cancer, keeping your blood glucose levels under control (see page 201) can significantly reduce your risk. Good control of your blood sugar can also reduce your risk for the serious complications that can result from uncontrolled diabetes.

Cervical cancer

Cervical cancer forms in the tissues of the cervix (the lower portion of the uterus that opens into the vagina). It is usually a slow-growing cancer that may not produce symptoms but that can be detected with regular Pap tests (see page 188). Each year, more than 11,000 new cases of cervical cancer are diagnosed in the United States and nearly 4,000 deaths are attributed to the cancer.

A group of viruses called the human papillomaviruses (HPVs) are the No. 1 cause of cervical cancer. There are more than 100 HPVs that cause warts. Some warts commonly grow on the hands and feet, and different types of HPVs cause growths in the genital area called genital warts.

Although most women with cervical cancer have the human papillomavirus infection, not all women with an HPV infection develop cervical cancer. Many different types of HPV can affect the cervix and only some of them produce abnormalities in cells that can become cancerous. Some HPV infections go away without treatment.

Before cervical cancer develops, the cells of the cervix go through changes called dysplasia, in which abnormal cells start appearing in the cervical tissue. The abnormal cells usually revert to normal, but sometimes they can become cancerous and spread more deeply into the cervix and to surrounding areas. Cervical dysplasia occurs more often in women in their 20s and 30s. Death from cervical cancer is rare in women younger than 30 and in women of any age who have regular screenings with the Pap test.

Women who do not have regular Pap tests face an increased risk of developing cervical cancer. The risk of death from cervical cancer increases with age. It is highest for white women between the ages of 45 and 70 and for black women in their 70s. However, widespread screening with the Pap test has caused the number of deaths from cervical cancer to decrease dramatically in the United States.

RISK FACTORS

Women are fortunate that there is an effective, reliable screening test available that can detect early, potentially precancerous changes in cells in the cervix and allow doctors to remove the abnormal cells and prevent the cancer from developing. Having regular Pap tests can significantly reduce a woman's risk of developing the cancer. Following are the major risk factors for cervical cancer:

- **HPV infection** Infection in the cervix with HPV is the major risk factor for cervical cancer. About 30 types of HPV can be transmitted through sexual activity and infect the cervix; about half of these have been linked to cervical cancer.

- **Having many sexual partners** Women who have had many sexual partners have an increased risk for HPV infection and cervical cancer. Using condoms and other barrier methods of birth control provides some protection but does not fully protect against HPV, because no barrier contraceptive completely covers the outer genital area.

- **Having first sexual intercourse at a young age** Women who become sexually active at a young age and have many sexual partners have a high risk for HPV infection and cervical cancer.

- **Failure to have regular Pap tests** HPV infection is widespread in the population among both males and females, and the virus spreads easily during sexual activity. Regular Pap tests can detect HPV infection and precancerous changes and enable a woman to avoid cervical cancer.

- **Having a weakened immune system** Women with a weakened immune system, such as from HIV/AIDS or from taking immune-suppressing drugs after a transplant, have an increased risk for cervical cancer because they are more vulnerable to HPV infection. Also, precancerous changes can develop more quickly into cancer in a woman with a weakened immune system.

- **DES exposure** Between 1940 and 1971, many doctors prescribed the hormone diethylstilbestrol (DES) to pregnant women to prevent miscarriage. It was later found that the hormone raised the risk for cervical cancer and cancer of the vagina in the daughters of these women. About 1 out of every 1,000 women whose mother took DES develops cancer of the cervix or vagina. If you were born between 1940 and 1972 and you think you may have been (or don't know if you have been) exposed to DES, ask your doctor how to find out your exposure risk and what screening tests you should have.

- **Smoking** Cigarette smokers have twice the rate of cervical cancer of nonsmokers. Cancer-causing substances in cigarette smoke are carried in the bloodstream throughout the body; by-products of tobacco have been found in the cervical mucus of women who smoke. These substances may contribute to the development of cervical cancer by damaging the genetic material of cells in the cervix.

- **Family history** Cervical cancer may run in some families, but the reasons for this are not clearly understood. If a woman's mother or sister had cervical cancer, her risk of developing the cancer is doubled or tripled compared with women who don't have a family history of the cancer.

PREVENTION

To protect against cervical cancer, take the following precautions:

- **Consider having the HPV vaccination.** A vaccination against HPV (see page 171) is available that is highly effective in preventing infection with the two "high-risk" strains of HPV that cause 70 percent of all cervical cancers, and the types that cause 90 percent of all genital warts. Talk to your doctor about having the vaccination.

- **Have regular Pap smears.** Having gynecological exams and Pap tests helps to prevent cervical cancer. The Pap test finds early abnormal changes in the cervix so they can be treated before cancer develops. Women who don't have Pap tests regularly are at increased risk for cervical cancer.

- **Avoid having multiple sex partners.** The more sex partners you have, the more likely you are to be exposed to HPV, the major cause of cervical cancer.

- **Practice safe sex.** If you are not in a mutually monogamous relationship, use a condom correctly every time you have sex, including oral and anal sex. Although HPV infection can occur in genital areas that are not covered by a condom, condom use has been linked to a lower rate of cervical cancer.

Vaginal and vulvar cancer

Cancer that forms in the tissues of the vagina is rare; only about 2,000 cases are diagnosed each year in the United States, usually in women over age 60. The most common type of vaginal cancer is squamous cell carcinoma, which starts in the thin, flat cells (squamous cells) that line the vagina. Another type of vaginal cancer is adenocarcinoma, which begins in glandular cells in the lining of the vagina.

Cancer of the vulva (the external female genital organs, including the clitoris, vaginal lips, and opening to the vagina) is also rare; only about 3,500 cases occur each year in the United States. Vulvar cancer tends to develop slowly over a number of years.

RISK FACTORS

Your risk for vaginal or vulvar cancer is higher if you have ever had a human papillomavirus (HPV; see page 170) infection, which causes genital warts. HPV infection can cause abnormal changes in genital cells that can become cancerous.

You are also at increased risk for vaginal cancer if your mother took diethylstilbestrol (DES) when she was pregnant with you. DES, a synthetic form of estrogen, was prescribed between 1938 and 1971 to treat some complications of pregnancy. In 1971, DES was linked to clear cell adenocarcinoma in a small number of daughters of women who had used DES during pregnancy. This uncommon cancer is usually diagnosed between ages 15 and 25 in DES-exposed daughters. Although clear cell adenocarcinoma is extremely rare, it's important that DES-exposed daughters be aware of the risk and have regular pelvic examinations.

PREVENTION

Prevention strategies for vaginal and vulvar cancer include the following:

- **Avoid having multiple sex partners.** The more sex partners you have, the higher your exposure to the HPV viruses and potential cancers in the genital area.

- **Practice safe sex.** Use a condom every time you have sex. Latex condoms protect against HPV and many other sexually transmitted diseases.

- **Have regular Pap tests.** A Pap test (see page 188) can detect abnormal changes in the genital area that can become cancerous. Have a Pap test as often as your doctor recommends.

Men's cancers

Men can develop a number of different types of cancer, including cancer of the prostate, the testicle, and the penis. Men are well known for avoiding the doctor's office and ignoring symptoms, but early detection and treatment of these cancers can dramatically improve their chances of survival. If something seems suspicious, don't wait. See your doctor promptly for a diagnosis and early treatment.

Prostate cancer

Prostate cancer is the most common cancer in American men and is the second leading cause of cancer deaths in American men, after lung cancer. Doctors diagnose more than 200,000 new cases of prostate cancer each year in the United States. Although the number of men with this disease is large, the number of men who are expected to die of the disease is considerably smaller.

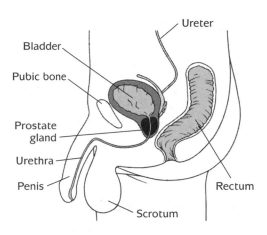

Cancer that forms in tissues of the prostate usually occurs in older men. What causes prostate cancer and why one man develops it and another does not are not fully understood.

RISK FACTORS

Most men who have known risk factors such as the following do not develop prostate cancer. Conversely, men who develop prostate cancer often have none of the known risk factors, except for growing older.

- **Age**   The chance of developing prostate cancer goes up sharply as a man gets older. In the United States, most men with prostate cancer are over age 65. The cancer is rare in men younger than age 45.

- **Family history**   A man's risk is higher if his father or brother had prostate cancer.

- **Changes in prostate cells**   Men with abnormal prostate cells called high-grade prostatic intraepithelial neoplasia (PIN) may be at increased risk for prostate cancer. These prostate cells look abnormal under a microscope.

- **Race**   The risk for prostate cancer is high among blacks, moderately high among whites, and lowest among native Japanese. Studies have shown a link between high levels of testosterone and prostate cancer risk.

- **Diet** Some studies suggest that men who eat a diet high in animal fat or meat may be at increased risk for prostate cancer. Men who eat a diet rich in fruits and vegetables seem to have a lower risk.

PREVENTION

You can help protect against prostate cancer by minimizing the risk factors you can control. That means consuming plenty of fruits and vegetables, eating less red meat, and avoiding animal fat. Some studies suggest that eating foods with the antioxidant lycopene, such as tomatoes and some other fruits and vegetables, may help reduce the risk for prostate cancer. Some researchers are studying whether the mineral selenium and vitamin E can also help reduce prostate cancer risk.

Testicular cancer

Testicular cancer is the most common cancer in young men ages 15 to 35. However, the cancer is rare, accounting for only about 1 percent of all cancers in men. It is much more common in whites than in blacks. The incidence of testicular cancer has risen over the last century, although the reasons for this are not clear. Most testicular cancers are found by men themselves, but doctors usually examine the testicles during routine physical exams.

RISK FACTORS

Risk factors for testicular cancer include the following:

- Having an undescended testicle
- History of cancer in one testicle
- Family history of testicular cancer
- Exposure to some chemicals (such as Agent Orange during the Vietnam War)
- Having a rare condition in which the testicles don't develop normally

PREVENTION

There is little you can do to prevent testicular cancer. However, finding it early, when it is most treatable, provides the best chances for a good outcome. That's why you should perform a testicle self-exam at least every month (it's easiest after you shower or bathe), get regular checkups that include a testicle exam, and see your doctor right away if you notice anything unusual.

Cancer of the penis

Cancer of the penis is very rare. Only about 1,300 new cases and 300 deaths occur each year in the United States. Most penile cancers are squamous cell cancers, which begin in the skin around the glans (head) of the penis. The cause is unknown.

RISK FACTORS

Infection with the human papillomavirus (HPV; see page 170) may be a risk factor for cancer of the penis. The virus is sexually transmitted and is recognized as the major cause of cervical cancer in women. Having many sexual partners is a risk factor for HPV infection. Studies have shown a lower incidence of penis cancer from HPV in men who have been circumcised. Risk factors include the following:

- Being age 60 or older
- Having phimosis (a condition in which the foreskin cannot be pulled back over the head of the penis; see page 509)
- Having poor personal hygiene
- Having many sexual partners
- Using tobacco products

10

PREVENTING INFECTIONS

INFECTIONS ARE CAUSED BY MICROORGANISMS—including bacteria, viruses, fungi, and protozoa—that can invade the body and multiply inside. Your immune system is a group of organs, cells, and proteins that can recognize these foreign invaders, seek them out, and destroy them. The immune system attacks with white blood cells or with proteins called antibodies. The symptoms you have from an infection—such as fever, pain, and inflammation—are the result of this immune-system response.

The steps you need to take to prevent an infection depend on how the infection is spread, but a few commonsense steps can help protect you and others in many situations. Wash your hands frequently, especially before you eat and after you use the toilet. Keep your children home from school when they have a cold, the flu, or any other contagious disease. Cook and handle foods properly to make sure you don't spread a food-borne infection. This chapter covers infectious diseases, including common infections like colds and the flu; infections transmitted by insects, animals, and pets; and food-borne infections.

Common bacterial and viral infections

Bacteria and viruses are the two kinds of microorganisms that cause most infections. Bacteria live everywhere, and many beneficial bacteria live in and on the human body. Problems arise when harmful bacteria enter the body or when beneficial bacteria multiply in greater-than-normal numbers. Some bacteria produce toxins that damage cells. Antibiotics effectively treat most bacterial infections.

Viruses cause infection by invading cells and taking over the cells' machinery to make copies of themselves. In the process, the cells they invade are usually destroyed. The newly produced viruses then invade other cells, continuing the cycle of multiplication and cell destruction. Antibiotics do not work against viruses, but some viral infections can be treated with antiviral drugs.

The common cold

Sneezing, a scratchy throat, a runny nose—everyone is familiar with the first signs of a cold. Although the common cold is usually mild, with symptoms lasting from one to two weeks at most, it is a leading cause of doctor visits and missed days from school and work. According to some estimates, Americans experience 1 billion colds every year. Cold viruses spread in two ways: by touching virus-contaminated surfaces such as telephones or doorknobs and then touching your eyes, nose, or mouth; and by inhaling virus-containing droplets of mucus from an infected person's cough or sneeze.

Children have six to ten colds a year on average. One reason colds are so common in children is that they are often in close physical contact with other children in day care centers and schools. Adults average about two to four colds a year, although the range varies widely. Women, especially those between ages 20 and 30, have more colds than men, probably because of their closer contact with children. On average, people older than 60 have fewer than one cold a year—perhaps because they have already been exposed to many of the viruses that cause colds.

In the United States, most colds occur during the fall and winter. Beginning in late August or early September, the rate of colds increases slowly for a few weeks and remains high until March or April, when it declines. The seasonal variation may relate to the opening of school and to cold weather, which prompt people to spend more time indoors, increasing the chances that viruses will spread from person to person.

Seasonal changes in humidity also affect the prevalence of colds. The most common cold-causing viruses survive better when humidity is low, especially during the colder months of the year. Cold weather can also make the inside lining of the nose drier and more vulnerable to viral infections.

More than 200 different viruses are known to cause the common cold. Colds always spread from one person to another. You can't get a cold from exposure to cold weather or from getting chilled or overheated. Nor do factors such as exercise, diet, or enlarged tonsils or adenoids cause colds. On the other hand, research suggests that psychological stress and allergic diseases affecting the nose or throat can increase the risk for colds.

PREVENTION

Here are some steps you can take to avoid getting a cold or passing a cold to others. Make sure you teach your children how to protect themselves—and remind them of the following whenever necessary:

- Wash your hands often with soap and water. When water isn't available, use an alcohol-based hand sanitizer.
- Keep your hands away from your eyes, mouth, and nose.
- Avoid getting close to people who have colds.
- If you have a cold, avoid getting close to people.
- If you sneeze or cough, cover your nose or mouth, and then wash your hands.

Some people have tried the following measures for preventing and treating colds, and some have made claims that they help relieve their symptoms:

- **Echinacea** Echinacea is a dietary herbal supplement that some people use to relieve cold symptoms. The herb may be somewhat helpful if taken in the early stage of a cold, but it won't help prevent you from getting a cold.
- **Vitamin C** Many people are convinced that taking large doses of vitamin C will prevent colds or relieve cold symptoms, but the scientific evidence for this is nonconclusive and contradictory. Some research has shown that taking vitamin C can shorten a cold or even prevent colds. Other studies have suggested that vitamin C has no

effect on a cold's severity or length, but that it can limit how often a person gets colds.

The bottom line is that vitamin C may help a cold only if a person has insufficient levels of the vitamin to begin with. Also, the effects may vary by individual. Taking vitamin C over long periods in large amounts may be harmful, especially in people with kidney disease. Also, taking excessive amounts of vitamin C can cause diarrhea.

- **Zinc** Zinc lozenges became popular after medical research showed they could reduce the severity and length of colds. But many zinc studies are not scientifically sound. Zinc seems to be most effective when taken as a lozenge within a day of the onset of cold symptoms.

- **Humidity** Cold viruses flourish in dry air and in the parched mucous membranes of the nose and throat. Use a humidifier to add humidity to your surroundings, but change the water daily and clean the humidifier every other day to prevent the buildup of mold, fungi, and bacteria—which can make you even sicker.

- **Saltwater gargle** To ease a sore throat, dissolve ½ teaspoon of salt in an 8-ounce glass of warm water and gargle nightly while your throat is sore.

- **Saline nasal spray** Over-the-counter saline nasal sprays can help relieve a stuffy nose. Saline sprays are safe for children, too.

- **Chicken soup** Your mother was right: chicken soup may help relieve some of the discomfort of colds and the flu. It seems that chicken soup may reduce inflammation and increase the rate at which mucus moves through the nasal passages, reducing congestion. If nothing else, warm liquids often help relieve cold symptoms temporarily.

What has been proven *not* to work against colds? The following have no effect on colds or the flu:

- **Antibiotics are not for colds.** Colds and the flu are caused by viruses; antibiotics work only against bacterial infections. Taking antibiotics for a cold or the flu can be harmful because doing so can contribute to the development of strains of bacteria that are resistant to the effects of antibiotics (see box on page 303). Do not expect your doctor to prescribe an antibiotic for a cold.

- **Over-the-counter cough syrups are not for colds.** Do not take cough syrup when you have a cold—and don't give it to your children.

Coughing is beneficial because it clears mucus from the lower part of the airways. Suppressing a cough can make cold symptoms worse. And the ingredients in some cough syrups may be harmful to children.

- **Don't "starve a cold."** The longtime message to starve a cold is not good advice. Not eating when you have a cold will not shorten the duration of your cold or make the symptoms any better. In fact, a lack of nutrition may worsen or prolong a cold by weakening your immune system.

Influenza

Influenza, or flu for short, is a very contagious infection that causes high fever, chills, a dry cough, sore throat, runny or stuffy nose, headache, prominent muscle aches, and extreme fatigue. The flu is more severe and long-lasting than a cold and can be life-threatening in infants, older adults, and people with respiratory problems such as asthma.

PREVENTION

The same preventive methods that work for a cold (see page 297) can help protect against the flu. But with the flu, there is a very effective prevention option: a yearly flu shot. Flu viruses change from year to year, which is why you need to have a flu shot every year. To give your body time to build up anti-flu defenses, you should have the shot between September and mid-November, before flu season starts. Side effects from the flu shot are mild for most people, including soreness, redness, or swelling at the site of the shot. About 5 to 10 percent of people have minor side effects such as headache or a low-grade fever, which last for about a day after the shot. You should not get the vaccination if you are highly allergic to eggs or latex (components of the vaccine).

The flu vaccine also comes in the form of a nasal spray. This option is available for some people who can't tolerate a shot. The nasal spray is not recommended for infants or people with asthma.

Pneumococcal disease

You may have heard of pneumococcal pneumonia, which affects the lungs, but the bacteria that cause this type of pneumonia can also attack other parts of the body. When the pneumococcal bacteria invade the lining of the brain, they cause meningitis. Entering the bloodstream, they can cause septic shock, which may lead to organ failure. They can also cause middle ear and sinus infections.

PREVENTION

All people 65 years of age and older should have the pneumococcal vaccination. In addition, adults and children older than 2 years who have certain chronic diseases should be vaccinated. Check with your doctor to see if you would benefit from having the pneumococcal vaccination. The shot is safe and can be given at the same time as the flu shot. Most people need only a single dose of the penumococcal vaccine, but the protective effect can wear off over time, so a booster may be needed after 5 or 10 years. The vaccine can protect against the most common strains of pneumococcal bacteria.

About half of people who get the pneumococcal shot have minor side effects such as temporary swelling, redness, and soreness at the site on the arm where the shot was given. A few people have fever, muscle pain, or more severe swelling and pain in the arm.

Tetanus, diphtheria, and pertussis

Tetanus (sometimes called lockjaw) is caused by toxins produced by bacteria called Clostridium tetani. The bacteria can enter the body through a tiny pinprick or scratch, but they most often enter through deep puncture wounds or cuts such as those made by nails or knives. Tetanus bacteria are commonly present in soil, dust, and manure. The disease cannot spread from person to person. Common initial signs of tetanus are headache and

---

TDAP VACCINATION NOW RECOMMENDED FOR TEENS AND ADULTS

Recent epidemics of pertussis in the United States have caused the Centers for Disease Control and Prevention (CDC) to recommend that adults have at least one Tdap booster shot to help prevent the spread of this dangerous infection. In 2004, there were more than 25,000 cases of pertussis diagnosed in the United States. More than 8,000 of these were among adolescents, and more than 7,000 were among adults. Up to 2 in 100 adolescents and 5 in 100 adults with pertussis are hospitalized or have complications. Talk to your doctor about having the Tdap booster shot.

muscle stiffness in the jaw, followed by stiffness in the neck, difficulty swallowing, muscle spasms, sweating, and fever.

Diphtheria is an infection that affects the tonsils, throat, nose, or skin. Like tetanus, it is caused by the toxins of bacteria (in this case, Corynebacterium diphtheriae), but this infection can spread from an infected person to the nose or throat of another person. Diphtheria can cause breathing problems, heart failure, paralysis, and sometimes death. Other symptoms include a low-grade fever and enlarged lymph nodes in the neck. Diphtheria is sometimes mistaken for a severe sore throat. A second form of diphtheria causes sores on the skin that can be painful, red, and swollen.

Pertussis (whooping cough) is a serious bacterial infection of the respiratory system that makes the air passages inflamed, narrowed, and clogged with thick mucus. The infection is spread by inhaling droplets that have been sneezed or coughed into the air by an infected person. The severe coughing bouts that are characteristic of the infection can cause permanent damage to an infant's lungs or brain.

PREVENTION

Vaccination is the best way to protect against tetanus, diphtheria, and pertussis. Most people receive a series of five vaccinations during childhood in the form of a combined tetanus-diphtheria-pertussis vaccine (Tdap). A combination vaccination against tetanus and diphtheria, called a Td booster, is given to teens and adults. (A newer vaccination is now recommended that includes the pertussis vaccine; see box on previous page.) You need to have a Td shot every 10 years throughout your life. It is especially important to have a booster shot if you have a severe cut or puncture wound and have not had a booster in the past 5 to 10 years. When side effects from the shot occur, they usually are minor and include soreness, redness, or swelling at the site of the shot.

Methicillin-resistant Staphylococcus aureus

Staphylococcus aureus, often referred to simply as "staph," are bacteria that commonly live on the skin and in the nose without causing health problems. But sometimes staph can cause infections. Staph bacteria are one of the most common causes of skin infections in the United States. Most of these skin infections, such as pimples and boils, are minor and can be treated without antibiotics. But staph bacteria also can cause more serious infections, such as surgical wound infections, bloodstream infections, and pneumonia, which require treatment with antibiotics.

Methicillin-resistant Staphylococcus aureus (MRSA) is a type of bacteria that is resistant to certain antibiotics. That means some commonly prescribed antibiotics cannot eliminate it. These antibiotic-resistant bacteria can be spread from person to person through casual contact or through contaminated objects. Staph infections, including MRSA, occur most frequently among people who have a weakened immune system, such as those in hospitals, nursing homes, and dialysis centers.

However, MRSA infections are becoming more widespread in healthy people outside the hospital setting. These infections can occur among young people who have cuts or wounds and have close contact with one another, such as members of sports teams and schoolchildren. They are usually skin infections, such as abscesses, boils, pimples, and other pus-filled sores.

RISK FACTORS

Risk factors for hospital-acquired MRSA include the following:

- Current or recent hospitalization
- Living in a nursing home or other long-term care facility
- Having an invasive procedure such as surgery or insertion of a tube (catheter) into the body
- Recent or long-term antibiotic use

Risk factors for MRSA acquired outside the hospital include the following:

- Young age—because of incomplete development of the immune system
- Participation in contact sports
- Sharing towels, razors, or athletic equipment
- Having a weakened immune system, such as from HIV/AIDS
- Living in crowded or unsanitary conditions, such as in a prison

PREVENTION

To prevent a MRSA infection, follow the same good hygiene practices for avoiding any infection, including a cold or the flu (see page 297). Follow these guidelines to prevent the spread of infection:

- Keep your hands clean by washing thoroughly with soap and water or using an alcohol-based hand sanitizer.
- Keep cuts and scrapes clean and cover them with a bandage until they're healed.
- Avoid contact with other people's wounds or bandages.
- Never share personal items such as towels, razors, or athletic equipment.

WHAT CAUSES ANTIBIOTIC RESISTANCE?

Antibiotics should be used only to treat bacterial infections; they do not work against the viruses that cause the common cold, coughs, runny nose, most sore throats (other than strep, which is bacterial), the flu, or most cases of bronchitis. Don't expect your doctor to prescribe an antibiotic when you have a cold or the flu because taking antibiotics unnecessarily can be harmful. Every time a person takes an antibiotic, bacteria that are sensitive to the effects of the antibiotic are killed, but tougher, resistant bacteria can survive and multiply. As a result, commonly prescribed antibiotics can become powerless against these drug-resistant bacteria, infections become harder to eliminate, and some infections can become fatal in at-risk people, especially the very young, the very old, and people with a weakened immune system. Follow these guidelines for proper use of antibiotics:

- Do not take an antibiotic for a viral infection such as a cold, a cough, or the flu.
- If the doctor prescribes an antibiotic for a bacterial infection, take the antibiotic exactly as instructed. Do not skip doses, and complete the prescribed course of treatment, even if you are feeling better.

- Never save any antibiotics for the next time you get sick. If you have any leftover medication, discard it once you have completed your prescribed course of treatment.
- Never take antibiotics that are prescribed for someone else. The antibiotic may not be appropriate for your illness, and taking the wrong medication may delay appropriate treatment and allow bacteria to multiply and become resistant.

If you are a parent:

- Do not insist that your child's doctor prescribe an antibiotic after he or she has determined it is not needed.
- Ask your child's doctor about antibiotic resistance.
- Do not give your children antibiotics for a viral infection such as a cold, a cough, or the flu. Antibiotics should be used only to treat bacterial infections.
- Make sure that your children take all medication exactly as prescribed, even if they no longer have any symptoms. If treatment stops too soon, some bacteria may survive and cause a reinfection that is harder to treat.

Adult vaccinations

Some vaccinations are essential for most adults, especially older people. Others are appropriate only for people who have specific risk factors. The following list catalogs the diseases that can be prevented in adults by vaccination. Check the list and make sure all your vaccinations are up-to-date.

Diphtheria

Haemophilus influenzae
    type b (Hib)

Hepatitis A

Hepatitis B

Herpes zoster (shingles)

Human papillomavirus (HPV)

Influenza (flu)

Measles

Meningococcus
    (bacterial meningitis)

Mumps

Pneumococcus (pneumonia)

Pertussis (whooping cough)

Polio

Rubella (German measles)

Tetanus (lockjaw)

Varicella (chicken pox)

A vaccination, like any medication, can cause problems such as severe allergic reactions in some people, but for the vast majority of people this risk is extremely small. If you have any unusual symptoms such as a high fever after having a vaccination, tell your doctor right away. Signs of a serious allergic reaction can include difficulty breathing, hoarseness or wheezing, hives, pale skin, weakness, a fast heartbeat, or dizziness.

If you think you or someone you're responsible for might be experiencing a reaction to a recent vaccination, call your doctor, take the person to a doctor right away, or call 911. Tell the doctor what happened, the date and time it happened, and when the vaccination was given. Ask the doctor, nurse, or health department to report the reaction by filing a Vaccine Adverse Event Reporting System (VAERS) form, which enables the government to keep track of adverse reactions to vaccinations.

Infections from insects, animals, and pets

The most common insects known to spread disease are mosquitoes and ticks. Fleas can spread plague, but this disease is uncommon among humans in the United States. It's important to know the basics of infection prevention: what insects pose a problem and why, how to keep them away, and what to do if they bite.

Pets can add fun, companionship, and a feeling of safety to your life. But before getting a pet, think carefully about which animal is best for your family. Who will take care of the pet? Does anyone in the household have pet allergies? What type of animal suits your lifestyle and budget? Once you own a pet, keep it healthy and know the signs of health problems in your pet. Pets can transmit a number of infections, so always wash your hands after handling your pets, especially after cleaning up their droppings or stool.

Salmonella

Salmonella is a bacterial disease caused by Salmonella bacteria. Many different kinds of salmonella can make people sick. People usually get salmonella from eating contaminated food, such as chicken or eggs, but they can also acquire it through contact with animal feces. Reptiles (including lizards, snakes, and turtles), baby chicks, and ducklings are especially likely to pass salmonella to people. So can dogs, cats, birds (including pet birds), horses, and farm animals. Symptoms of salmonella usually include diarrhea, fever, and stomach pain that start one to three days after exposure. These symptoms usually go away after about a week.

PREVENTION

The best advice is to wash your hands with soap and water after you touch a pet or any farm or zoo animal, and after contact with animal feces, such as when changing a cat litter box. Be especially careful to wash your hands after touching reptiles or any objects or surfaces that a reptile has touched. Carry an alcohol-based sanitizer with you in case you don't have easy access to soap and water. If you have a weakened immune system, avoid contact with reptiles, baby chicks, and ducklings. Be extra cautious when visiting farms and touching farm animals, including animals at petting zoos.

Toxoplasmosis

A single-celled parasite called Toxoplasma gondii causes a disease known as toxoplasmosis. The parasite is found throughout the world, and more than 60 million Americans have the infection. Of those, very few have symptoms because a healthy person's immune system usually prevents the parasite from causing illness. However, the infection can cause serious health problems in pregnant women and people with a weakened immune system.

Toxoplasmosis can be acquired in the following ways:

- Accidentally swallowing cat feces from an infected cat. This can happen if you accidentally touch your hands to your mouth after gardening, cleaning a cat litter box, or touching anything that has come into contact with cat feces.

- Eating contaminated raw or partly cooked meat, especially pork, lamb, or venison; or by touching your hands to your mouth after handling undercooked meat.

- Contaminating food with knives, utensils, cutting boards, or other foods that have had contact with raw meat.

- Drinking water contaminated with Toxoplasma.

- Before birth. Most infants who were infected before birth have no symptoms, but they can develop symptoms later in life. A small percentage of infected newborns have serious eye or brain damage at birth.

- Rarely, from an infected organ transplant or blood transfusion.

PREVENTION

Here are some steps you can take to reduce your risk for toxoplasmosis:

- Wear gloves when you garden or do anything outdoors that involves handling soil. Wash your hands well with soap and water after any outdoor activities, especially before you eat or prepare food.

- Cover your children's sandbox to prevent contamination by outdoor cats.

- When preparing raw meat, wash thoroughly with soap and hot water any cutting boards, sinks, knives, and other utensils that might have touched the raw meat to avoid cross-contaminating other foods. Wash your hands well with soap and water after handling raw meat.

- Cook all meat thoroughly—to an internal temperature of 160°F—until it is no longer pink in the center or until the juices become colorless. Don't taste meat before it's fully cooked.

- If you are pregnant, don't change a cat litter box. Avoid gardening unless you wear gloves, and wash your hands thoroughly afterward.

Cats, which can pass the parasite in their feces, often use gardens and sandboxes as litter boxes.

Cat scratch disease

Cat scratch disease is a bacterial disease transmitted through the bite or scratch of an infected cat. Most people with the disorder develop a mild infection at the site of a cat bite or scratch. Lymph nodes, especially those around the head, neck, and upper limbs, usually become swollen. A person can also experience fever, headache, fatigue, and loss of appetite.

Pet cats can spread the disease to people. Kittens are more likely to be infected and pass the bacterium to people than are adult cats. About 40 percent of cats carry the bacterium that causes the disease at some time in their life. Affected cats don't show any signs of illness, so you can't tell which cats can spread the disease.

PREVENTION

You can reduce your risk of acquiring cat scratch disease by taking the following precautions with cats:

- Avoid rough play with cats, especially kittens, to avoid scratches and bites.
- Wash cat bites and scratches immediately and thoroughly with running water and soap.
- Don't allow cats to lick any open wounds you have.
- Fleas can also transmit cat scratch disease. Control fleas on your pet cats and avoid petting outdoor cats.
- Keep your pet cat inside to reduce its chances of getting infected or getting fleas.

If you develop an infection (with pus and swelling) where you were scratched or bitten by a cat, or if you have symptoms such as fever, headache, swollen lymph nodes, or fatigue, contact your doctor right away.

Rabies

Rabies is a life-threatening infection caused by a virus. Rabies is mainly a disease of animals, but humans can get rabies when they're bitten by infected animals. At first, rabies might not cause any symptoms. But weeks, or even years after a bite, rabies can cause pain, fatigue, headaches, fever, and irritability. These symptoms can be followed by seizures, hallucinations, and paralysis. Rabies is ultimately fatal. Wild animals—especially bats—are the most common source of human rabies infection in the United States.

PREVENTION

A rabies vaccination can prevent rabies. If you have been exposed to the rabies virus, you should have the vaccination as soon as possible. People who are at high risk of exposure to rabies—including veterinarians, animal handlers, laboratory workers, and people who often explore caves—should also have the rabies vaccination.

For most people, the most effective way to prevent rabies is to stay away from and refrain from touching or handling stray cats or dogs, or wild animals you might come into contact with. If you have been bitten by an animal, or if you see a bat in your home, hotel room, or sleeping quarters, see a doctor immediately. Bat bites are so small that you may not know you've been bitten. If you have been exposed to the rabies virus and have never been vaccinated against it, you should receive five doses of the vaccine—one dose right away, and additional doses on the 3rd, 7th, 14th, and 28th days after the first dose. You will also be given a shot of rabies immune globulin at the same time as the first dose for immediate protection. If you have been exposed to the virus and have been previously vaccinated, you should get two doses of rabies vaccine—one right away and another three days later.

Tick-borne infections

Ticks are parasites that feed on the blood of animals such as deer, mice, rabbits, or raccoons. Ticks, which are usually found in wooded areas or tall grass, can transmit viruses and bacteria as they feed. Several different types of ticks exist and each can transmit a different disease. The most common tick-borne diseases in the United States are Rocky Mountain spotted fever and Lyme disease.

ROCKY MOUNTAIN SPOTTED FEVER

Rocky Mountain spotted fever is caused by an organism that is spread to humans in the bites of infected ticks. The infection is a severe and frequently reported illness in the United States. Although the disease was first

PREVENTING TICK-BORNE INFECTIONS

Reducing your exposure to ticks is the best defense against tick-borne infections. You and your family can protect yourselves by taking the following steps, especially if you live in or near or visit an area where there are deer, such as a forest, open prairie, or farmland:

- **Wear a long-sleeved shirt and long pants and light-colored clothing.** Tuck your pant legs into your socks so ticks can't travel up your legs. Light-colored clothing lets you see ticks that may be crawling on your clothing.

- **Use tick repellent.** Take special precautions from May through July, when ticks are most active. Spray repellents containing permethrin (see page 311) on your boots and clothing; the protection will last for several days. Repellent containing DEET can be applied to the skin, but will last only a few hours before you have to apply it again. Use DEET with caution and in low concentrations on children (see page 313).

- **Do a self-check.** Each night, check your pants, arms, and legs—and those of your children—for ticks. The bugs can be as small as the period at the end of this sentence and are usually black. Carefully check clothing, pets, and hair. Inspect your entire body using a handheld or full-length mirror. (See right for how to remove a tick.)

- **Use landscaping to provide a tick-safe zone around your home.** Ticks thrive in humid, wooded areas and die in sunny, hot environments. Place wood chips or gravel between your home and lawn. Mow frequently. Remove leaf litter, brush, and tall grass from around your home.

- **Discourage deer.** Never feed deer on your property. Learn about deer-resistant plants. Construct physical barriers to discourage deer from entering your yard.

- **Control ticks around your home and community.** Check with local health officials about the best time to apply tick pesticide in your area, or contact a professional pesticide company to apply pesticides on your property.

How to remove a tick

If you or someone else has been bitten by a tick, follow these steps for removing it:

- Use fine-tipped tweezers to grasp the tick as close to the skin surface as possible and pull upward with steady, even pressure. Don't twist or jerk the tick, or its mouthparts could break off and remain in the skin. If this happens, remove the mouthparts with tweezers.

- After removing the tick, thoroughly clean the bite site with an antiseptic such as rubbing alcohol and wash your hands with soap and water.

- Don't squeeze, crush, or puncture the body of the tick because its fluids can contain infectious microorganisms that could make you sick. Disinfect with rubbing alcohol any part of the skin that was accidentally exposed to tick fluids or wash the area with soap and water.

- Save the tick for identification in case you become sick. Seeing the tick could help your doctor make an accurate diagnosis. Place the tick in a sealable plastic bag and put it in the freezer. Write the date of the bite on a piece of paper and put it in the bag.

discovered and recognized in the Rocky Mountain area (hence the name), few cases are reported from that area now. The disorder occurs throughout the United States during the months of April through September. Over half of all cases occur in the south-Atlantic region, in Delaware, Maryland, Virginia, West Virginia, North Carolina, South Carolina, Georgia, Florida, and Washington, D.C. The highest incidence is in North Carolina and Oklahoma. The infection also occurs in Mexico and in Central and South America.

Initial symptoms of Rocky Mountain spotted fever include a sudden onset of fever, headache, and muscle pain, followed by a rash, joint pain, and diarrhea. The infection can be difficult to diagnose in the early stages because the symptoms resemble those common to many other diseases. But if you have a persistent fever, headache with neck stiffness, and/or a new rash, see your doctor immediately; without proper treatment, the infection can be fatal.

LYME DISEASE

Lyme disease is a bacterial infection transmitted by the deer tick. Within one to two weeks of being infected, affected people usually develop a rash with fever, headache, and muscle or joint pain. The disease sometimes produces a telltale bull's-eye rash, but this symptom does not always appear. Some people have Lyme disease and don't have any early symptoms. After several days or weeks, the bacteria spread throughout the body, producing symptoms such as rashes in other parts of the body, pain that seems to move from joint to joint, and signs of inflammation of the heart or nerves. If the disease remains untreated, it can cause swelling and pain in major joints such as the knees, or mental changes, even months after the initial infection. Lyme disease can also cause long-term heart problems.

Mosquito-borne infections

Mosquito bites can transmit diseases such as West Nile fever, malaria, dengue fever, and yellow fever. West Nile fever is the mosquito-borne disease most prevalent in the United States. Most mosquitoes are not infected and the chances of getting a bite from an infected mosquito are small. But you can take the measures described in this section to reduce the risks even more.

WEST NILE FEVER

West Nile fever is a potentially serious disease caused by a virus that is spread in the bites of infected mosquitoes. In northern climates, most cases appear in late summer and early fall. In southern climates, the virus can be transmitted throughout the year. Mosquitoes become infected with the West Nile virus when they feed on infected birds, and they can then spread the virus to humans and other animals when they bite. The virus does not appear to be spread from person to person or from animals to people. In a few cases, the virus has been spread through blood transfusions, organ transplants, and breast milk, and during pregnancy from mother to fetus.

Most infected people—about 80 percent—have no symptoms. Up to 20 percent have symptoms such as fever, headache, body aches, nausea, vomiting, and sometimes swollen lymph glands or a skin rash on the chest, stomach, or back. Symptoms sometimes last only a few days, but even healthy people have become sick for several weeks. About 1 in 150 infected people develops a severe illness with symptoms such as high fever, headache, neck stiffness, stupor, disorientation, coma, tremors, convulsions, muscle weakness, vision loss, and numbness and paralysis. These symptoms can last for several weeks, and the nervous system effects may be permanent. People usually develop symptoms between 3 and 14 days after the virus-spreading mosquito bite.

PREVENTING WEST NILE VIRUS

People over the age of 50 are more likely to develop serious symptoms of West Nile fever and should take extra care to avoid mosquito bites. The more time you are outdoors, the higher your risk of being bitten by an infected mosquito. When you are outdoors, use insect repellent (see below) containing DEET and wear long-sleeved shirts and long pants when mosquitoes are present, especially at dusk. Be sure to also protect your children. If you find a dead bird, don't handle it with your bare hands. Contact your local health department for instructions on how to report and dispose of it. Usually health department workers will dispose of a dead bird after they log a report to monitor the presence of the West Nile virus in the community.

Using insect repellents

Mosquitoes become attracted to people by their skin odor and by the carbon dioxide from their breath. The ingredients in insect repellents make you less attractive for feeding. Repellents work only at short distances, so you may still see mosquitoes flying around you. Remember that repellents don't kill mosquitoes—they help reduce your exposure to mosquitoes that might carry viruses or other parasites that can cause serious and sometimes life-threatening illnesses.

Apply repellent whenever you're going to be outdoors so you don't have to worry so much about mosquito bites. Even when you don't see any mosquitoes, there's a good chance that they're around. Many of the mosquitoes that carry disease-causing organisms bite between dusk and dawn. If you're outdoors during this time, it is especially important to apply repellent.

You should reapply repellent if you're being bitten by mosquitoes. Always follow the directions on the product you're using. If you sweat, swim, or get caught in heavy rain, you may have to reapply repellent more frequently. Repellents containing a higher concentration (higher percentage) of active ingredients typically provide longer-lasting protection. Products containing DEET (diethyltoluamide) and picaridin usually provide longer-lasting protection than other repellents. DEET is probably the most common effective ingredient found in insect repellents.

Permethrin is another long-lasting repellent that works well, but you can use it only on clothing, shoes, bed nets, and camping gear—not directly on the skin. Permethrin is highly effective as both an insecticide and a repellent. Permethrin-treated clothing repels and kills ticks, mosquitoes, spiders, centipedes, and other insects, and permethrin retains its insect-killing effects after repeated laundering. Always apply permethrin insecticide according to the instructions on the label. Some commercial products, such as bed netting, are available pretreated with permethrin.

Oil of lemon eucalyptus, a plant-based repellent, is fairly effective and it doesn't contain any harmful chemicals. In medical studies, when oil of lemon eucalyptus was tested against mosquitoes found in the United States, it provided protection similar to repellents with low concentrations of DEET.

Choose a repellent that protects you for the

DON'T BE AN INSECT MAGNET: USE INSECT REPELLENTS

Follow these guidelines for safely and effectively using insect repellents:

- Use enough repellent to cover all exposed skin or clothing; heavy application is not necessary to achieve protection.
- Don't apply repellent to skin that is under clothing.
- Don't apply repellent to cuts, wounds, or irritated skin.
- After returning indoors, wash the repellent-treated skin with soap and water. This precaution may vary depending on the product; check the label.
- Don't spray aerosol or pump products in enclosed areas.
- Don't spray aerosol or pump products directly into your or anyone else's face; spray your hands and then rub them carefully over your face, avoiding your eyes and mouth.

amount of time you'll be outdoors. A product with a higher percentage of active ingredients is a good choice if you'll be outdoors for several hours, while one with a lower concentration can be used for shorter periods. If you are concerned about the health effects of using chemical-based insect repellents, talk to your doctor. Depending on your health status, it may be better to be exposed to potentially harmful chemicals for a short time than to be bitten by a mosquito that carries a potentially serious disease.

Insect repellents can sometimes cause reactions such as skin irritation. Eye irritation can occur if a repellent gets in the eyes. If you suspect you are having a reaction to a product, stop using it, wash the affected skin area, and call the doctor. If some of the product gets in your eyes, flush them with water right away and call your doctor. If you go to the doctor, take the product with you.

Insect repellents can be used safely by pregnant or nursing women. Other than the routine precautions described in the box on page 312, you don't have to take any additional protective measures for using registered repellents if you are pregnant or breastfeeding. Talk to your doctor if you have questions.

USING INSECT REPELLENTS ON CHILDREN

Most insect repellent products can be used safely on children, but manufacturers are required to state any age restrictions on the label. If you don't see any restrictions, you can assume the product can be used safely on children. Oil of lemon eucalyptus products should never be used on children under the age of 3.

Because DEET is the most widely available repellent, it provokes the most questions about its use on children. No studies have been done to determine what concentration of DEET is safe for children, because researchers are reluctant to test potentially harmful chemicals on children. However, no serious illness has been linked to the use of DEET in children when it is used according to the manufacturer's recommendations. In general, insect repellents containing DEET that have a concentration of up to 10 percent seem to be safe when used according to the package directions. Repellents with DEET should not be used on infants younger than 2 months. When choosing the type and concentration of repellent to use on your child, take into account the amount of time he or she will be outdoors, the potential for exposure to mosquitoes, and the risk of any mosquito-transmitted diseases in the area.

If you are concerned about using repellents on your children, talk to your children's doctor. Using repellents is not the only way to avoid mosquito bites. Often the best defense is a barrier. Children—like adults—should wear clothing with long pant legs and long sleeves while outdoors. Use mosquito netting over infant carriers and strollers.

Here are some guidelines for safely using insect repellent on children:

- Always follow the recommendations on the product label.
- When using repellent on a child, apply it to your hands and then rub it on your child. Avoid children's eyes and mouth and use repellent sparingly around their ears.
- Don't apply repellent to a child's hands because children tend to put their hands in their mouth.
- Never allow young children to apply insect repellent to themselves.
- Keep repellents out of the reach of children.
- Don't apply repellent under your child's clothing. If you apply repellent to clothing, wash the clothing before letting your child wear it again.

Fungal infections

If you've ever had athlete's foot or a vaginal yeast infection, you can blame a fungus. A fungus is actually a primitive vegetable. The fungus family includes mushrooms, mold, and mildew. Fungi live in the air, in soil, on plants, and in water. Some live in the human body. Only about half of all types of fungi are potentially harmful.

You are more likely to develop a fungal infection if you have a weakened immune system or take antibiotics (which reduce the helpful bacteria that are normally present in the body and prevent fungi from growing). Fungal infections can be difficult to eliminate.

Athlete's foot

Athlete's foot is a common fungal infection caused by a tinea fungus that can be found in areas that are damp, dark, and warm, especially in public locker rooms and showers. Athlete's foot can last for a short or long time and may come back after treatment. The infection is very contagious—it can be transmitted through direct contact with someone else's infection, or from contact with contaminated items such as shoes, stockings, and shower or pool surfaces.

The most common symptoms of athlete's foot are cracked, flaking, and peeling skin between the toes. The affected area is usually red and itchy. You may feel burning or stinging, and have blisters, oozing, or crusting in the area. In addition to the toes, the symptoms can also appear on the heels, palms of the hands, and between the fingers. If the fungus spreads to the nails, they can become discolored and thick, and they may crumble.

PREVENTION

Take these steps to avoid athlete's foot:

- Keep your feet clean and dry, especially between the toes.
- Wash your feet thoroughly with soap and water and dry them carefully and completely at least twice a day.
- Wear clean, cotton socks, and change your socks and shoes as often as needed to keep your feet dry.
- Do not walk barefoot near public pools, showers, locker rooms, or dressing rooms.
- Wear shoes that let air circulate to help keep your feet dry.

Ringworm

Ringworm is a skin and scalp disease caused by a tinea fungus that can grow on skin, hair, or nails. Ringworm on the scalp usually produces a bald patch of scaly skin. People with ringworm on other parts of their skin can have a ring-shaped rash that is reddish and may be itchy. The rash can be dry and scaly or wet and crusty. As its name implies, the rash sometimes looks like a ring—red around the edges and clear in the middle.

You can get ringworm from infected people through skin-to-skin contact and from touching their personal items, such as towels, combs, or razors, or in shared showers and pools. Many different kinds of animals can transmit ringworm to people, through direct contact with an infected animal's skin or hair. Dogs and cats (especially puppies and kittens), cows, goats, pigs, and horses can have ringworm and pass it on to people.

Taking the following steps can help you reduce your exposure to the fungus that causes ringworm:

- Keep your skin and feet clean and dry.
- Shampoo your hair regularly, especially after having a haircut.
- Never share clothing, towels, hairbrushes, combs, headbands, hats, baseball caps, or personal-care items.
- Wear flip-flops in gym locker rooms and at swimming pools.
- Don't touch pets that have bald spots.

Vaginal yeast infections

A yeast infection in the vagina is caused by an overgrowth of the yeast Candida. Yeast normally live in the vagina in small numbers, but when the normal bacteria that are present in the vagina are out of balance (such as can result from taking antibiotics for a bacterial infection), more yeast can grow and cause an infection. Vaginal yeast infections are common; three out of four women have a vaginal yeast infection at some time in their life. Almost half of women have two or more yeast infections. The most common symptom of a yeast infection is extreme itchiness in and around the vagina. Other symptoms include the following:

- Burning, itching, redness, and swelling of the vagina and the area around it
- Pain when urinating
- Pain or discomfort during sex
- A thick, white vaginal discharge that looks like cottage cheese and does not have a bad odor

A woman can develop a vaginal yeast infection from having sex, but this is rare. Many factors, including the following, can change the normal acidity of the vagina and raise the risk for a yeast infection.

- Stress
- Lack of sleep
- Illness
- Poor diet, or excess intake of sugary foods

- Pregnancy
- Having your period
- Taking birth-control pills
- Taking antibiotics
- Taking steroid medications
- Having a disease that weakens the immune system, such as poorly controlled diabetes and HIV/AIDS

PREVENTION

The following tips can help you avoid vaginal yeast infections:

- Do not use douches.
- Avoid scented hygiene products such as bubble bath, sprays, pads, and tampons.
- Change tampons and pads often during periods.
- Do not wear tight underwear or clothes made of synthetic fabrics.
- Wear cotton underwear and pantyhose with a cotton crotch.
- Change out of wet swimsuits and exercise clothes as soon as possible.
- Avoid eating sugary foods.

Food-borne infections

Raw foods of animal origin are those most likely to be contaminated and to transmit infections to people. Especially risky are raw meat and poultry, raw eggs, unpasteurized milk, and raw shellfish. Also risky are foods that mix the meat or dairy products of many animals—such as bulk raw milk, pooled raw eggs, or ground beef—because an organism present in one of the animals can contaminate the batch. It is hard to imagine, but true, that a single hamburger can contain meat from hundreds of animals, that one restaurant omelet can contain eggs from hundreds of chickens, or that a glass of milk can contain milk from hundreds of cows. Manufacturing processes can expose food to potentially dangerous organisms as well. For example, a broiler chicken carcass can be exposed to the drippings and juices of the many thousands of other birds that have gone through the same equipment.

Plant foods—especially raw fruits and vegetables—can also be contaminated. Outbreaks have been traced to fresh fruits and vegetables that were processed under less-than-sanitary conditions. These outbreaks highlight the importance of the quality of the water used for washing and chilling produce after harvest. Using unclean water can contaminate many boxes of produce. Fresh manure used to fertilize vegetables can also contaminate the vegetables with dangerous Escherichia coli (E. coli) bacteria and other organisms. Alfalfa and other raw sprouts can be especially dangerous because the conditions under which they are grown are also ideal for growing microbes, and because sprouts are eaten raw; a few bacteria present on the seeds can multiply into millions on the sprouts. Unpasteurized fruit juice can also become contaminated by germs present in or on the fruit used to make it.

Washing produce can lower the amount of contamination, but not eliminate it. It's a good idea to soak your produce in a sinkful of water to which you've added a healthy splash of white vinegar, which kills bacteria, mold, and viruses. Rinse the produce thoroughly and pat or air dry.

Common symptoms of food-borne illness include diarrhea, abdominal cramping, fever, headache, vomiting, and severe exhaustion. Symptoms can come on as quickly as half an hour after eating the contaminated food, but they may not develop for several days or weeks. Symptoms usually last only a day or two, but in some cases can persist for a week to 10 days. For most healthy people, food-borne illnesses are not long-lasting or life-threatening. The illnesses can be severe in older people, however, because the immune system tends to weaken with age.

PREVENTION

Taking the following simple precautions can reduce your risk for food-borne diseases:

- **Cook meat, poultry, and eggs well.** Use a thermometer to measure the internal temperature of meat to make sure it is cooked sufficiently to kill bacteria. For example, pork and ground beef should be cooked to an internal temperature of 160°F. Eggs should be cooked until the yolk is firm. Fish should be cooked until it is opaque and flakes easily with a fork.

- **Do not cross-contaminate one food with another.** Wash your hands, utensils, and cutting boards after they've been in contact with raw meat or poultry and before they touch other food. After cooking meat, put it on a clean plate, not on the surface that held it when it was raw.

Separate raw meat, poultry, and seafood from other foods in your grocery shopping cart and in your refrigerator. Use different cutting boards for raw meat products and produce.

- **Refrigerate leftovers promptly.** Bacteria can grow quickly at room temperature, so refrigerate leftover foods if you won't be eating them within four hours. Large quantities of food will cool more quickly if you divide them into several shallow containers for refrigeration. Set your refrigerator no higher than 40°F and the freezer unit at 0°F.

- **Wash your produce.** Rinse fresh fruits and vegetables under running tap water to remove visible dirt and grime, and then immerse them in a bath of vinegar and water. Remove and discard the outermost leaves of a head of lettuce or cabbage. Bacteria can grow on the cut surface of fruit or vegetables, so be careful not to contaminate them while

---

AVOIDING INFECTIONS WHEN YOU SWIM

A number of infections can be acquired from wading or swimming in the ocean, freshwater lakes, rivers, and swimming pools. Water can be contaminated by other swimmers and by sewage, animal waste, and wastewater runoff. Diarrhea and other serious infections can spread when disease-causing organisms from human or animal feces are introduced into the water. Accidentally swallowing even small amounts of water contaminated with feces can cause illness.

To reduce your risk of acquiring a waterborne infection while swimming or engaging in other water activities, it's especially important to avoid swallowing water. To avoid contaminating water and spreading an infection to others, do not go swimming if you have diarrhea. You should also avoid swimming or wading in the following situations:

- Beaches that may be contaminated with human sewage or animal feces (such as from cattle, sheep, or dogs)

- Beaches located near storm drains
- Any beach after a heavy rainfall
- Freshwater streams, canals, and lakes in areas of the Caribbean, South America, Africa, and Asia where the infection schistosomiasis is present
- Bodies of water that may be contaminated with urine from animals infected with the Leptospira bacterium
- If you have any open cuts or abrasions that could serve as entry points for disease-causing organisms

Generally, pools that contain chlorinated water can be considered safe to swim in. However, some organisms (such as Giardia, hepatitis A, norovirus, and Cryptosporidium) are resistant to chlorine levels commonly found in chlorinated swimming pools. For this reason, you should also avoid swallowing chlorinated water in swimming pools.

slicing them up on the cutting board. Avoid leaving cut produce at room temperature for too long.

- **Do not be a source of food-borne illness.** Wash your hands with soap and water before preparing food and after using the toilet, changing diapers, and handling pets. Wash your cutting boards, dishes, utensils, and countertops with hot, soapy water before and after preparing each food item. If you use cloth towels to wipe up the counter after preparing food, wash them in the hot cycle of your washing machine before reusing them. Avoid preparing food for other people if you have diarrhea.

- **Report suspected food-borne illnesses.** Let your local health department know about any incident of food poisoning. Calls from people in the community are often how outbreaks are first detected. If a public health official contacts you to find out more about an illness, cooperate fully. In public health investigations, it can be as important to talk to healthy people as to those who are sick.

Feeding your baby safely

When your baby eats, harmful bacteria can be introduced into food or bottles, where it can grow and multiply even after refrigeration and reheating. If your baby doesn't finish a bottle, don't put the bottle in the refrigerator for another time. And if you feed a baby from a jar of baby food, don't put the unfinished jar in the refrigerator for later; saliva on the spoon can contaminate the remaining food. Don't give your baby perishable items such as milk, formula, or food that's been out of the refrigerator for longer than two hours.

When traveling with your baby, transport bottles and food in an insulated cooler. Place the ice chest in the passenger compartment of the car (it is cooler there than in the trunk). Use frozen gel packs to keep food or bottles cold on long outings. Don't keep bottles or food in the same bag with dirty diapers.

Follow the manufacturer's recommendations for preparing bottles before filling them with formula or milk. Don't use formula past its expiration date. If you make homemade baby food, use a brush to clean the areas around the blades of the blender or food processor; old food particles can harbor harmful bacteria that could contaminate other foods. Use soap and hot water to wash and rinse all utensils (including the can opener) that come in contact with your baby's food.

To freeze homemade baby food, put the mixture in an ice cube tray. Cover it with heavy-duty plastic wrap until the food is frozen. Then pop the food cubes into a clean freezer bag or airtight container and date it; you can store it up for to three months. You can also use small jars for freezing, but make sure you leave about a half inch of space at the top (because food expands when frozen).

If you buy commercial baby foods, check to see if the safety button on the lid is down. If the jar lid doesn't pop when you open it, don't use the food. Discard any jars with chipped glass or rusty lids.

Never use honey as a sweetener to entice your baby to drink water or milk from a bottle. Honey is not safe for children younger than 1 year because it can contain the botulinum organism that could cause infant botulism poisoning or death. Don't give raw or unpasteurized milk to infants or children, because it can contain dangerous bacteria or other organisms.

Sexually transmitted diseases

You can find discussions of the different types of sexually transmitted diseases (STDs) in chapter 5. This section of the book focuses on preventing STDs. Sexual abstinence is the only foolproof way to prevent STDs, but abstinence is not always practical—or desirable. Practicing safer sex is the second-best way to avoid STDs. Safer sex means taking the measures during sex that can prevent you from acquiring or transmitting an STD. The most common STDs are genital herpes, genital warts (HPV), chlamydia, gonorrhea, syphilis, hepatitis B, and HIV/AIDS.

STDs are contagious infections that can be passed from person to person through sexual intercourse or other sexual contact, including oral and anal sex. Many of the microorganisms that transmit STDs can live on the penis, vagina, anus, mouth, and on nearby skin surfaces. Most STDs are spread by skin-to-skin contact with a sore on a partner's genitals or mouth, but some are spread through contact with body fluids, such as semen or blood.

Some STDs can also be transmitted through nonsexual contact with infected tissues or fluids, such as infected blood. For example, intravenous drug users can acquire HIV or hepatitis B from sharing needles. HIV and hepatitis B can also be transmitted to a fetus during pregnancy. The following factors raise your risk of acquiring an STD:

- Not knowing if a sexual partner has an STD.
- Having sex with someone who has had an STD in the past.
- Having sex without using a male or female condom.
- Using drugs or alcohol when sex could take place.
- Having sex with an intravenous drug user.
- Engaging in anal intercourse.

The safest strategy is to remain in a mutually monogamous sexual relationship with a person you know has tested negative for STDs. Having unprotected sex with a new partner poses a high degree of risk. Before having sex, you and your partner should both get tested for STDs—including HIV and hepatitis B—and disclose the results to each other. If such a strategy fails, use a condom each and every time you have sex. Both male and female condoms can significantly lower the risk of contracting or spreading an STD—but they are not foolproof, and don't fully protect against all STDs, such as herpes and genital warts, which can be present on genital areas not protected by a condom. Keep in mind that condoms can only be effective against STDs if you use them consistently and correctly every time you have sex. (For more detailed instructions on how to use a condom correctly, see page 177.) Follow these guidelines for using a condom properly:

- Put the condom on from start to finish of sexual activity.
- Use a condom each time you have sex, and use it only once.
- Use only water-based lubricants. Never use oil-based or petroleum-based lubricants because these materials can weaken and tear latex.
- Don't use condoms containing the spermicide nonoxynol-9 because this spermicide has been linked to an increased risk of acquiring HIV.

Here are some additional safer-sex measures:

- **Don't have multiple sex partners.** Having sex with someone is like having sex with everyone that person has ever had sex with. Having multiple partners exponentially raises your risk for STDs.
- **Be in a committed relationship.** Before starting a sexual relationship, develop a committed relationship that nurtures trust and commu-

nication. You need to be able to talk about any previous STDs you have had.

- **Stay sober.** Using alcohol and other drugs impairs judgment, weakens resolve, and reduces your ability to use a condom correctly.

- **Be open and honest.** Some STDs last a lifetime. If you have an incurable STD, such as herpes, tell a potential sex partner. If you both agree on having sex, be sure to use a latex condom to protect your partner every time you have sex.

- **Take precautions during pregnancy.** If you have an STD, educate yourself about the risk to your baby—ideally, before getting pregnant. Ask your doctor how to prevent the fetus from becoming infected. If you are HIV-positive, do not breastfeed.

11

KEEPING YOUR BONES AND JOINTS HEALTHY

YOUR BONES AND JOINTS work together to perform many critical functions, from running a 10-mile race to tying your shoes. It's important to take care of your bones and joints to maintain their flexibility and range of motion, and to help you stay independent as you get older. The best way to do this is to be physically active. Osteoporosis (which affects the bones) and osteoarthritis (which affects the joints) are two of the most common and debilitating disorders among older Americans.

Osteoporosis

Osteoporosis, which means "porous bone," is a disorder characterized by low bone mass and the deterioration of bone tissue, causing the bones to become fragile and increasing the risk for fractures, especially of the hip, spine, and wrist. Osteoporosis affects both males and females, but nearly 70 percent of affected people are women. Osteoporosis can occur at any age, but is most common in people over age 50. The disorder is responsible for more than 1.5 million fractures each year, including 300,000 hip fractures,

700,000 vertebral fractures, 250,000 wrist fractures, and more than 300,000 fractures at other sites.

Throughout life, the body removes old bone—a process called resorption—and adds new bone to the skeleton. During childhood and adolescence, new bone is added faster than old bone is removed, allowing the bones to grow larger, thicker, and heavier. Bone formation outpaces resorption until bone reaches its highest density and strength—called peak bone mass—at around age 30. After that, bone resorption slowly begins to outpace bone formation.

If you don't build up enough bone during your childhood and adolescence, you will have less in reserve to compensate for the loss of bone density that tends to occur with aging. It's like putting money in the bank for later. The more bone mass you build up for the future, the stronger your bones will be as you get older and the more you can afford to lose before your bones reach a level at which they can easily fracture.

For women, bone loss is the greatest during the first few years after menopause (when estrogen production decreases), and it continues into the years after menopause. Osteoporosis develops when bone resorption occurs too quickly, or when bone formation occurs too slowly. The disorder is more likely to develop in women whose bone density did not reach its full potential density during the younger bone-building years.

Osteoporosis is often called a "silent" disease because bone loss occurs without symptoms, although some people may notice that they are shorter than they used to be, their posture is somewhat stooped, or their shoulders are rounded (because the bones in their spine have weakened). People often don't know they have osteoporosis until their bones become so weak that a sudden strain, bump, or fall causes a fracture.

RISK FACTORS

Certain risk factors, such as the following, increase your risk for osteoporosis. However, some people who develop osteoporosis have no known risk factors.

- Being female
- Being older
- Having low bone density
- Having a fracture after age 50
- Having a family history of osteoporosis or fractures

- Being thin, having a low body mass index (BMI; see page 85), or having small bones
- Deficiency of the female hormone estrogen (which strengthens bones) at menopause, especially early or surgically induced menopause, or from an abnormal absence of periods (such as from extreme weight loss or anorexia)
- Low lifetime intake of calcium and vitamin D
- Long-term use of some medications (such as corticosteroids, some chemotherapy drugs, and some antiseizure drugs)
- Having a digestive disorder that can interfere with the body's ability to absorb calcium, such as a peptic ulcer (see page 341) or lactose intolerance (see page 338)
- Being a male with a low testosterone level
- Being inactive
- Smoking cigarettes, or having a history of smoking
- Drinking alcohol excessively

PREVENTION

To reach your best possible peak bone density and keep your bones strong as you age, adopt the following lifestyle measures:

- **Get enough calcium.** An inadequate intake of calcium throughout life contributes to the development of osteoporosis. Many Americans consume less than half the amount of calcium they need (see the chart on the next page) to build and maintain healthy bones. The body's demand for calcium is greater during childhood and adolescence, when the skeleton is growing rapidly, and during pregnancy and breastfeeding. Postmenopausal women and older men also need to consume more calcium because the body becomes less efficient at absorbing calcium and other nutrients with age. Ask your doctor how much calcium you should get every day.

  Good sources of calcium include low-fat dairy products; dark green leafy vegetables; sardines and salmon with bones; tofu; almonds; and foods fortified with calcium, such as orange juice, breakfast cereals, and breads. Depending on how much calcium you consume each day from food, you may also need to take a calcium supplement.

Daily recommended calcium intakes

	Calcium (in milligrams)
Children and adolescents	
1 through 3 years	500
4 through 8 years	800
9 through 18 years	1,300
Women and Men	
19 through 49 years	1,000
50 years and older	1,200
Women who are pregnant or lactating	
18 years and younger	1,300
19 years and older	1,000

- **Get enough vitamin D.** Vitamin D plays an important role in bone health by helping the body absorb calcium. Your skin makes vitamin D through exposure to sunlight. While many people are able to obtain enough vitamin D naturally, others cannot. Vitamin D production decreases with age and from lack of exposure to the sun (especially during the winter in northern latitudes, and in people who are housebound). Depending on your situation, you may need to take vitamin D supplements to ensure an adequate daily intake. Ask your doctor how much vitamin D you should be getting every day. The National Osteoporosis Foundation recommends that, for maintaining bone density and preventing osteoporosis, adults under age 50 get 400 to 800 international units (IUs) of vitamin D3 daily, and adults age 50 and older get 800 to 1,000 IUs of vitamin D3 daily. Vitamin D3 is the form of vitamin D that best supports bone health. It is also called cholecalciferol. Food sources include fortified milk, egg yolks, saltwater fish, and liver.

- **Be physically active.** Like muscle, bone is living tissue that responds to exercise by becoming stronger. Weight-bearing exercise is the best for bones because it forces the bones to work against gravity. Examples of weight-bearing exercise include walking, hiking, jogging, stair climbing, weight training, skipping rope, playing tennis, and dancing.

MEDICATIONS THAT CAN PREVENT OSTEOPOROSIS

A number of medications are available for both preventing and treating osteoporosis. Doctors currently use alendronate, raloxifene, risedronate, and ibandronate to prevent and treat postmenopausal osteoporosis. Teriparatide is used for treating osteoporosis in both postmenopausal women and men at high risk for fractures. Hormone replacement therapy (HRT; see page 520) is also used for preventing osteoporosis after menopause.

- **Bisphosphonates** Alendronate, risedronate, and ibandronate are in a class of drugs called bisphosphonates, which are used to prevent bone loss after menopause. Alendronate and risedronate have been shown to increase bone mass and reduce the incidence of spine, hip, and other fractures. Ibandronate reduces the incidence of spinal fractures. Some bisphosphonates are fortified with calcium and vitamin D.

- **Raloxifene** Raloxifene is a member of a class of drugs called selective estrogen receptor modulators (SERMs) that prevent bone loss, especially in the spine and hip. Raloxifene has beneficial effects on bone mass and bone turnover and can reduce the risk for fractures in the vertebra. While side effects are uncommon, those reported include hot flashes and blood clots in the veins.

- **Calcitonin** Calcitonin is a naturally occurring hormone that promotes calcium regulation and bone growth. In women who are at least five years past menopause, calcitonin slows bone loss, increases spinal bone density, and relieves the pain of bone fractures. Calcitonin reduces the risk for spinal fractures and possibly also hip fractures. The drug is available as an injection or nasal spray. Injectable calcitonin may cause an allergic reaction and unpleasant side effects including flushing of the face and hands, frequent urination, nausea, and skin rash. The only side effect reported with nasal calcitonin is a runny nose.

- **Teriparatide** Teriparatide is an injectable form of human parathyroid hormone. Teriparatide stimulates new bone formation in both the spine and the hip. It also reduces the risk for fractures in postmenopausal women. In men, the drug cuts the risk for fractures of the vertebra. Side effects include nausea, dizziness, and leg cramps.

- **Hormone replacement therapy** HRT has been shown to lower bone loss, increase bone density in the spine and hip, and reduce the risk for spine and hip fractures in postmenopausal women. It is most commonly administered in pills or skin patches. Side effects include irregular vaginal bleeding, breast tenderness, and blood clots in the veins. Taking estrogen alone can increase the risk for endometrial cancer (see page 284). Long-term use may raise the risk for breast cancer, stroke, and heart attack in some women.

PREVENTING FRACTURES

If you already have osteoporosis, avoiding fractures is a major concern. Falls can increase your risk of breaking a bone in the hip, wrist, spine, or other parts of your body. Objects in your environment, such as toys on the stairs, can cause falls, but falls can also result from weakened vision or balance, or from taking certain medications, such as sedatives and anti-depressants. Be aware of any physical changes that affect your balance or the way you walk, and talk about these changes with your doctor. Here are some tips to help you eliminate the environmental factors that could cause falls:

Outdoors

- Use a cane or a walker for added stability.
- Wear rubber-soled shoes for traction.
- Walk on grass when sidewalks are slippery.
- In winter, sprinkle salt or kitty litter on slippery sidewalks.
- Be careful on highly polished floors that can become slick when wet.

Indoors

- Keep rooms free of clutter, especially on floors.
- Wear supportive, low-heeled shoes, even at home.
- Avoid walking in socks, stockings, or slippers.
- Be sure carpets and area rugs have skid-proof backing or are tacked to the floor.
- Keep stairwells well lit and make sure stairs have handrails on both sides.
- Install grab bars on bathroom walls near the tub, shower, and toilet.
- Use a rubber bath mat in the shower or tub.
- Keep a flashlight and fresh batteries beside your bed.
- Add ceiling fixtures to rooms lit only by lamps.
- Consider carrying a cell phone with you, even when you're at home, so you don't have to rush to answer the phone when it rings. And if you fall, you can use your cell phone to call for help.

Osteoarthritis

The term "arthritis" means inflammation of a joint. There are several different forms of arthritis. Osteoarthritis is by far the most common, especially among older people. Osteoarthritis is the wear-and-tear form of arthritis that develops when the surface layer of cartilage (the slick tissue that covers the ends of bones where they meet to form a joint) breaks down and wears away. An estimated 12 percent of the U.S. population (nearly 21 million Americans) age 25 and older have osteoarthritis. Although osteoarthritis is more common in older people, younger people can also develop it—usually after a joint injury. Both men and women can develop the disorder, but it is more likely to occur in people who are overweight and in those who have jobs that overuse certain joints. Osteoarthritis is a leading cause of disability in the United States.

Healthy cartilage allows bones to glide easily over one another. Cartilage also absorbs the shock of physical movement. When cartilage degenerates, the bones underneath it start to rub together, causing pain, swelling, and loss of motion in the joint. Over time, the joint may become misshapen. Small deposits of bone—called osteophytes, but commonly known as bone spurs—sometimes grow on the edges of the joint. Bits of bone or cartilage can break off and float inside the joint space, causing even more pain and damage. Unlike some other types of arthritis, such as rheumatoid arthritis, osteoarthritis affects only the joints and does not affect the skin or any other parts of the body.

The most common symptoms of osteoarthritis include joint pain and stiffness. The erosion of the joints often leads to loss of mobility. The joints most often affected are those near the tips of the fingers, the thumb, neck, knees, lower spine, and hips.

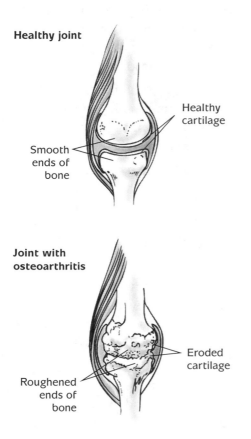

Healthy joint

Healthy cartilage

Smooth ends of bone

Joint with osteoarthritis

Eroded cartilage

Roughened ends of bone

How osteoarthritis damages joints

In a healthy joint (top), healthy cartilage cushions the bones, enabling them to glide easily against each other. In a joint damaged by osteoarthritis (bottom), the cartilage has worn down, causing the bones to rub against each other, producing inflammation and pain. The ends of the bones become rough, and bits of bone can break off and float inside the joint, causing even more pain.

RISK FACTORS

Doctors believe that osteoarthritis is the result of many interrelated factors, including wear and tear on the joints over time, joint injury, and inherited factors that cause changes in cartilage at the molecular level—not simply the consequence of age-related cartilage degeneration. Following are the most common risk factors for osteoarthritis:

- **Obesity**   Excess weight puts added stress on the joints. Every 2-pound increase in weight increases the risk for arthritis by 9 to 13 percent. A weight loss of as little as 11 pounds can cut in half a woman's risk of developing osteoarthritis in the knee.

- **On-the-job overuse**   Repetitive, forceful, or prolonged exertion of the hands; frequent or heavy lifting, pushing, pulling, or carrying heavy objects; jobs requiring kneeling or squatting or prolonged awkward postures; and vibration all take their toll on the joints.

- **Sports injuries**   Sports such as football, which produce intense, direct joint impact from contact with other players, playing surfaces, or equipment, pose the highest risk for osteoarthritis. Sports such as soccer or baseball pitching, which involve both repetitive joint impact and twisting, also increase the risk. Regular, moderate running poses a moderate risk.

- **Heredity**   Genetic researchers have discovered more than one gene linked to an increased risk for osteoarthritis, showing that the disorder has a strong genetic component. These genetic abnormalities lower the threshold at which physical stress on the joints can cause osteoarthritis.

- **Age**   Although osteoarthritis is not an inevitable part of aging, most people who have the disorder are over age 45, and most people over age 60 have some degree of osteoarthritis.

- **Weak muscles**   Weakness of the quadriceps muscle in the front of the thigh is common in people with osteoarthritis. Doctors think that the muscle weakness comes first and contributes to the development of osteoarthritis.

PREVENTION

You can take several steps to prevent or delay the onset of osteoarthritis, including the following:

- **Keep your weight down.** Achieving a healthy weight lowers your risk of developing osteoarthritis in the knees and hips. It can also slow the progression of arthritis in people who already have it and delay costly knee replacement surgery.

- **Perform strength-training exercises.** Strengthening your thigh muscles can reduce your risk of developing osteoarthritis in your knees. In fact, some doctors now think that weak leg muscles may be a risk factor for the disorder. Walk up stairs and do leg crunches to build up your quads. See page 52 for a discussion of strength training and its benefits.

- **Work smart.** Many cases of osteoarthritis in men result from work activities, especially heavy lifting and kneeling. When you lift heavy objects or people, be sure to bend your knees and use your legs instead of your back to bring the load up (see box).

PROPER LIFTING TECHNIQUE

During an average workday, many workers are responsible for physically moving containers by lifting, lowering, filling, emptying, or carrying them. Many health-care workers must lift heavy people in and out of bed. If your job involves heavy lifting, plan your workflow to eliminate unnecessary carrying as much as you can. Ask someone to help you, and wear protective gear such as a waist belt to lessen the stress on your back and other joints. Follow these additional guidelines to reduce your risk of developing work-related osteoarthritis:

- Slide, push, or roll instead of carrying whenever you can.
- Carry only as much as you can safely handle by yourself.
- Use extra caution when lifting loads that may be unstable.
- Get a secure grip; wearing gloves with rubber dots can improve your hold.

- Avoid jerking by using smooth, even motions.
- When lifting a heavy object, keep the load close to your body. Bend from your hips and knees, not your back. Keep your back straight; don't arch it. Try to keep the load between your shoulders and your waist, and use your legs to push up and lift the load—not your upper body or back.
- If you carry items on your shoulder, wear a shoulder pad and switch shoulders often.
- Don't twist your body; step to one side or the other to turn.
- Alternate heavy lifting or forceful exertion tasks with less physically demanding ones.
- Take rest breaks.

12

KEEPING YOUR DIGESTIVE SYSTEM HEALTHY

WHEN YOU TAKE A BITE of an apple, your body begins a process of breaking down the food into smaller and smaller pieces that allow it to be absorbed and distributed to all the cells in your body. This process of breaking down food into a usable form is called digestion. The human digestive system can accommodate a wide variety of diets—after all, people throughout the world have to depend on the food that is available to them.

Although Americans can choose from a huge variety of foods, convenient packaged and fast foods with little nutritional value often replace natural foods such as fresh fruits and vegetables. The typical American diet lacks adequate amounts of important nutrients such as fiber and can contain potentially harmful elements such as saturated fat, salt, and added sugars. Over time, the effects of a poor diet can take their toll in the form of digestive disorders such as heartburn and diverticular disease. Long-term excessive drinking can lead to liver disease. This chapter discusses ways in which you can avoid many of the most common digestive disorders.

Gas and bloating

As embarrassing as it can be, gas affects everyone. Most people produce about 1 to 4 pints of gas a day and pass gas about 14 times a day. Many people who think they are passing excessive amounts of gas are in reality passing normal amounts. Gas is made up of odorless vapors—carbon dioxide, oxygen, nitrogen, hydrogen, and sometimes methane. The unpleasant odor comes from bacteria in the large intestine that release small amounts of gases that contain the ingredient sulfur.

Gas in the digestive tract—the esophagus, stomach, small intestine, and large intestine—comes from two sources: swallowed air and the normal breakdown of some undigested foods by harmless bacteria that are naturally present in the large intestine (colon). Swallowed air is a common cause of gas in the stomach. Swallowing small amounts of air when you eat and drink is normal, but sometimes more air can be taken in from, for example, eating or drinking quickly, chewing gum, smoking, or wearing loose dentures.

Burping (or belching) is the way most swallowed air—which contains nitrogen, oxygen, and carbon dioxide—leaves the stomach. The remaining gas moves into the small intestine, where it becomes partially absorbed. A small amount travels into the large intestine for release through the rectum.

The body does not digest and absorb some carbohydrates (the sugar, starches, and fiber found in many foods) in the small intestine because of a shortage or absence of certain enzymes. This undigested food then passes from the small intestine into the large intestine, where normal, harmless bacteria break down the food, producing hydrogen, carbon dioxide, and, in about one third of people, methane. Eventually these gases exit through the rectum. People who make methane don't necessarily pass more gas, and it is not known why some people produce methane and others don't.

Foods that produce intestinal gas in one person may not cause gas in another. Most foods that contain carbohydrates can cause gas. By contrast, fats and proteins cause little gas. Foods that can cause intestinal gas include the following:

- Dried peas and beans (legumes)
- Some vegetables (including broccoli, cabbage, Brussels sprouts, onions, artichokes, and asparagus)
- Some fruits (including pears, apples, and peaches)
- Whole grains (including whole wheat and bran)

- Soft drinks and fruit drinks
- Milk and milk products (such as cheese and ice cream)
- Packaged foods prepared with the milk sugar lactose (including some breads, cereals, and salad dressings)
- Foods containing the sugar substitute sorbitol (such as dietetic foods and sugar-free candies and gums)

PREVENTION

Experience has shown that the most successful ways to reduce the discomfort of gas are to change your diet, take anti-gas medications, and reduce the amount of air you swallow. Doctors tell people to eat fewer foods that cause gas, but for some, this advice may mean cutting out healthy foods such as beans, fruits and vegetables, whole grains, and dairy products. Doctors sometimes also suggest limiting high-fat foods to reduce bloating and discomfort, which helps the stomach empty faster, allowing gases to move into the small intestine. Because the amount of gas produced by certain foods varies from person to person, you need to learn through trial and error which foods affect you and how much of these foods your digestive system can handle.

Many over-the-counter medications are available to help reduce gas-related symptoms, including antacids with simethicone (a foaming agent that joins together gas bubbles in the stomach to be more easily belched away). But these medications have no effect on intestinal gas. Digestive enzymes, such as lactase supplements, help digest carbohydrates and may allow you to eat foods that would normally cause gas. The enzyme lactase, which helps people with lactose intolerance (see next page) digest the sugar lactose in milk, is available in caplet and chewable tablet form without a prescription. Chewing lactase tablets just before eating helps the body digest foods containing lactose, such as dairy products. You can also find lactose-reduced milk and other dairy products at many grocery stores. Most grocery and drug stores also carry an over-the-counter natural enzyme supplement that can help digest the sugar in beans and many vegetables. The enzyme comes in liquid and tablet form.

To reduce belching, doctors often suggest ways to reduce the amount of air swallowed, such as avoiding chewing gum and hard candy, eating at a slow pace, and checking with a dentist to make sure that your dentures fit properly.

LACTOSE INTOLERANCE

Lactose intolerance is the inability to digest lactose, the main sugar found in milk and other dairy products. People with lactose intolerance have a shortage of the enzyme lactase, which is produced by cells lining the small intestine. Lactase breaks down milk sugar into two simpler forms of sugar called glucose and galactose, which then get absorbed into the bloodstream. Not all people who are deficient in lactase have the symptoms commonly brought on by lactose intolerance, but those who do are said to have lactose intolerance.

Between 30 and 50 million Americans are lactose intolerant. Some ethnic and racial populations are more likely to be affected than others. Up to 80 percent of African Americans, 80 to 100 percent of Native Americans, and 90 to 100 percent of Asian Americans are lactose intolerant. In fact, people of northern European descent are the only group that is relatively unaffected by the condition. Babies who are born prematurely are also likely to be lactose intolerant, because lactase levels don't increase until the third trimester of pregnancy.

People sometimes confuse lactose intolerance with cow's milk intolerance because the symptoms can be similar, but lactose intolerance and cow's milk intolerance are unrelated. Being intolerant to cow's milk is an allergic reaction triggered by the immune system.

People with lactose intolerance may feel very uncomfortable when they digest milk products. Common symptoms, which range from mild to severe, include nausea, cramps, bloating, gas, and diarrhea. Symptoms usually appear from 30 minutes to two hours after eating or drinking lactose-containing foods. The severity of symptoms depends on many factors, including the amount of lactose a person can tolerate and the person's age, ethnicity, and digestion rate.

Milk and other dairy products are a major source of calcium in the American diet, so people who are lactose intolerant need to find alternate sources of this essential mineral. Yogurt with active cultures is a good source of calcium for many people with lactose intolerance. Even though yogurt is fairly high in lactose, the bacterial cultures used to make it produce some of the lactase enzyme needed for proper digestion. Other good sources of calcium include calcium-fortified orange juice, sardines, and lactose-free milk and other dairy products.

Gastroesophageal reflux disease

Gastroesophageal reflux disease (GERD) is a chronic form of heartburn. GERD occurs when the lower esophageal sphincter (a ring of muscle that constricts the opening from the esophagus into the stomach) opens spontaneously or doesn't close properly, allowing the stomach contents to rise up into the esophagus. GERD is also called acid reflux or acid regurgitation, because digestive juices (acids) flow back up out of the stomach, sometimes with food.

When acid reflux occurs, you can taste food you have eaten or fluid in the back of your mouth. When refluxed stomach acid touches the lining of the esophagus, it can cause a burning sensation in the chest or throat, which people commonly call heartburn or acid indigestion. Occasional heartburn is common and does not necessarily mean you have GERD. But persistent reflux that occurs more than twice a week is considered to be GERD. People of all ages can have GERD, including children.

Persistent reflux can lead to inflammation, ulceration, and the formation of scar tissue that can make the esophagus narrower. Left untreated, GERD can increase the risk for cancer of the esophagus. Over time, the backup of stomach acids can irritate the esophagus and cause a condition called Barrett's esophagus, in which the cells lining the lower part of the esophagus change or become replaced with abnormal cells that could eventually become cancerous.

The reason some people develop GERD and others don't is unclear, but research has found that in people with GERD, the lower sphincter relaxes while the rest of the esophagus is working. Anatomical abnormalities such as a hiatal hernia sometimes contribute to GERD. A hiatal hernia occurs when the upper part of the stomach and the lower esophageal sphincter move above the diaphragm (the muscle wall that separates the stomach from the chest). Normally the diaphragm helps the sphincter keep acid from rising up into the esophagus. When a hiatal hernia is present, acid reflux can occur more easily. A hiatal hernia can develop at any age, but is most often found in otherwise healthy people over age 50. Most of the time, a hiatal hernia produces no symptoms.

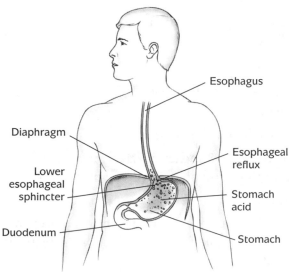

Esophagus

Diaphragm

Lower esophageal sphincter

Duodenum

Esophageal reflux

Stomach acid

Stomach

What causes GERD?

The esophagus is the tube that carries food from the mouth to the stomach. The lower esophageal sphincter is a ring of muscle at the bottom of the esophagus that acts like a valve between the esophagus and the stomach. Gastroesophageal reflux occurs when the sphincter malfunctions, allowing food and stomach acid to flow back up into the esophagus. The acid irritates the lining of the esophagus, causing heartburn. Left untreated, GERD can raise the risk for esophageal cancer.

RISK FACTORS

Anyone, including infants and children, can have GERD. Factors that contribute to GERD include the following:

- Obesity
- Pregnancy
- Smoking

The following common foods can trigger or worsen reflux symptoms:

- Citrus fruits
- Chocolate
- Drinks with caffeine or alcohol
- Fatty and fried foods
- Garlic and onions
- Mint flavorings
- Spicy foods
- Tomato-based foods such as spaghetti sauce, salsa, chili, pizza, and soups

PREVENTION

Prevention of GERD involves making one or more of the following lifestyle changes:

- If you smoke, stop.
- Avoid foods and beverages that worsen symptoms—including alcohol and spicy, fatty, or acidic foods.
- Lose weight if you need to.
- Eat small, frequent meals instead of three large ones.
- Wear loose-fitting clothes.
- Avoid lying down for three hours after a meal.
- Raise the head of your bed 6 to 8 inches by securing wood blocks under the bedposts. Just using extra pillows will not help.
- Don't eat close to bedtime.

If you have heartburn or GERD, your doctor may recommend over-the-counter antacids or medications that block acid production or help the muscles that empty the stomach.

Peptic ulcers

A peptic ulcer is a sore in the lining of the stomach or duodenum (the beginning of the small intestine from the stomach). Peptic ulcers are common: one in ten Americans develops an ulcer at some time in his or her life. People of any age and gender can develop an ulcer.

Contrary to what many people believe, peptic ulcers are not caused by stress or by eating spicy food. Most ulcers are caused by infection with the bacterium Helicobacter pylori (H. pylori). The organism weakens the protective mucus coating of the stomach and duodenum, which allows acid to get through to the sensitive lining underneath. Both the acid and the bacteria can irritate the lining and cause an ulcer.

H. pylori infection is common in the United States. About 20 percent of people under 40 and half of those over 60 have it, although most infected people do not develop ulcers. Why H. pylori doesn't cause ulcers in every infected person is not known. Infection may depend on certain characteristics of the infected person, the type of H. pylori, and other factors yet to be discovered. How people contract H. pylori is also unknown, but doctors think it may be through food or water. The bacterium has been found in saliva, so it may also be spread through mouth-to-mouth contact, such as kissing. The good news is that ulcers caused by H. pylori can be cured in about two weeks with antibiotics.

Another common cause of peptic ulcers is the long-term use of nonsteroidal anti-inflammatory drugs (NSAIDs), such as aspirin and ibuprofen. NSAIDs can interfere with the stomach's natural ability to protect itself against exposure to stomach acid and other digestive juices, which can lead to ulcer formation. In rare cases, cancerous tumors in the stomach or pancreas can also cause ulcers.

RISK FACTORS

You may be at risk for peptic ulcers if you have any of the following risk factors:

- **Older age**   Older people tend to develop ulcers more often than younger people.
- **Infection with H. pylori**   The H. pylori bacterium is a common cause of peptic ulcers.

Sudden, severe abdominal pain

A sudden attack of ulcer pain can be a medical emergency. If you have any of the following symptoms, get immediate medical attention:

- Sharp, sudden, persistent stomach pain
- Bloody or black, tarry stools
- Bloody vomit or vomit that looks like coffee grounds

These symptoms could be a sign of one of the following life-threatening problems:

- Perforation—when the ulcer burrows through the wall of the stomach or intestine
- Bleeding—when acid or the ulcer breaks a blood vessel
- Obstruction—when the ulcer blocks the path of food trying to leave the stomach

- **Taking NSAIDs regularly** These common painkillers, including aspirin and ibuprofen, can irritate the stomach and intestinal lining, promoting the development of ulcers.

- **Family history** For people who have close relatives with ulcers, the lifetime chance of developing an ulcer is three times as great as that of the general population.

- **Poor sanitary conditions** Poor sanitation or living in areas without safe drinking water increases the risk for infection with H. pylori and peptic ulcers.

PREVENTION

One step you can take to lower your risk for peptic ulcers is to limit your use of aspirin, ibuprofen, and other NSAIDs. No one knows for sure how H. pylori spreads, so it is difficult to know how to prevent infection with the bacterium. Researchers are currently trying to develop a vaccine against H. pylori. If you have an ulcer caused by H. pylori, your doctor will treat you with a course of antibiotics to speed healing and prevent recurrences. However, you can be reinfected with H. pylori in the future.

Diverticular disease

The presence of small sacs, or out-pouchings, called diverticula, in the walls of the colon (large intestine) characterizes diverticular disease. Diverticular disease is made up of two conditions: diverticulosis and diverticulitis. Diverticulosis occurs when the pouches form and bulge out like weak areas of a tire. Diverticulitis occurs if the pouches become inflamed.

Doctors aren't sure what causes diverticular disease, but many think a diet low in fiber (see page 4) plays a major role. Fiber is a nutrient in food that the body does not digest; the fiber stays in the colon and absorbs water, which makes stool easier to pass. Diets low in fiber can cause constipation, in which stool is hard and difficult to pass. Constipation causes the muscles to strain during bowel movements. This straining may promote the development of diverticula in the colon. If stool or bacteria get into the pouches, they can produce inflammation in the pouches, causing diverticulitis.

RISK FACTORS

The major risk factor for diverticular disease is eating a diet that is low in fiber. The risk increases with age, starting at about age 40. Nearly half of people between ages 60 and 80 have diverticular disease, and almost everyone over 80 has it to some degree.

PREVENTION

Eating a high-fiber diet is the best way to prevent diverticular disease. Talk to your doctor about using high-fiber capsules or powdered drink mixes. Daily use can help you get the fiber you need if you can't get it through your diet. You should also ask your doctor about which food choices are best for

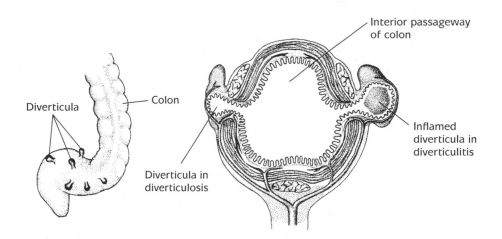

Diverticular disease

Diverticula, which are small pouches or sacs, can develop when the inner lining of the intestines bulges through the outer wall. The presence of these pouches is called diverticulosis, a condition that may not produce any symptoms. Diverticula are most likely to occur in someone who eats a low-fiber diet, which allows particles of stool to lodge in the intestinal lining. When the pouches become inflamed or infected, the condition is called diverticulitis, a more serious and painful condition that could cause an intestinal obstruction or an abscess, which could rupture and be life-threatening.

you. Eating foods high in fiber is simple and can help reduce diverticular disease symptoms and problems. Talk with your doctor about making changes in your diet. Learn how to include more high-fiber foods in your diet. Remember to drink plenty of water when you increase the fiber content of your diet, or you could actually become more constipated. See page 5 for how to increase the fiber in your diet.

Hemorrhoids

Hemorrhoids result when the veins around the anus or lower rectum become swollen and inflamed. Hemorrhoids can develop inside the anus (internal) or under the skin around the anus (external). Hemorrhoids usually are not life-threatening, and the symptoms usually go away within a few days.

Hemorrhoids are common in both men and women; one out of two people has had a hemorrhoid by age 50. Hemorrhoids can result from straining to have a bowel movement, having chronic constipation or diarrhea, or engaging in anal intercourse. Other risk factors include having a family history of hemorrhoids, getting little physical activity, and sitting for long periods.

Hemorrhoids are common during pregnancy, because of the extra pressure of the fetus on the abdomen, as well as hormonal changes during pregnancy that cause the hemorrhoidal blood vessels to enlarge. These blood vessels also undergo severe pressure during childbirth. For most women, hemorrhoids caused by pregnancy are temporary.

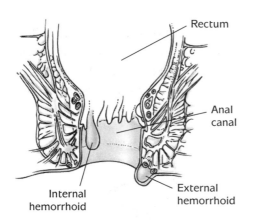

Hemorrhoids

Hemorrhoids are swollen veins in the lining of the anus. External hemorrhoids form on the rim of the anus. Internal hemorrhoids develop inside the anal canal but sometimes hang down out of the anus because of straining during bowel movements or during a vaginal delivery. Both types of hemorrhoids can cause itching, pain, and bleeding.

PREVENTION

The most effective way to prevent hemorrhoids is to keep your stool soft so it can pass easily and you don't have to strain to have a bowel movement. You should also empty your bowels as soon as possible when you have the urge. Here are some additional preventive measures:

- Increase your level of physical activity—walk more.
- Increase the fiber in your diet (see page 5) to help reduce constipation and straining during bowel movements.
- Don't strain during bowel movements.

Irritable bowel syndrome

Irritable bowel syndrome (IBS) is a common disorder that is characterized by cramping, abdominal pain, bloating, constipation, and diarrhea.

IBS causes a great deal of discomfort and distress, but it does not permanently harm the intestines and does not lead to a serious disease such as cancer. Most people with IBS can control their symptoms with diet, stress management, and prescribed medications. But for some people, IBS can be disabling. They may be unable to work, attend social events, or even travel short distances because of the discomfort.

Researchers have yet to discover any specific cause for IBS. One theory is that people who have IBS have a colon that is especially sensitive and reacts to certain foods and stress. Another idea is that people with IBS do not have normal bowel movements; the intestinal movement may occur in spasms or even stop working temporarily. (Spasms are sudden strong muscle contractions that come and go.) The immune system, which fights infection, may also contribute to IBS.

Some researchers believe that serotonin, a chemical (neurotransmitter) that delivers messages from one part of the body to the brain, plays a role in IBS. About 95 percent of the serotonin in the body is located in the intestinal tract; the other 5 percent is found in the brain. People with IBS seem to have abnormal levels of serotonin in their intestines, which can cause problems with bowel movements and sensation, making the intestines more sensitive to pain.

Some experts think that IBS could be caused by a bacterial infection in the intestinal tract. Studies show that people who have had gastroenteritis (inflammation of the stomach and intestines) sometimes develop IBS. Other research has found very mild celiac disease in some people with symptoms similar to IBS. People with celiac disease cannot digest gluten, a substance found in grains such as wheat, rye, and barley. When people with celiac disease eat these foods, they become very sick because their immune system responds by damaging the small intestine.

Stress may also stimulate colon spasms in people with IBS. The colon has many nerves that connect to the brain. These nerves control the normal contractions of the colon and cause abdominal discomfort at stressful times. People often experience cramps or "butterflies" when they are nervous or upset. In people with IBS, the colon can be overly responsive to even slight conflict or stress. Stress also makes the mind more aware of the sensations in the colon, making a person with IBS perceive these sensations as unpleasant.

RISK FACTORS

IBS can occur at any age, but often begins in adolescence or early adulthood. It is twice as common in women as in men, and is more common in young adults. Risk factors may include the following:

- Eating a low-fiber diet
- Experiencing emotional stress
- Overusing laxatives
- Having had infectious diarrhea
- Having had temporary bowel inflammation

PREVENTION

Some evidence suggests that IBS is affected by the immune system, which fights infection in the body; and stress usually affects the immune system. For all these reasons, stress management (see page 114) may play an important role in preventing IBS symptoms. Stress management options include the following:

- Stress reduction (relaxation) training and relaxation therapies such as meditation and yoga
- Counseling and support
- Regular exercise such as walking
- Lifestyle changes to reduce stressful situations
- Getting sufficient sleep

Other preventive measures that may be helpful include the following:

- Consuming more fiber
- Limiting the use of laxatives
- Not overeating at meals

Liver disorders

The liver is one of the most important organs in the body. It has numerous vital jobs, including transforming food into energy, cleansing toxins from the blood, fighting infection, stemming bleeding, and storing energy for when cells need it. Liver disease affects people of all ages, but is most common between the ages of 40 and 60. Liver disease can take many forms. Viruses—including hepatitis A, B, and C—cause some of them. Others result from taking illegal drugs or drinking alcohol excessively. If the liver forms scar tissue from damage, it is called cirrhosis. The most common preventable liver disorders include hepatitis, alcoholic and nonalcoholic fatty liver disease, and gallstones.

Hepatitis

Hepatitis means "inflammation of the liver." Inflammation can be caused by many things, but infections due to hepatitis viruses are a common cause. Hepatitis reduces the liver's ability to perform essential functions. Hepatitis can be sudden and temporary (acute) or long-term (chronic). If the virus stays in the blood for six months or longer after infection, doctors consider it to be chronic. Severe cases can cause life-threatening liver failure. Most acute cases are mild and last only a few weeks. At least five different viruses are currently known to cause hepatitis. In the United States, infection with the A, B, and C viruses are the most common. Here are descriptions of the five types of hepatitis:

- **Hepatitis A**   The hepatitis A virus is found in the feces of infected people and is spread by close contact with an infected person, or by consuming food or water contaminated with infected feces. In the United States, hepatitis A can occur in isolated cases or in widespread epidemics. It is often contracted in childhood or young adulthood as a mild illness that goes away on its own. The disease is especially common in developing countries with inadequate sanitation systems.

- **Hepatitis B**   Hepatitis B is spread by contact with the blood, semen, or vaginal secretions of an infected person. The virus can be spread through sexual activity, sharing contaminated intravenous needles, or using unsterilized needles for tattoos or body piercings. An infected pregnant woman can transmit the virus to her baby during a vaginal delivery. The virus is *not* transmitted in breast milk, so infected mothers can safely breastfeed. Hepatitis B virus can cause life-long infection, cirrhosis (scarring) of the liver, liver cancer, liver failure, and death.

- **Hepatitis C** Hepatitis C virus is transmitted through contact with an infected person's blood. Hepatitis C is more likely than the other hepatitis viruses to become chronic. The virus is transmitted most often through sharing intravenous drugs and having an unsanitary tattoo or body piercing. Less often, it is spread through sexual contact.

- **Hepatitis D** Hepatitis D virus is a defective virus that needs the hepatitis B virus to exist. Hepatitis D virus is also transmitted through infected blood.

- **Hepatitis E** Hepatitis E virus is transmitted in much the same way as the hepatitis A virus, but hepatitis E is uncommon in the United States.

RISK FACTORS

Following are the risk factors for the three most common types of viruses that cause hepatitis in the United States—hepatitis A, B, and C:

- **Hepatitis A** Anyone can get hepatitis A, but the following factors increase the risk:
  - Living with someone who has hepatitis A
  - Being a child in day care
  - Working in a day care center
  - Being male and having sex with males
  - Traveling to developing countries where hepatitis A is common

- **Hepatitis B** Hepatitis B spreads by contact with an infected person's blood, semen, or vaginal secretions. The following factors increase the risk for a hepatitis B infection:
  - Having unprotected sex with an infected person
  - Sharing intravenous drug needles
  - Having a tattoo or body piercing performed with tools previously used on someone with hepatitis B
  - Being pricked with a needle that has hepatitis B–infected blood on it (Health-care workers can get hepatitis B in this way.)

○ Living with someone who has hepatitis B

○ Sharing a toothbrush or razor with an infected person

○ Traveling to countries where hepatitis B is common

○ Being born to a woman with hepatitis B

You *cannot* get hepatitis B in the following ways:

○ Shaking hands with an infected person

○ Hugging an infected person

○ Sitting next to an infected person

● **Hepatitis C**   Hepatitis C is spread by contact with an infected person's blood. You could contract hepatitis C in the following ways:

○ Sharing intravenous drug needles

○ Being pricked with a needle that has infected blood on it (Health-care workers can get hepatitis C this way.)

○ Being born (in a vaginal delivery) to an infected mother

○ Having a tattoo or body piercing with unsterilized tools, in rare cases

○ Having unprotected sex with an infected person, especially if either partner has other sexually transmitted diseases

You *cannot* get hepatitis C in the following ways:

○ Shaking hands with an infected person

○ Hugging an infected person

○ Kissing an infected person

○ Sitting next to an infected person

Before 1992, when a test became available for screening donor blood and blood products for hepatitis C, some people acquired hepatitis C from blood transfusions or organ transplants. If you received a blood transfusion or organ transplant before 1992 or blood products (such as clotting factors) before 1987, talk to your doctor about being tested for the hepatitis C virus. You could be infected and have no signs or symptoms.

PREVENTION

You can protect yourself from hepatitis A and B by having a vaccination. The hepatitis B vaccination is required for all American children (see page

444) and is recommended for adults who are at risk for exposure to the virus. People who may be at risk include those who have several sex partners, health-care workers, college students who live in dormitories, or someone who lives with an infected person. Ask your doctor about having a hepatitis B vaccination. Children ages 2 to 18 and adults receive three shots, spread out over a year. You need all of the shots to be protected.

If you are planning a trip to a developing country where hepatitis A is often widespread, ask your doctor about having the hepatitis A vaccination. An injection of immune globulin (infection-fighting proteins) can provide immunity to the virus for two to three months. The two-shot vaccination against hepatitis A provides even more protection after the second shot, although exactly how long the protection lasts is unknown. Make sure you get all the shots before you go. If you miss a shot, call your doctor or clinic right away to set up a new appointment.

You can protect yourself and others from hepatitis A in the following ways:

- Always wash your hands after using the toilet and before preparing food or eating.
- Wear gloves if you have to touch another person's stool. Wash your hands well afterward.
- Drink and brush your teeth with bottled water when you're in an underdeveloped country. Don't use ice cubes, and don't wash fruits and vegetables in tap water. You may even have to be careful not to open your mouth and take in water during a shower.

You can protect yourself and others from hepatitis B by taking the following measures:

- Always use a condom when you have sex.
- Don't share intravenous drug needles with anyone.
- Wear gloves if you have to touch someone else's blood.
- Don't use an infected person's toothbrush, razor, or anything else that could have blood on it.
- Make sure that a tattoo or body piercing is done with clean tools.

You can protect yourself and others from hepatitis C by taking the following measures:

- Don't share intravenous drug needles with anyone.

- Wear gloves if you have to touch someone else's blood.

- Don't use an infected person's toothbrush, razor, or other personal item that could have the person's blood on it.

- If you get a tattoo or body piercing, make sure it's done with clean tools.

- Always use a condom during sex, especially if you have multiple sex partners.

HEPATITIS A AND B: WHO SHOULD GET VACCINATED?

People who are at high risk for hepatitis A or B should get immunized against the viruses. You may not think you're at risk, but simply traveling to a foreign country may place you at risk. Doctors recommend that all infants, children, and adolescents have the hepatitis B vaccination. See below to find out if you should be immunized against hepatitis.

Hepatitis A

- Travelers to developing countries with high rates of hepatitis A, including Mexico

- Men who have sex with men

- Users of illegal drugs

- People who work with hepatitis A virus in research settings

- People who work with infected monkeys and other nonhuman primates

- People who receive clotting factor concentrates (such as people with hemophilia)

- People with chronic liver disease

Hepatitis B

- All infants, children, and adolescents

- People with multiple sex partners and those who have been recently diagnosed with a sexually transmitted disease

- Sex partners and household contacts of hepatitis B virus carriers

- Men who have sex with men

- People with occupational exposure to blood, such as health-care workers

- Household contacts of adoptees from countries with high rates of hepatitis B, including nannies

- Injection drug users

- Travelers to countries with high rates of hepatitis B (if you're staying longer than six months)

- Clients and staff in institutions for the developmentally disabled

- People with chronic kidney failure (including those on regular hemodialysis)

- People receiving clotting factor concentrates

- Prison inmates

Nonalcoholic fatty liver disease

Nonalcoholic fatty liver disease is a common, but often "silent," liver disease. It's the same disorder as alcoholic liver disease (see next page), but it occurs in people who drink little or no alcohol. The major characteristic of the disorder is fat in the liver, along with inflammation and liver damage. Most people with fatty liver disease feel fine and are not aware they have a liver problem, even if their liver is inflamed and becoming enlarged.

Nonalcoholic fatty liver disease affects 10 to 20 percent of all people in the United States. Although nonalcoholic fatty liver disease is becoming increasingly common, its underlying cause is not clear. It most often occurs in people who are middle-aged and overweight or obese. Many people with nonalcoholic fatty liver disease have elevated blood fat levels (especially of cholesterol and triglycerides), and many have diabetes (see chapter 8) or prediabetes. However, not every obese person or every person with diabetes develops nonalcoholic fatty liver disease. In addition, some people with nonalcoholic fatty liver disease are not obese, don't have diabetes, and have normal blood cholesterol and other fats. The disorder can occur without any apparent risk factors and can even occur in children.

While the underlying cause of the liver injury that leads to nonalcoholic fatty liver disease is not known, the following factors seem to play a role:

- Insulin resistance (a condition in which the cells are less sensitive to the effects of the hormone insulin)
- Release of toxic inflammatory proteins by fat cells
- Inflammatory damage inside liver cells

Of all of these factors, insulin resistance seems to have the strongest link.

RISK FACTORS

Following are the factors that seem to increase the risk of developing nonalcoholic fatty liver disease:

- **Being overweight or obese** The more you weigh, the higher your risk. More than 70 percent of people with nonalcoholic fatty liver disease are obese (have a BMI of 30 or higher; see page 85).
- **Diabetes** When insulin becomes unable to maintain normal blood sugar levels, liver damage results. Up to 75 percent of affected people have diabetes.

- **High cholesterol and triglyceride levels**   Eight out of 10 people with nonalcoholic fatty liver disease have high levels of these fats in their blood.

Other, less important risk factors include the following:

- **Abdominal surgery**   Surgical procedures performed on the small intestine, including gastric bypass surgery to treat obesity, produce quick weight loss, but can raise the risk for nonalcoholic fatty liver disease.

- **Medications**   Taking some medications such as corticosteroids and hormone replacement therapy (HRT; see page 520) can also boost risk.

PREVENTION

The best protection against nonalcoholic fatty liver disease is keeping your weight within the healthy range and maintaining healthy cholesterol and blood sugar levels. Your doctor will recommend that you avoid alcohol and avoid exposure to chemicals and other substances that could damage your liver.

Alcoholic liver disease

Your body cannot store alcohol, and either eliminates it in urine, breathes it out, or converts it into a chemical called acetaldehyde in the liver. Acetaldehyde is a poison that disrupts the metabolism of fat in the body, causing fat to build up in the liver—a condition called fatty liver. When fat builds up in the liver, it eventually causes scarring (cirrhosis).

Alcoholic liver disease progresses through stages of increasing severity, from the accumulation of fat inside the liver (fatty liver), to sudden but short-term inflammation of the liver (alcoholic hepatitis). People with alcoholic fatty liver disease or alcoholic hepatitis will eventually develop cirrhosis if they continue to drink. In a person with cirrhosis of the liver, scar tissue replaces normal, healthy tissue, blocking the flow of blood through the liver and preventing it from working as it should. Cirrhosis is the 12th leading cause of death in the United States, killing about 26,000 people each year.

The final stage of alcoholic liver disease usually develops after more than a decade of heavy drinking. The amount of alcohol that can injure the liver varies greatly from person to person. In women, as few as two to three drinks per day have been linked to cirrhosis; in men, as few as three to four drinks per day can lead to cirrhosis. Alcohol injures the liver by blocking the normal metabolism of protein, fats, and carbohydrates.

RISK FACTORS

Following are the most important risk factors for alcoholic liver disease:

- **Alcohol abuse**   Chronic heavy drinking or binge drinking are the major risk factors for alcoholic liver disease.

- **Age**   The effects of alcoholic hepatitis are most likely to show up after years of heavy drinking, but symptoms of the disease can develop in people as young as 20.

- **Acetaminophen**   Taking medications, including over-the-counter drugs, that contain the pain reliever acetaminophen can cause liver damage in people who drink alcohol excessively or take excessive amounts of acetaminophen.

- **Gender**   Women are two to three times more susceptible to liver damage from alcohol than men, partly because of their smaller size and partly because they lack certain stomach enzymes that help break down alcohol, so their liver endures the higher blood levels of alcohol for longer periods of time. When liver disease occurs in women, it worsens more quickly than in men.

- **Genes**   Medical science has uncovered some genetic mutations that influence the way the body breaks down alcohol. If you have such a mutation, your chances of developing alcoholic liver disease are increased.

PREVENTION

The only sure way to prevent alcoholic hepatitis is to drink very lightly, or not at all. People vary greatly in their sensitivity to alcohol, and even occasional social drinkers risk liver damage. The current recommendation for moderate drinking is no more than two drinks per day for men and no more than one drink per day for women. One drink is usually defined as 12 ounces of beer, 5 ounces of wine, or 1.5 ounces of distilled spirits—each contains 15 grams of alcohol. However, because people differ greatly in their sensitivity to alcohol, these recommendations may be too high for some people. And it is never safe to "save up" your daily drink to have seven on a weekend night.

People who should not drink alcohol at all include pregnant women and people who have pancreatitis (inflammation of the pancreas), advanced nerve damage, or alcohol dependence (see page 142). If you have been diagnosed with alcoholic hepatitis, you should never drink alcohol again.

Care should also be taken with pain medications, including over-the-counter drugs, especially acetaminophen. The liver detoxifies and eliminates drugs from the body, and many medications, including nonprescription drugs, can damage liver cells, especially if they are taken excessively or with alcohol. Be extra careful not to mix acetaminophen with alcohol—the combination can cause liver failure. Talk to your doctor about the effect on your liver of any medications you take.

Gallstones

Gallstones are small, pebble-like formations that develop in the gallbladder (a small, pear-shaped pouch that sits below the liver in the upper right abdomen). Gallstones form when the digestive liquid bile hardens into pieces of stone-like material. Bile is made in the liver, then stored in the gallbladder until the body needs it. The gallbladder contracts and pushes the bile into a tube, called the common bile duct, which carries the bile to the small intestine, where the bile helps with digestion. Bile contains water, cholesterol, fats, bile salts, proteins, and bilirubin (a waste product).

The two types of gallstones are cholesterol stones and pigment stones. Cholesterol stones form when bile contains too much cholesterol, too much bilirubin, or not enough bile salts. The reason these imbalances occur is unclear. Cholesterol stones, which account for about 80 percent of all gallstones, are made up mostly of hardened cholesterol.

Although the cause of pigment stones is not fully understood, they tend to form in people who have liver cirrhosis, biliary tract infections, or inherited blood disorders such as sickle cell anemia, in which the liver makes too much of the pigment bilirubin; bilirubin is the substance that forms pigment stones.

Common sites of gallstones

Gallstones may stay inside the gallbladder or pass easily through the common bile duct into the upper part of the small intestine (duodenum) without causing symptoms. However, problems can develop if a gallstone gets trapped inside the cystic duct or bile duct. If a stone blocks the cystic duct, pressure builds up in the gallbladder, causing pain and infection. If a stone blocks the common bile duct, it prevents bile from draining out of the liver to the intestine, producing jaundice and fever.

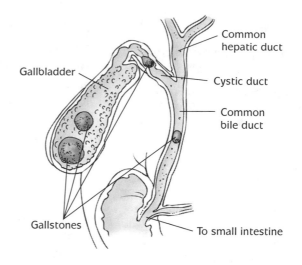

Gallstones can be as tiny as a grain of sand or as large as a golf ball. The gallbladder can develop just one large stone, hundreds of tiny stones, or a combination of these. Gallstones can block the normal flow of bile if they travel from the gallbladder and lodge in any of the ducts that transport bile from the liver to the small intestine. Bile trapped in these ducts can cause inflammation in the gallbladder, the ducts, or in rare cases, the liver. Sometimes gallstones passing through the common bile duct produce inflammation in the pancreas—called gallstone pancreatitis—an extremely painful and potentially dangerous condition.

RISK FACTORS

The following people are at increased risk for gallstones:

- Women—especially women who are pregnant, use hormone replacement therapy, or take birth-control pills
- People over age 60
- Native Americans and Mexican Americans
- People who are overweight or obese
- People who fast or lose a lot of weight quickly
- People who eat a diet high in fat and cholesterol and low in fiber
- People with a family history of gallstones
- People with diabetes
- People who take certain types of cholesterol-lowering medications

Gallbladder attack

Notify your doctor immediately if you think you are having a gallbladder attack. Although the pain goes away as the gallstone moves, your gallbladder can become infected and rupture if a blockage remains. If any of the bile ducts stay blocked for a long time, the gallbladder, liver, or pancreas can be damaged or become infected. Left untreated, the condition can be fatal. If you have any of the following symptoms, you should seek medical help immediately:

- Prolonged pain (for more than five hours usually in the upper right abdomen)
- Nausea and vomiting
- Fever—even low-grade—or chills
- Yellowish color of the skin or whites of the eyes (jaundice)
- Clay-colored stool

PREVENTION

Eating a diet that is low in cholesterol and saturated and trans fats and losing weight may help prevent a gallbladder attack. But don't lose weight too quickly, or you could trigger an attack.

13

KEEPING YOUR URINARY TRACT HEALTHY

THE URINARY SYSTEM CONSISTS of the kidneys, ureters, bladder, and urethra. The kidneys remove excess liquid and waste from the blood and transform them into urine. The kidneys also balance salts and other substances in the blood, and produce a hormone needed for the formation of oxygen-carrying red blood cells. Narrow tubes called ureters carry urine from the kidneys to the bladder, which stores urine until it is eliminated from the body through the urethra during urination.

The average adult passes about 1½ quarts of urine each day, depending on the fluids and foods consumed. The amount of urine produced at night is about half that produced during the day. The most common urinary system disorders are infections, kidney disease, bladder cancer, and urinary incontinence.

Urinary tract infections

Infection of the urinary tract is one of the most common types of infection in the body. Urinary tract infections (UTIs) account for more than 8 million

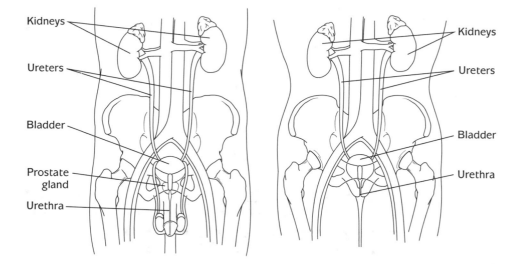

Male and female urinary tracts

The urinary tract consists of the kidneys, ureters, bladder, urethra, and prostate gland (in men). The kidneys filter the blood and eliminate waste products and excess water in urine. The ureters carry urine from the kidneys to the bladder, which holds the urine until it is eliminated through the urethra during urination. The male and female urinary tracts differ slightly. The male urethra is about 10 inches long and provides an outlet for semen as well as urine, while the female urethra is about 1½ inches long and lies, with the bladder, just in front of the reproductive organs.

doctor visits each year in the United States. Women are especially prone to having UTIs for reasons that are not fully understood; one in five women develops a UTI during her lifetime. Although UTIs in men are not as common, they can become very serious when they occur.

Urine is normally sterile—free of bacteria, viruses, and fungi—but it contains fluids, salts, and waste products. An infection can occur when bacteria, usually from the rectum, spread to the external opening of the urethra and begin to multiply. Most UTIs are caused by the bacterium Escherichia coli (E. coli), which normally lives in the colon.

An infection limited to the urethra is called urethritis. Bacteria that travel up to the bladder and multiply cause a bladder infection called cystitis. If the infection is left untreated, bacteria can travel farther up the ureters to infect the kidneys. A kidney infection is called pyelonephritis, and can be serious.

Microorganisms called Chlamydia and Mycoplasma can also cause UTIs in both men and women, but these infections tend to be limited to the urethra and reproductive system. Unlike E. coli, Chlamydia and Mycoplasma infections can be sexually transmitted and require treatment of both partners to avoid reinfections.

The urinary system is structured in a way that helps protect against infection. The ureters and bladder normally stop urine from backing up toward the kidneys, and the flow of urine from the bladder helps wash bacteria out of the body. In men, the prostate gland produces secretions that slow bacterial growth. In both sexes, immune system defenses also prevent infection. But despite the body's safeguards, infections can still occur, given the right conditions.

RISK FACTORS

Some people are more at risk of developing a UTI than others. Any abnormality of the urinary tract that obstructs the flow of urine (a kidney stone, for example) can set the stage for an infection. An enlarged prostate gland (see page 502) can also slow the flow of urine and raise the risk for infection. People with diabetes or other chronic diseases that can weaken the immune system (such as HIV/AIDS) are at increased risk for UTIs.

A common medical source of UTIs is the use of a catheter, a tube placed in the urethra and bladder to help a person who cannot pass urine. Some people, especially the elderly or those who have nervous system disorders that cause loss of bladder control, may need a catheter in place permanently. Because bacteria on the catheter can infect the bladder, it is especially important to take measures to keep the catheter clean to reduce the risk for infections.

In adult women, the rate of UTIs gradually increases with age. Scientists are not sure why women have more urinary tract infections than men. One possible explanation may be that a woman's urethra is shorter than a man's, allowing bacteria quicker access to the bladder. Also, a woman's urethral opening is closer to sources of bacteria from the anus and vagina. In young women, sexual intercourse often triggers a urinary tract infection, a phenomenon sometimes called "honeymoon cystitis." Women who use a diaphragm are more likely to develop UTIs than those who use other forms of birth control. Many women experience frequent UTIs.

Pregnant women seem no more prone to UTIs than other women, but when a UTI occurs during pregnancy, it is more likely to travel to the kidneys, where it is more serious. According to some reports, about 2 to 4 percent of pregnant women develop a UTI. Scientists think that hormonal changes and shifts in the position of the urinary tract during pregnancy make it easier for bacteria to travel up the ureters to the kidneys.

In men, UTIs are often caused by an obstruction (such as a kidney stone or enlarged prostate) or from a medical procedure involving a catheter. UTIs in older men are frequently linked to a prostate infection, which can have serious consequences if not treated immediately. Prostate infections are difficult to cure because antibiotics cannot easily penetrate infected prostate tissue. For this reason, men with prostatitis often need a long course of antibiotic treatment.

PREVENTION

Doctors recommend the following steps to avoid UTIs, especially if you are a woman:

- Drink plenty of water every day.
- Urinate when you feel the need; don't resist the urge.
- If you are a woman, wipe from front to back to prevent bacteria around the anus from entering the vagina or urethra.
- Take showers instead of tub baths.
- Clean your genital area before and after sexual intercourse.
- Urinate after having sex.
- Avoid using feminine hygiene sprays and douches, which can irritate the urethra.
- Drink cranberry juice to flush out your urinary tract. The juice has antibacterial properties.
- If you develop UTIs frequently and use spermicides, talk to your doctor about using another form of birth control.
- Wear underwear with a cotton crotch.

Kidney disease

The kidneys are bean-shaped organs, each about the size of a fist, located near the middle of the back, just below the rib cage. The main job of the kidneys is to filter blood, by tiny units inside the kidneys called nephrons. One kidney has about 1 million nephrons, which remove waste products and extra water as urine. Urine flows from the kidneys through tubes called ureters to the bladder, which stores the urine until it is released from the body during urination.

The wastes in the blood come from the normal breakdown of active tissues and from eaten food. After the body has taken what it needs from food, waste is sent to the blood. The kidneys remove these wastes from the blood. Kidney disease occurs when the nephrons become damaged and can no longer effectively filter wastes from the blood. The damage usually occurs very gradually over many years, in both kidneys, and does not cause any obvious symptoms; for this reason, kidney disease is often not detected at an early stage.

The major causes of kidney disease are diabetes, high blood pressure, and inherited factors. Some over-the-counter medications, when taken regularly over a long period of time, and exposure to some poisons can cause kidney disease.

RISK FACTORS

You are at risk for kidney disease if you have diabetes or high blood pressure or a family history of kidney disease. Talk to your doctor about getting tested. Here are the most common risk factors:

- **Diabetes**   When diabetes (see chapter 8) is not controlled, elevated levels of sugar (glucose) in the blood can damage the nephrons, a condition called diabetic nephropathy. Keeping blood sugar levels in the healthy range can help people with diabetes delay or prevent this serious complication. Diabetes is the most frequent cause of kidney failure, accounting for almost 45 percent of new cases.

- **High blood pressure**   High blood pressure (see page 235) can damage the small blood vessels in the kidneys, reducing the kidneys' ability to filter wastes from the blood. If you have high blood pressure, be sure to take any medications your doctor prescribes. Blood pressure medications called angiotensin-converting enzyme (ACE) inhibitors and angiotensin receptor blockers (ARBs) have been found to be especially protective of the kidneys.

- **Heredity**   Some kidney diseases result from inherited factors, and can run in families. If you have a family history of any kind of kidney problems, you may be at risk for kidney disease, and you should talk to your doctor about it. Polycystic kidney disease (PKD), for example, is a genetic disorder in which many cysts grow in the kidneys; the cysts can slowly replace much of the mass of the kidneys, reducing kidney function and leading to kidney failure.

- **Being African American** African Americans are four times more likely to have kidney failure than whites. Diabetes and high blood pressure are the two leading causes of kidney failure in African Americans. Many African Americans know they have diabetes or high blood pressure, but don't know they may also have kidney disease.

- **Being Native American or Hispanic** Scientists cannot explain the higher rates of kidney disease among Native Americans and Hispanics, but like African Americans, these groups also have an elevated risk of developing type 2 diabetes and high blood pressure.

- **Some over-the-counter medications** Products that combine aspirin, acetaminophen, and other painkillers such as ibuprofen have been found to be especially harmful to the kidneys if taken regularly for a long time. If you take painkillers regularly, check with your doctor to make sure you are not putting your kidneys at risk.

- **Injury** An injury such as a direct and forceful blow to the kidneys can lead to kidney dysfunction.

PREVENTION

The best ways to prevent kidney disease are to keep blood sugar levels and blood pressure within the normal ranges. Follow these guidelines:

- **Control your blood pressure.** If you have high blood pressure, take any medications your doctor prescribes. Medications that are used for lowering blood pressure can significantly slow or prevent kidney disease.

- **Eat a healthy diet and exercise regularly.** A healthy diet (see chapter 1) and regular physical activity will help control or prevent high blood pressure and type 2 diabetes, which can lead to kidney disease.

- **If you already have diabetes, keep your blood sugar levels normal.** Check your blood sugar levels as often as your doctor recommends, and take your diabetes medication exactly as prescribed, based on your food intake and physical activity. Follow a healthy diet and be physically active, and see your doctor regularly for checkups.

- **Limit your intake of over-the-counter pain relievers.** Ask your doctor about which pain relievers could cause kidney problems, especially those that combine acetaminophen, aspirin, and medications such as ibuprofen.

- **Ask your doctor to test your blood and urine for kidney disease.** If the tests show that you have kidney disease, your doctor may prescribe a medication such as an ACE inhibitor or angiotensin receptor blocker (ARB).

- **Limit your intake of protein to the recommended daily allowance for your gender and age.** People who already have diabetes or kidney disease should consume the recommended dietary allowance for protein (see page 6), but avoid high-protein diets. For people with greatly reduced kidney function, a diet containing low amounts of protein may help delay the onset of kidney failure.

Urinary incontinence

Urinary incontinence, the unintentional loss of urine, is a problem for more than 13 million Americans, affecting half of all people over the age of 65, mostly women. Although about half of all older people living at home or in long-term care facilities have episodes of incontinence, bladder problems are not a natural consequence of aging, and they are not exclusively a problem of older people. Urinary incontinence can be improved in 8 out of 10 cases, but fewer than half of people with bladder problems ever discuss the condition with their doctor, often allowing the condition to go untreated.

Incontinence has several causes. Women are most likely to develop incontinence during pregnancy and childbirth, or after the hormonal changes of menopause, because of weakened pelvic muscles (see page 497). Older men can become incontinent as the result of prostate surgery. Pelvic injury, spinal cord damage, consuming excess caffeine, and taking some medications (including cold remedies or over-the-counter diet pills) can also cause episodes of incontinence. There are a few different types of urinary incontinence.

- **Stress incontinence** Stress incontinence occurs when the bladder muscle cannot handle the increased pressure from high-impact exercises such as running or jumping, or from coughing, sneezing, or lifting something heavy. Chronic lung conditions that cause persistent coughing can also contribute to incontinence. This kind of incontinence occurs mostly in women under age 60 and in men who have had prostate surgery.

- **Urge incontinence**   In urge incontinence, also called irritable bladder, the bladder contracts uncontrollably, triggering a sudden urge to urinate. A person may leak a small amount of urine before reaching the toilet. This form of incontinence is more common in older adults.

- **Mixed incontinence**   Mixed incontinence is a combination of stress and urge incontinence, and is most common in older women.

- **Overflow incontinence**   In overflow incontinence, the bladder becomes too full because it cannot empty completely. This form of incontinence is caused by a bladder obstruction or injury. In men, it can result from an enlarged prostate (see page 502).

- **Functional incontinence**   People with functional incontinence may have problems thinking, moving, or speaking that keep them from reaching a toilet in time. For example, a person with Alzheimer's disease may not be able to plan a trip to the bathroom in time to urinate, or a person in a wheelchair may be unable to get to the toilet in time. Sometimes disorders such as arthritis make it hard to get to the toilet in time and can make it even harder to control urine leakage.

- **Incontinence caused by illness or infection**   Bladder infections and infections in the vagina can cause temporary incontinence. Bladder control returns when the illness goes away. Being unable to have a bowel movement or taking certain medications can also reduce bladder control.

Other factors, such as mental impairment or taking some medications, can also cause incontinence. Sometimes incontinence is a long-term, ongoing problem resulting from factors such as the following:

- Inability of the bladder to empty completely
- Weakening of the muscles that help to hold or release urine
- A blocked urinary passage
- Damage to the nerves that control the bladder

Urine leaking during pregnancy can result from the following:

- Pressure of the pregnancy on the bladder and pelvic muscles
- Vaginal delivery

- Damage to bladder-control nerves
- Episiotomy (an incision between the vagina and anus sometimes performed to ease delivery)

If you lose bladder control after having a baby, don't worry—the problem usually goes away on its own. Your muscles may just need time to recover after the delivery. If you still have bladder problems six weeks after giving birth, talk to your doctor. Without treatment, lost bladder control can become a long-term problem.

Some women have bladder-control problems after they enter menopause. After your periods end, your body stops making the female hormone estrogen. Some experts think the loss of estrogen may weaken bladder tissue.

RISK FACTORS

Urinary incontinence is very common. The following factors raise your risk:

- **Being female** Women have stress incontinence far more often than men; pregnancy, childbirth, and menopause are potential factors. Men who have prostate gland disorders are more likely to develop urge incontinence or overflow incontinence.

- **Age** As you age, the muscles in your pelvis begin to weaken, as they can in other parts of your body. This weakening lowers the amount of urine your bladder can hold.

- **Being overweight** Carrying extra weight puts excess pressure on the bladder and its adjoining muscles. The muscles lose strength and can release urine each time you cough or sneeze.

- **Smoking** Long-term smokers who have a chronic cough are at increased risk of developing stress incontinence. Persistent coughing strains the ring of muscle that constricts the opening of the urethra, making it less able to prevent urine from leaking.

- **Peripheral artery disease** Blocked arteries raise the risk for incontinence if they cause injury to the nerves that control the bladder.

- **High-impact exercise** High-impact activities, such as jumping, running, and playing basketball, can trigger incontinence. Such energetic activities place abrupt but powerful pressure on the bladder, allowing urine to leak out.

- **Certain medical conditions** Having kidney disease, diabetes, or arthritis can raise the risk of having episodes of incontinence.

PREVENTION

The most effective thing you can do to strengthen your pelvic muscles and prevent incontinence is to perform Kegel exercises (see page 498). In the beginning, it may be easier to do these exercises lying down. When your pelvic muscles get stronger, you can do the exercises sitting or standing at any time—for example, while sitting at your desk, in the car, waiting in line, doing the dishes. Be persistent. It may take three to six weeks before you see results.

14

CONTROLLING ALLERGIES

THE IMMUNE SYSTEM is a network of cells, tissues, and organs whose major job is to defend the body against outside invaders, primarily infection-causing microorganisms such as bacteria, viruses, parasites, and fungi. But sometimes the immune system reacts abnormally, or excessively. For example, the immune system may mistake the body's own cells or tissues for foreign invaders and launch an attack against them. This is what occurs in autoimmune diseases such as rheumatoid arthritis. In another abnormal immune reaction, the immune system overresponds to what is normally a harmless substance, such as ragweed pollen. The result is an allergic reaction. People can have an allergic reaction to something they inhale or eat, to something that comes in contact with their skin, to a medication, or to wasp or bee venom. Allergies are common, affecting an estimated 40 million to 50 million Americans.

Allergic rhinitis

Allergic rhinitis is an allergic reaction that produces inflammation of the mucous membrane that lines the nose. Allergic rhinitis is a collection of symptoms, predominantly in the nose and eyes, in people who are allergic to airborne particles of dust, dander, mold, or plant pollens. When the allergic rhinitis is seasonal, the condition is commonly called hay fever. Allergic reactions that last all year are known as perennial allergic rhinitis. Allergies result from an overly sensitive immune system response to a normally harmless substance that doesn't cause an immune response in most people.

The pollens that cause hay fever differ from person to person and from region to region. Large, visible pollens seldom cause hay fever. The main offenders are small, hard-to-see pollens. Hot, dry, windy days are more likely to have increased amounts of pollen in the air than cool, damp, rainy days, when most pollen gets washed to the ground. The following are some of the plants that are frequently blamed for hay fever:

- Trees (deciduous and evergreen)
- Grasses
- Ragweed

RISK FACTORS

The most important risk factor for allergic rhinitis, as with most allergies, is having a family history of allergies. You don't necessarily inherit a specific type of allergy, such as hay fever, but the inclination to develop allergies often runs in families. If both of your parents have allergies, you are likely to have them as well. For unknown reasons, the chances are greater if your mother has allergies than if just your father has them.

PREVENTION

Symptoms of allergic rhinitis can sometimes be prevented by avoiding known allergy triggers. During the pollen season, people with hay fever should remain indoors in an air-conditioned area whenever possible. Pollen seasons can differ among plants:

- Most trees produce pollen in the spring.
- Grasses usually produce pollen during the late spring and summer.
- Ragweed and other late-blooming plants produce pollen during late summer and early fall.

People who are sensitive to indoor allergens, such as house dust, should cover their mattresses and pillows with dust mite covers. See page 383 for more tips on ways to make your bedroom dust-free.

People who are allergic to animals, usually cats or dogs, should avoid close contact with them. Check to see if a friend has a cat or dog before going to visit. If your child has a significant animal allergy, try to make sure his or her friends' homes are animal-free. If contact does happen, wash your hands frequently and try to avoid touching your nose and eyes.

Food allergies

A food allergy is an abnormal response of the body's immune system to a specific food. The reaction usually occurs immediately or within a few hours after eating the food. Allergic reactions to food can cause serious illness and even death in severe cases. If you have a food allergy, it is extremely important for you to work with your doctor to find out which food or foods cause your allergic reaction. Food allergies can last a lifetime, but many food allergies diagnosed during childhood go away as the person gets older.

Some people have abnormal reactions such as indigestion to certain foods or beverages, but these are not allergic reactions because they don't involve the immune system. A more common food reaction is not actually a food allergy but a food intolerance, such as lactose intolerance (an adverse reaction to milk and other dairy products; see page 338), even though the symptoms can look and feel similar to those of a food allergy. Some substances, including sulfites in wine or monosodium glutamate (MSG) in food, can cause chemical disturbances in the body but are not true allergens.

If you have a true food allergy, your immune system mistakenly recognizes a certain food as a harmful substance. In response, your immune system produces a protein that fights the specific food. This protein, called a food-specific antibody, circulates through the blood and attaches to cells in your nose, throat, lungs, skin, stomach, or intestinal tract, triggering allergy symptoms. The next time you eat the same food, even in a small amount, it interacts with the antibody on the surface of the cells and causes those cells to release chemicals such as histamine. Depending on the part of the body in which histamine is released, it will produce the various symptoms of food allergy. In adults, the foods that most often cause allergic reactions include the following:

- Shellfish such as shrimp, crayfish, lobster, and crab
- Peanuts

- Tree nuts such as walnuts
- Fish
- Eggs

The following foods are most likely to cause allergies in children:

- Wheat
- Milk
- Peanuts
- Tree nuts such as walnuts
- Soybeans

Chocolate, often named a culprit by parents, hardly ever causes food allergies. Peanuts and tree nuts are the leading causes of the potentially deadly food allergy reaction called anaphylaxis (see next page). Children are more likely to outgrow allergies to milk, egg, or soy than allergies to peanuts. The foods to which adults or children are likely to be allergic are those foods they eat most often. In Japan, for example, rice allergy is common, while in Scandinavia, codfish allergy is common.

RISK FACTORS

The following are the most common risk factors for food allergy:

- **Family history** Allergies tend to run in families, so your immune system will form antibodies to a food if you come from a family in which allergies are common—not necessarily food allergies but any allergies, including allergic rhinitis (see page 369) or asthma (see page 380). If you have two parents with allergies, you are more likely to develop a food allergy than someone with one parent with allergies.

- **Age** Food allergies most frequently affect children, especially infants and toddlers.

PREVENTION

The only way to prevent an allergic reaction to food is to avoid the food that triggers the reaction. Once you and your doctor have identified the food (or foods) to which you are sensitive, you must remove the food from your diet. To do this requires reading the ingredient lists on the labels of all foods you are considering eating. Many allergy-causing foods, such as peanuts, eggs, and milk, are present in foods in which you might not expect to find them.

Peanuts, for example, are used as a protein source in many baked goods, and eggs are sometimes used in salad dressings.

If you have a food allergy, you need to be prepared for unintentional exposures. Even people who know exactly what food they are allergic to are occasionally unknowingly exposed to the food. If you have had an

---

WARNING

Anaphylactic shock

Anaphylactic shock, or anaphylaxis, is a severe and potentially fatal allergic reaction that requires emergency medical treatment. An anaphylactic reaction is characterized by the following symptoms:

- Severe itching or a rash over several areas of the body
- Swelling of the lips, tongue, or throat (feeling a lump in your throat that makes breathing difficult)
- Excessive sweating or cold, clammy skin
- Difficulty swallowing
- Difficulty breathing
- Difficulty speaking
- Vomiting
- Confusion, dizziness, light-headedness, or fainting

If you have any of the above symptoms for the first time, particularly after eating a new food, after an insect bite or sting, or after having an injection of a medication, call 911 or your local emergency number. If you have already had a severe allergic reaction, you should always wear a medical-alert bracelet or necklace and carry a self-injecting device containing epinephrine (adrenaline), often referred to as an epi-pen, for which your doctor can give you a prescription. If you think you are having an anaphylactic reaction, use the epi-pen to give yourself an injection. Seek medical help immediately, even if you have already given yourself an injection, by calling 911. Anaphylactic reactions can be fatal even when they start off with mild symptoms, such as tingling in the mouth and throat.

If you are with someone who is having an anaphylactic reaction, call 911 immediately. If the person becomes unconscious, lay him or her down with legs raised to improve circulation to the heart and brain. Don't try to take the person to the hospital yourself—it could delay lifesaving treatment from the paramedics.

CONTROLLING ALLERGIES   **373**

allergic reaction to a food, you should take the following potentially life-saving steps:

- Wear a medical-alert bracelet or necklace at all times stating that you have a food allergy and can have a severe reaction.
- Carry a self-injecting device (such as epi-pen) containing epinephrine so you can inject yourself when you feel symptoms coming on.

If your child has a food allergy, follow these guidelines to ensure his or her safety:

- Notify all your child's teachers and babysitters that your child has a food allergy.
- Explain food allergy symptoms to your child, caregivers, and teachers.
- Write up an action plan of care for your child's caregivers and for the school in case your child has a reaction. Make sure there is an epi-pen available and that caregivers know how to use it in case of an emergency.
- Have your child wear a medical-alert bracelet.

EXERCISE-INDUCED FOOD ALLERGY

Exercise-induced food allergy is an allergic reaction that occurs when exercising after eating a specific food. Some people get this reaction from many foods, and others get it only after eating a specific food. As exercise continues and body temperature rises, itching and light-headedness can occur. Allergic reactions such as hives may appear, and anaphylaxis (see previous page) may even develop. Preventing exercise-induced food allergy is simple—avoid foods that seem to cause this if you will be active, or avoid exercising for a couple of hours after eating the food.

Medication allergies

Allergies to medications account for 5 to 10 percent of all harmful drug reactions in the United States. The antibiotic penicillin is the drug that most often causes reactions, and is responsible for 400 deaths every year in the United States. If you are allergic to a medication, the first time you take the medication, your immune system mistakenly initiates a response against it. When you take the medication again, your immune system remembers it as an "enemy" and produces antibodies and histamine to fight it, producing the symptoms of an allergic reaction.

Most medication allergies are not serious, causing minor skin rashes and hives. But in some cases, they can cause more serious symptoms, including anaphylactic shock (see page 373), which can be fatal. Some people confuse an uncomfortable but not serious side effect of a medication, such as nausea, with a true drug allergy, which can be much more serious.

Following are the most common allergy-causing drugs:

- Penicillin
- Sulfa drugs
- Anticonvulsants
- Insulin (especially from animal sources)
- Local anesthetics
- X-ray contrast dyes

RISK FACTORS

The most important risk factor for a drug allergy is a family history of allergies. Allergies can run in families—not necessarily drug allergies but any allergies, including allergic rhinitis (see page 369) and asthma (see page 380). If you have two allergic parents, you are more likely to develop a drug allergy than someone with one allergic parent. Of course, you need to be exposed to the medication before you can develop an allergic reaction to it.

PREVENTION

If you know you are allergic to a certain medication, avoid taking it. Your doctor may tell you to also avoid similar medications. For example, if you are allergic to penicillin, you should also avoid the antibiotics amoxicillin or ampicillin. Sometimes doctors approve the use of a necessary medication for a person who has an allergy to it, after pretreating the person with corticosteroids and antihistamines to suppress the immune system reaction. But you should never attempt to pretreat yourself in this way, without a doctor's supervision.

Venom allergies

Thousands of people are stung by insects each year in the United States, but only about one or two out of every thousand are allergic to insect venom. From 40 to 50 Americans die each year as a result of allergic reactions to venom. If you have an allergy to the venom of a stinging insect, your immune system reacts to the venom as if it were a life-threatening substance. After the first sting, your immune system becomes sensitized to the venom and begins to produce antibodies and histamine that trigger the familiar symptoms of allergy. Honeybees, yellow jackets, hornets, wasps, and imported fire ants are the insects most likely to carry venom that could cause allergic reactions.

RISK FACTORS

You may have an increased risk for allergy to stinging insect venom in the following circumstances:

- **You have been frequently stung by bees.** The majority of people who are allergic to bees are beekeepers or their families, or people who live near beekeepers.
- **You have ever been stung by a wasp.** Sensitization to wasp venom needs only a few stings, and can even occur after a single sting.

PREVENTION

If you have an allergy to stinging insect venom, you should always wear a medical-alert tag and carry a hypodermic self-injecting device (epi-pen) containing epinephrine (adrenaline) in case of a sting. See your doctor about getting these items. An insect venom allergy can cause anaphylactic shock (see page 373), which can be fatal. Self-injecting epinephrine often reverses the reaction, but it does not always work. For this reason, you should still get medical help after an allergic reaction to a sting, even if you've given yourself an injection of epinephrine. Call 911.

You might also want to talk to your doctor about having venom immunotherapy, the process of injecting venom in slowly increasing doses to desensitize the immune system to the venom and prevent future allergic reactions.

It's always a good idea to stay away from stinging insects, even if you don't have an allergy. Most bees will not attack if you leave them alone, but if provoked, a bee will sting to defend itself or its nest. You can recognize wasps' nests by their papier-mâché-like appearance, often built in overhanging structures such as the eaves of buildings and under patio umbrellas. Allergic reactions to wasp stings seem to occur more often in the southern parts of the United States. Yellow jackets have alternating yellow and black body stripes and usually nest in the ground, where they can be easily stepped on or disturbed by activities such as lawn mowing. Yellow jackets are highly aggressive and often hover near sugary soft drink cans, food, and garbage. Imported fire ants are found in the southern United States. They sting repeatedly in a half-moon pattern. Within a day, the stings become a small pimple full of pus.

Take the following precautions to avoid stinging insects:

- Wear light-colored clothing that covers as much of your body as possible.

- Use unscented soaps, shampoos, deodorant, and cosmetics.

- Avoid flowering plants.

- Check for new nests during the warmer hours of the day in July, August, and September, when bees are very active.

- Keep areas clear of food. Social wasps thrive in places where people discard food, so clean up picnic tables, grills, and other outdoor eating areas.

- If a single stinging insect is flying around, remain still or lie facedown on the ground. The face is the most likely place for a bee or wasp to sting. Don't swing or swat at an insect or it could sting you in defense.

- If you're attacked by several stinging insects at the same time, run to get away from them. Bees release a chemical when they sting. This chemical alerts other bees to follow. Go indoors or jump into water if you can. Outdoors, it's better to run to a shaded area than to an open area.

- If a bee enters your vehicle, stop slowly, and open all the windows.

WHAT TO DO IF SOMEONE IS STUNG

- Have someone stay with the person to make sure he or she doesn't have an allergic reaction. If the person is having a severe reaction such as trouble breathing, call 911 immediately.
- Wash the site with soap and water.
- Remove the stinger by wiping a 4-inch by 4-inch piece of gauze over the site or by scraping a fingernail over the site. Never squeeze the stinger or use tweezers because doing so can cause more venom to enter the skin and could injure the muscle.
- Apply ice to reduce the swelling.
- Don't scratch the sting, because scratching can cause the site to swell and itch more, and increase the risk for infection.

15

KEEPING YOUR LUNGS HEALTHY

YOU BREATHE NEARLY 25,000 TIMES each day. When you inhale, your lungs get oxygen from the air and transfer it to your bloodstream, which carries the oxygen to all the cells in your body. A slice of normal lung looks like a pink sponge filled with tiny bubbles or holes. These bubbles, surrounded by a fine network of tiny blood vessels, give the lungs a large surface area to exchange oxygen (into the blood where it's carried throughout the body) and carbon dioxide (out of the blood). This process is called gas exchange.

In people with lung disease, this process doesn't work as it should. Every breath can be difficult. Millions of people in the United States have lung disease, and if all types of lung disease were counted together, it would be the No. 3 killer in the United States. Pneumonia (see page 299), an acute infection in the air spaces of the lungs, is common, and some types of pneumonia can be prevented with a vaccination. Two of the most common chronic lung diseases are asthma and chronic obstructive pulmonary disease. Asthma is not, for the most part, considered a preventable disease, but people who have asthma can prevent asthma attacks. Chronic obstructive pulmonary disease, on the other hand, is preventable—smoking is one of its primary causes.

Asthma

Asthma is a condition in which the airways in the lungs become inflamed and tighten, making it hard to breathe. The airways are the tubes that carry air in and out of the lungs. The inflammation and tightening usually occur only when a person with asthma has a respiratory infection or comes in contact with something he or she is sensitive to, such as a cat or a dog, cigarette smoke, cold air, grass, or flowers. Asthma is a chronic disease—it tends to last for years, and the symptoms usually occur in episodes, or "flares."

More than 22 million people in the United States have asthma, including 6.5 million children under age 18. Without appropriate treatment, asthma can greatly limit a person's activities and result in asthma attacks, which can require hospitalization and even be fatal; about 4,000 Americans die from asthma attacks each year. It's essential to treat underlying inflammation that causes the airways to tighten. Asthma can run in families. It often begins in childhood, but can start at any age. Sometimes asthma clears up on its own as a person gets older.

Asthma causes repeated episodes of wheezing, breathlessness, chest tightness, and nighttime or early morning coughing. Mucus production also increases and further clogs the airways. When asthma symptoms become worse than usual, it is called an asthma attack. In a severe asthma attack, the airways can narrow so much that vital organs don't get enough oxygen.

Asthma symptoms often get worse at night, waking a person because of difficulty breathing. Everyone's lungs work better during the day than at night, but for people with asthma, the nightly dip in lung function is even more exaggerated. At night, people might also be around more of the things—such as dust mites in bedding, feathers in pillows, and dander on pets—that can trigger asthma attacks. Stomach acid that can flow up into the mouth when a person is lying down (gastroesophageal reflux disease; see page 338) can trickle into the lungs and trigger an attack. Many people with asthma may experience anxiety during an asthma attack, because breathing is so difficult that it causes fear and a sense of impending doom.

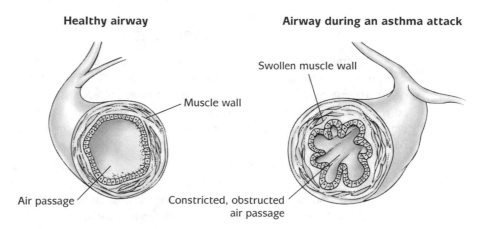

Healthy airway

Muscle wall

Air passage

Airway during an asthma attack

Swollen muscle wall

Constricted, obstructed
air passage

What happens during an asthma attack

An asthma attack occurs when the smooth muscle walls of the airways become swollen from inflammation and constrict, obstructing the airway. Mucus production also increases, further blocking the airways. Breathing becomes difficult and the body tissues get less oxygen.

RISK FACTORS

The following factors can increase a person's chances of developing asthma:

- Living in a city, especially the inner city
- Exposure to secondhand smoke
- Exposure to workplace triggers such as farm and laboratory animals, birds, insects, paint, plastics and resins, fish and seafood, plants, wood dust, metals, drugs, chemicals, dyes, and flour
- Having at least one parent with asthma
- Having many upper respiratory infections during childhood
- Being overweight
- Having chronic gastroesophageal reflux disease (GERD)

The following are risk factors for developing asthma during childhood:

- Premature birth
- Low birth weight
- Family history of asthma
- Inhaling tobacco smoke at home
- Being around things that trigger asthma (see box on next page)

ASTHMA TRIGGERS

An asthma attack can be triggered by exposure to certain things in the environment, such as dust mites and tobacco smoke. These factors are called asthma triggers. If you have asthma, be aware of your asthma triggers so you can avoid them as much as possible, and be alert for a possible attack when you can't avoid your triggers. Here are some of the most common triggers:

- **Secondhand smoke**   Secondhand smoke is the smoke breathed out by a smoker. Parents, friends, and relatives of children with asthma should try to stop smoking and should never smoke around anyone with asthma. Never allow others to smoke in your home or car.

- **Dust mites**   Dust mites are everywhere—they feed on human skin flakes and are found in mattresses, pillows, carpets, upholstered furniture, bedcovers, clothes, stuffed toys, and fabric-covered objects. Washing bedding frequently can help reduce exposure.

- **Outdoor air pollution**   Exposure to pollution from industrial emissions and vehicle exhaust can cause an asthma attack. If air pollution aggravates your asthma, pay attention to air quality forecasts on the radio and television and plan your activities for when air pollution levels will be low.

- **Cockroaches**   Cockroaches and their droppings can trigger asthma attacks in some people. Cockroaches are usually found where food is eaten and crumbs are left behind. Remove as many water and food sources as you can. Use roach traps or gels to reduce the number of cockroaches in your home.

- **Pets**   Furry pets are often triggers of asthma attacks. If the family pet triggers an asthma attack, you might consider finding a new home for your pet. At least keep the pet out of the bedrooms.

- **Mold**   When mold is inhaled or breathed in, it can cause an asthma attack. Eliminate mold in all areas of your home. Keep the humidity level in your home between 35 and 50 percent. In hot, humid climates, it may be helpful to use an air conditioner or a dehumidifier, or both. Fix water leaks, which allow mold to grow behind walls and under floors.

- **Other triggers**   Exposure to pollen; having a cold or the flu; strenuous physical exercise; some medications; severe weather such as thunderstorms, high humidity, or freezing temperatures; and some foods and food additives can trigger asthma attacks. Strong emotional states can also lead to hyperventilation (rapid breathing) and an asthma attack.

PREVENTION

You can control your asthma by knowing the warning signs of an attack, staying away from things that trigger your attacks, and following the advice of your doctor. When you control your asthma, you won't have symptoms such as wheezing or coughing, you'll sleep better, you won't miss work or school, you can participate in physical activities, and you won't have to go to the hospital for emergency treatment. Take the following steps to get your asthma under control:

- **Have an action plan.** If you have asthma, ask your doctor to develop an asthma action plan to help you prevent attacks. As part of the action plan, ask your doctor to write down how many times a day you should take your medication, and when. He or she will probably give you a list of triggers to avoid. Don't be afraid to ask your doctor to explain anything you don't understand.

  Your action plan should include specific goals that will help you determine how well your asthma is under control. Your goals should include the following:
  - Preventing asthma attacks
  - Leading an active life without having symptoms
  - Sleeping through the night without having breathing problems
  - Not having side effects from your asthma medication

- **Have a flu shot every year.** Getting a flu shot every year is especially important for people with asthma because they have a high risk of developing serious complications from the flu. However, only about one third of all adults with asthma get a flu shot each year.

- **Keep your bedroom trigger-free.** Wash sheets, blankets, and other bedclothes frequently in water that is at least 130° F. (Lower temperatures won't kill dust mites.) Encase box springs and mattresses in a zippered, dust-proof cover. Keep bedroom furniture and furnishings to a minimum to minimize dust. Use an air filter to remove allergens from the air. Keep all animals with fur or feathers out of the bedroom.

- **Watch for sulfites.** Sulfites are food additives that can trigger asthma symptoms and attacks. Ask if sulfites have been added to dishes when dining in restaurants. Check food and wine labels for the terms sodium bisulfite, potassium bisulfite, sodium sulfite, sulfur dioxide, and potassium metabisulfite.

Omega-3s may protect against asthma

Omega-3 fatty acids (see page 8) seem to reduce asthma symptoms in adults and may help prevent the development of asthma in children. In one study, the healthy fats improved lung function by 64 percent in adults who had exercise-induced asthma, by reducing airway inflammation. Other studies have suggested that greater consumption of fatty fish, which contain high amounts of omega-3s, can enhance lung function and protect children against asthma. In addition, pregnant women with asthma who consume fatty fish that are high in omega-3s may significantly reduce their child's risk of developing asthma.

If you have asthma, you can try eating three servings of fatty fish—such as salmon, mackerel, and sardines—every week. Ask your doctor about taking omega-3 fatty acid supplements.

- **Minimize pet dander.** Bathe pets weekly and keep them outside as much as possible. If you have a furry pet, vacuum often. If your floors have a hard, uncarpeted surface, damp-mop them every week.

- **Prevent exercise-induced attacks.** Warm up before a workout. Wear a face mask in cold weather. Don't exercise for two hours after a meal. Use an inhaler 20 minutes before you exercise. Stay away from pollen or animals. Exercise indoors if the weather is cold and dry.

Chronic obstructive pulmonary disease

Chronic obstructive pulmonary disease (COPD) is a term that refers to two common lung disorders: chronic bronchitis (inflammation of the airways) and emphysema (damage to the air sacs in the lungs). These disorders damage the lungs and airways, making it hard to breathe. In people with COPD, the airways (the tubes that carry air in and out of the lungs) are partly obstructed, making it difficult for air to get in and out. The walls in the tiny air sacs in the lungs also break down, reducing the surface area needed to exchange oxygen and carbon dioxide in the lungs.

Your airways branch out like an upside-down tree; at the end of each branch are many small, balloon-like air sacs called alveoli. In healthy people, each airway is clear and open. The air sacs are small and delicate, and both the airways and air sacs are elastic and springy. When you breathe in, each air sac fills up with air like a small balloon; when you breathe out, the balloon deflates and the air goes out. COPD makes the airways and air sacs lose their shape and become floppy. Less air gets in and less air goes out for the following reasons:

- The airways and air sacs lose their elasticity, like an old rubber band.
- The walls between many of the air sacs break down.
- The walls of the airways become thick and inflamed (and swollen).
- Cells in the airways make more mucus than usual, which clogs the airways.

COPD is a major cause of disability and the fourth leading cause of death in the United States. There is no cure for COPD because the damage to the airways and lungs cannot be reversed, but there are measures that can slow the damage.

Cigarette smoking is the most common cause of COPD. Most people with COPD are smokers or former smokers. Pipe, cigar, and all other types of tobacco smoke can also cause COPD, especially if the smoke is inhaled. Breathing in other kinds of lung irritants, such as pollution, dust, or chemicals, over a long period of time can also cause or contribute to COPD. The lungs and airways are highly sensitive to these irritants, which can cause inflammation and narrowing of the airways, and destroy the elastic fibers that enable the lungs to stretch and return to their resting state. This damage is what makes breathing air in and out of the lungs more difficult. Other factors that can irritate the lungs and play a part in the development of COPD include the following:

- Working around certain chemicals and breathing in their fumes or dust over many years
- Having heavy exposure to air pollution
- Being around secondhand smoke

RISK FACTORS

Most people with chronic obstructive pulmonary disease are smokers or former smokers. People with a family history of COPD are more likely to develop it if they smoke. The chances of developing COPD are also greater in people who have spent many years breathing in lung irritants, such as air pollution, and chemical fumes, vapors, or dusts in the workplace. A person who has had frequent and severe lung infections, especially during childhood, is at increased risk of having lung damage that can lead to COPD; however, the use of antibiotics for bacterial lung infections has significantly lowered this risk. COPD is usually diagnosed in people over age 40.

IF YOU HAVE COPD

If your doctor has told you that you have severe COPD, here are some things you can do to improve your breathing and ease your daily life:

- Ask your friends and family for help.
- Do things slowly.
- Do things while sitting down.
- Put things you need in an easy-to-reach place.
- Find simple ways to cook, clean, and do other chores. Some people use a small table or cart with wheels to move things around. Using a pole or tongs with long handles can help you reach things.
- Keep your clothes loose.
- Wear clothes and shoes that are easy to put on and take off.
- Ask for help moving things so that you don't need to climb stairs as often.

If you're finding that it's becoming more difficult to catch your breath, your coughing has gotten worse, you're coughing up more mucus, or you have signs of infection (such as a fever), call your doctor right away. Your doctor may prescribe an antibiotic if you have an infection. In the following situations, you may need to be hospitalized:

- You have extreme difficulty catching your breath.
- You have a hard time talking.
- Your lips or fingernails turn blue or gray.
- You are not mentally alert.
- Your heartbeat is very fast.
- Home treatment of your worsening symptoms has not helped relieve the symptoms.

If you smoke, the most important thing you can do to prevent COPD is to quit smoking (see page 135). Ask your doctor about local smoking-cessation programs; many hospitals offer these programs. It's also important to stay away from people who are smoking and places where people smoke, such as bars. If you have a job that exposes you to dangerous fumes, vapors, or dust, consider finding another job. If that's not possible, take every precaution available at work, such as wearing a mask and other protective gear.

It's also important to keep the air in your home clean. Here are some steps that can help you breathe more easily at home:

- Keep smoke, fumes, and strong smells out of your house.
- If your house is painted or sprayed for insects, have it done when you can stay elsewhere.
- Cook near an open door or window.
- If you heat with wood or kerosene, keep a door or window open.
- Keep your windows closed and stay at home when air pollution or dust levels are high.

Here are some other tips to help improve your breathing and reduce your risk for problems:

- Get a flu shot and pneumonia vaccination.
- Learn breathing exercises.
- Walk and exercise regularly.
- Eat healthy foods.

Occupational lung diseases

People can be exposed to poisonous substances in the form of gases, vapors, fumes, particles, or powders while on the job, whether they work in an office or factory or on a farm. Many of these substances can damage the respiratory tract or cause lung diseases. The sources of some occupational lung diseases (such as inhaling a toxic gas that instantly makes breathing difficult) are obvious. Other causes—such as exposure to asbestos (an insulating building material) or coal dust—can take from 10 to 25 years to cause disease. Pneumoconiosis ("dust lung") is the name for lung diseases that occur from long-term exposure to metallic or mineral dusts such as asbestos (asbestosis), beryllium (berylliosis), coal (coal miners' lung, also called black lung disease), and silica (silicosis).

If your lungs are repeatedly exposed to harmful substances, the chronic inflammation can lead to permanent scarring of lung tissue and potentially fatal respiratory failure. Exposure to some substances increases the risk for lung cancer, especially in smokers.

PREVENTION

If you are exposed to potentially harmful substances, change jobs if possible. If you cannot change jobs, try to avoid the toxic material or fumes in the following ways:

- Avoid unventilated areas.
- Wear a canister face mask while working.
- If you smoke, stop (see page 135). Smoking increases the risk of developing other lung disorders.

16

HEADING OFF HEADACHES

WHAT HURTS WHEN YOU HAVE A HEADACHE? The bones of the skull and tissues of the brain cannot feel pain because they lack pain-sensitive nerve fibers. But the network of nerves that extends over the scalp, and certain nerves in the face, mouth, and throat can hurt badly. Also sensitive to pain are the muscles of the head and the blood vessels along the surface and at the base of the brain, because they contain delicate nerve fibers.

Stress, muscle tension, dilated blood vessels, and other triggers of headaches can set the ends of these pain-sensitive nerves into spasms of pain. Once stimulated, a nerve sends a message up the length of the nerve fiber to the nerve cells in the brain, signaling that a part of the body hurts. For example, when you stub your toe, nerves in the toe send a message to the brain that says, "Ouch! My toe hurts." In the same way, nerves in a dilated blood vessel send pain messages to the brain during a headache.

Most headaches do not require medical attention. But some types of headaches, such as the following, signal more serious disorders and require immediate medical attention.

- Sudden, severe headache
- Sudden, severe headache with a stiff neck

- Headache with fever
- Headache with convulsions
- Headache accompanied by confusion or loss of consciousness
- Headache following a blow to the head
- Headache with pain in the eye or ear
- Persistent headache in a person who was previously headache-free
- Recurring headaches in children
- Headache that interferes with normal life

Tension headaches

It's 4:00 p.m. and your boss has just asked you to prepare a 20-page briefing paper. Due date: tomorrow. You're already stressed-out and tired, and the more you think about the assignment, the tenser you become. Your teeth clench, your brow wrinkles, and soon you have a splitting tension headache. Tension headaches are the most common type of headache, named for the contraction of the neck, face, and scalp muscles brought on by stressful events. Tension headaches are a more severe but temporary form of muscle-contraction headaches. The pain is mild to moderate and feels like pressure is being applied to the head or neck. The headache usually disappears after the period of stress is over. Ninety percent of all headaches are classified as tension or muscle-contraction headaches.

Chronic muscle-contraction headaches can last for weeks, months, and sometimes years. The pain of these headaches is often described as a tight band around the head or a feeling that the head and neck are in a cast. The pain is steady, and usually occurs on both sides of the head. Chronic muscle-contraction headaches can make the scalp feel sore; even combing your hair can be painful.

Scientists used to think that the main cause of chronic muscle-contraction headache pain was sustained muscle tension, but a growing number of experts believe that, for many people, chronic muscle-contraction headaches are caused by depression and anxiety. The headaches tend to occur in the early morning or evening, when an affected person is anticipating conflicts at home or at work.

However, emotional factors are not the only triggers of muscle-contraction headaches. Some physical postures that tense the head and neck muscles—such as looking down while reading—can cause head and neck pain. So can prolonged writing under poor light, sitting in front of a computer screen all day, holding a phone between the shoulder and ear, and even prolonged gum-chewing.

More serious problems that can cause muscle-contraction headaches include degenerative arthritis of the neck and temporomandibular joint dysfunction (a disorder in the joint between the temporal bone above the ear and the lower jaw bone). The disorder results from a misaligned bite and jaw-clenching.

RISK FACTORS

Tension headaches are so common that almost everyone has had one, but the disorder is more common in women, whites, and people between ages 20 and 50. Unlike migraines, muscle-contraction headaches are not linked to hormones or foods and don't have a strong hereditary connection. Risk factors include the following:

- Poor posture
- Being overworked
- Having a cold or the flu
- Insomnia or sleep apnea
- Being overweight
- An underactive thyroid gland
- Dental problems
- Allergies
- Drinking alcohol excessively
- Temporomandibular joint dysfunction

PREVENTION

If you have tension headaches, you can try to prevent them using a variety of techniques. For example, keeping your posture erect when sitting or standing for long periods can prevent compression of the muscles and nerves in your neck, which could contribute to tension headaches. You could also try relaxation techniques (see page 122) or counseling to help you reduce and manage your stress. Cervical collars are sometimes recommended to encourage good posture. People who have infrequent tension headaches may benefit from taking a hot shower or applying moist heat to the back of their neck. Physical therapy, massage, and gentle neck exercises may also be helpful.

Migraine headaches

A migraine headache is severe head pain that is usually felt on only one side of the head, most often in the front of the head around the temples or behind one eye. The pain can be accompanied by nausea and vomiting and sensitivity to light, loud sounds, or certain odors. Migraines can strike at any time, but they often start in the morning. The pain can last a few hours or up to one or two days.

Medical science does not fully understand what causes migraine headaches. One theory focuses on blood vessel activity in the brain. Blood vessels can narrow and expand. Narrowing can constrict blood flow, causing problems with sight or dizziness. When the blood vessels expand, they press on nearby nerves, causing pain, according to the theory. Another theory focuses on chemical changes in the brain. When brain chemicals transmit messages from one cell to another—including the messages that tell blood vessels to narrow or expand—the messages can get interrupted, triggering a migraine.

More recently, genes have been linked to migraines. People who get migraines may inherit abnormal genes that control the functions of certain brain cells. Then, when the person comes in contact with a substance to which his or her body is sensitive, the substance triggers a headache.

Most people who get migraines know that specific things can trigger their headaches. Triggers can vary from person to person. One person's response to triggers can also vary from headache to headache. Some common triggers for recurring migraines include the following:

- Hunger
- Lack of sleep
- Bright light
- Loud noise
- Certain odors, such as exhaust fumes or perfume
- Hormone changes during the menstrual cycle
- Stress or anxiety

- Weather changes
- Alcohol, especially red wine
- Nicotine
- Certain foods, such as chocolate or aged cheeses
- Some food additives, such as MSG (monosodium glutamate) or the sulfites in wine

RISK FACTORS

Migraines often become less severe and less frequent with age. The following risk factors are common in people who have migraines:

- **Age**   Migraines most often affect people between ages 15 and 55.
- **Family history**   Many people who have migraines have parents or siblings with recurring migraines.
- **Gender**   Migraines are more common in women than in men.

HEADACHES IN CHILDREN

Migraine headaches often begin in childhood or adolescence, especially as kids enter adolescence and experience the challenges of puberty and secondary school. Children with migraines often have nausea and excessive vomiting. Some children have periodic vomiting but no headache (called an abdominal migraine), but then go on to develop headaches when they're older.

Childhood headaches can also be a sign of depression. If your child develops headaches along with other symptoms, such as a change in mood or sleep habits, talk to your child's doctor. Antidepressant medication and psychotherapy can be effective in treating childhood depression and related headaches.

The following factors can cause headaches in children:

- **Lack of sleep**   Make sure your child gets enough sleep. Encourage quiet activities before bed and keep the same bedtime and wake-up time every day.
- **Eye strain**   Limit screen time and keep TVs and computers out of your child's room.
- **Hunger**   Make sure that your child gets enough to eat throughout the day.
- **Migraine triggers**   Find out what triggers migraines in your child and help your child avoid those triggers. Watch for MSG (monosodium glutamate), caffeine, food dyes, and additives in foods (check labels), and loud noises and bright light.
- **Infection**   Watch for the signs of a sinus infection, including headache, feeling of pressure in the sinuses, fever, and bad breath.
- **Stress**   Talk with your child to find out if something is troubling him or her.

PREVENTION

The best way to prevent migraines is to find out what events or lifestyle factors, such as stress or certain foods, trigger your headaches. You might find it helpful to keep a headache diary to pinpoint your personal headache triggers. Each time you have a migraine, write down the time of day, the point in your menstrual cycle, where you are at the time, and what you were doing when the migraine began. Try to avoid or limit your triggers as much as you can. Because migraine headaches tend to be more common during stressful times, find healthy ways to cope with stress (see page 114). Talk with your doctor about starting an exercise program or taking a class to learn relaxation skills.

If your doctor has prescribed medication to help prevent your migraines, take it exactly as prescribed. Ask your doctor what you should do if you miss a dose and for how long you should take the medication. If you use headache medications too often or take more than the doctor prescribes, the medication can actually cause a condition called "rebound headaches"—the medication no longer relieves the pain and instead is causing headaches. Let your doctor know if the amount of medication he or she prescribed is not helping your headaches.

17

KEEPING YOUR EARS, NOSE, AND THROAT HEALTHY

YOUR EARS, NOSE, AND THROAT are complex, interconnected structures that enable you to make sounds, hear, keep your balance, smell, breathe, and swallow. A disorder in one of these areas often can affect the others. For example, many ear, nose, and throat problems can play a role in the development of headaches. Doctors who specialize in diagnosing and treating disorders of the ear, nose, and throat are otolaryngologists, informally referred to as ENTs.

Your ears

Your ears have two major functions: hearing and balance. The structures of the outer and middle ear collect sound and transmit it to the brain. The inner ear has tiny fluid-filled structures that are sensitive to position and movement and help in maintaining balance. The ear is susceptible to a variety of disorders—some that can lead to loss of hearing and others that can cause dizziness or loss of balance.

Hearing loss

Hearing loss is one of the most common conditions affecting older adults. Nearly one in three Americans ages 65 to 74 and almost half of those 75 and older experience some degree of hearing loss. Hearing loss can take many forms ranging from mild, in which a person misses certain high-pitched sounds (such as the voices of women and children), to a total loss. It can be hereditary or result from an underlying medical condition, an injury, taking certain medications, or long-term exposure to loud noise.

Hearing loss falls into two major categories: sensorineural and conductive. Sensorineural hearing loss is a permanent form of hearing loss that results from damage to the cochlea or to the auditory nerve that prevents it from transmitting sounds to the brain. Some degree of sensorineural hearing loss is common as people age. But it can also occur at any age from, for example, exposure to loud music or machinery noise, some viral infections, heredity, or as a side effect of some medications. Because this type of hearing loss can result from exposure to overly amplified music at rock concerts or by listening to music at high volumes through earphones, doctors have dubbed it "rock-and-roll deafness." About 30 million American workers are exposed to dangerous noise levels on the job.

Conductive hearing loss occurs when something interferes with the structures in the ear that conduct sound waves to the brain. Potential causes include impacted earwax, fluid in the middle ear, a perforated eardrum, or a cyst or tumor in the ear. These problems can usually be corrected with medical treatment.

Some hearing loss can be prevented. For example, vaccines can prevent some infections that can cause sensorineural hearing loss, such as meningitis or measles. Noise-induced hearing loss is 100 percent preventable. And since noise-induced hearing loss is permanent and irreversible, it's very important to take preventive measures early to protect your hearing. In the average person, aging does not cause impaired hearing until after age 60. People who have not been exposed to loud noise and are otherwise healthy can retain their hearing well into older age. But people who have been exposed to loud noise and have not protected their hearing can begin to lose their hearing earlier in life. For example, by age 25 the average carpenter has the hearing of a 50-year-old who has not had the same exposure to loud noise.

How do you know if a sound is loud enough to damage your ears? Use these two guidelines. First, if you have to raise your voice to talk to someone who is at arm's length from you, the noise is potentially hazardous to your hearing. Second, if your ears ring or sounds seem dull or flat after you leave a noisy place, you probably were exposed to dangerous noise levels. The effects of loud noise on your hearing depend on how loud the noise is and how long you have been exposed to it. But instead of wondering whether a sound may be dangerously loud, the safest course is to protect your ears by always wearing hearing protectors whenever you are around loud noise. If you already have hearing loss, it's still important to protect your hearing to reduce further loss; loud noises can continue to damage your remaining hearing.

RISK FACTORS

Age is an important risk factor for hearing loss because the inner and middle ear tend to gradually degenerate with age. The tiny hair cells in the cochlea die off and cannot grow back. But you can begin to lose your hearing earlier

SOUNDS AND HEARING

Scientists measure the volume of sound in decibels. Most otolaryngologists advise people to use earplugs or take other protective measures whenever they are exposed to sounds registering at 85 decibels and above. Hearing loss can be permanent if earsplitting sounds damage or destroy the fragile cells in the inner ear; these cells can never be restored. The following chart lists everyday sounds and their assigned sound levels.

Decibels	Type of sound	Effect on hearing
10	Barely audible	Safe
20	Ticking watch	Safe
30	Soft whisper at 16 feet	Safe
40	Suburban street (no traffic)	Safe
50	Interior of urban home	Safe
60	Normal conversation	Safe
70	Noisy restaurant	Safe
80	Loud music from stereo	Safe
90	Truck at 16 feet	Risk of injury
100	Rock concert	Risk of injury
110	Jet engine at 800 feet	Risk of injury
120	Jackhammer	Injury
130	Jet engine at 100 feet	Injury

in life if you expose yourself to extremely loud noise. You are probably at risk for hearing loss if you have been in the following circumstances:

- You have worked in a loud factory or operated loud equipment such as a jackhammer.
- You have attended rock concerts without wearing ear protectors.
- You have ridden loud subway trains.

PREVENTION

Noise-induced hearing loss is easy to prevent. Practice good hearing health in your everyday life by taking the following measures:

- Know which noises can cause damage to hearing (those at or above 85 decibels).
- Wear earplugs or other protective devices whenever you are exposed to loud noises. (Special earplugs and earmuffs are available at hardware and sporting goods stores.)
- Use MP3 players properly; make sure your children are listening at a safe volume.
- Be alert to hazardous noise in the environment, such as when you walk by a construction site where jackhammers and other loud equipment are being used.
- Protect the ears of young children.
- Make family, friends, and colleagues aware of the hazards of noise.

If you already have hearing loss and it is difficult for you to hear speech, ask your friends and family to face you when they talk so you can see their face. Seeing their expressions may help you understand them better. Ask people to speak more loudly, but not to shout. Tell them they don't have to talk slowly, just more clearly. Speaking with a lower pitch rather than a higher pitch may also help.

MP3 PLAYERS AND HEARING

The sound quality of MP3 players is high, and users tend to listen to their players a lot—often with the volume turned up high. Both the length of time you listen to an MP3 player and the volume you set it at can affect your hearing. Long-term use of MP3 players set at a high volume can cause hearing loss. You may not notice the hearing loss for years, but once the damage is done, it cannot be reversed. To make sure your hearing is protected, take these steps while listening to your favorite tunes:

- Keep the volume low enough to be able to have a conversation with your ear buds in.
- Never turn the volume all the way up—keep it below 60 percent of the maximum.

You'll know the music's too loud if you experience any of the following:

- You can't perceive conversations going on around you.
- People nearby can hear your music.
- You shout rather than speak in normal tones when you talk to someone nearby.

HOW TO PROTECT YOUR EARS FROM NOISE

The list below explains the most common types of ear protectors. Remember to use them whenever you're exposed to sounds above 85 decibels. Keep in mind that the best hearing protector is one that's comfortable and convenient enough that you'll wear it whenever you're in an environment with potentially damaging noise.

- **Expandable foam plugs** These plugs are made of a material designed to expand and conform to the shape of the wearer's ear canal.

- **Premolded, reusable plugs** Premolded plugs are made from silicone, plastic, or rubber, and come in "one-size-fits-all" or in different sizes. You may need a different size plug for each ear. The plugs should seal the ear canal without being uncomfortable. You may have to try different sizes before finding a good fit. Premolded plugs are inexpensive, reusable, washable, and convenient to carry.

- **Canal caps** Canal caps resemble earplugs on a flexible plastic or metal band. The earplug tips of a canal cap may be made from a foam or premolded material. Some are attached to bands that you can wear on your head, behind your neck, or under your chin. The main advantage of canal caps is convenience. When it's quiet, workers can leave the band hanging around their neck and then quickly insert the plug tips when hazardous noise starts again. Some people find the pressure from the bands uncomfortable, and not all canal caps have tips that adequately block all types of noise. The canal cap tips that resemble stand-alone earplugs seem to block the most noise.

- **Earmuffs** Earmuffs block out noise by completely covering the outer ear. You can get muffs with small or large ear cups depending on how much noise protection you need. Some muffs also include electronic components to help users communicate. Workers with heavy beards or sideburns or who wear glasses may not get good protection from earmuffs because hair and the arms of the glasses can break the seal of the earmuffs around the ear. For such workers, earplugs are best.

- **Other devices** Manufacturers have come up with new devices that are combinations of the traditional types of hearing protectors. Many people like the comfort of foam plugs, but don't want to roll them with dirty hands. They can use a new plug that's essentially a foam tip on a stem that is inserted like a premolded plug without having to be rolled.

Tinnitus

Do you hear a ringing, roaring, clicking, or hissing sound in your ears often or all the time? If you answered yes, you may have tinnitus. Tinnitus is a symptom, not a disease. The most common cause of tinnitus is hearing loss from damage to the hair cells of the cochlea (which convey sound information to the brain), which usually results from aging or exposure to loud noise. It also can result from an underlying condition such as an earwax blockage. Taking some medications—including nonsteroidal anti-inflammatory drugs, antidepressants, or some antibiotics—can also cause tinnitus. Some medical conditions, such as allergies, tumors that affect the auditory or facial nerves, or diabetes, can increase a person's risk for tinnitus. Up to 12 million Americans have tinnitus, and for about a million people, it is so severe that it interferes with daily life, making it difficult to hear, work, or even sleep.

The following factors can contribute to the development of tinnitus:

- **Hearing loss**   Scientists have discovered that people with different kinds of hearing loss can also have tinnitus.

- **Loud noise**   Too much exposure to loud noise can cause noise-induced hearing loss and tinnitus.

- **Some medications**   More than 200 medications, including aspirin (in higher doses), can cause or aggravate tinnitus. If you have tinnitus and you take medication, ask your doctor or pharmacist whether your medication could be the problem.

- **Other health problems**   Allergies, tumors, and problems in the heart and blood vessels, jaws, and neck can cause tinnitus.

IF YOU HAVE TINNITUS

If you already have tinnitus, see your doctor to determine the cause. He or she will check to see if your blood pressure, kidney function, diet, or allergies could be contributing to the problem, or if it is the result of a medication you are taking.

Try to think about some things that might help you cope with your tinnitus. Many people find that listening to music can make them forget about their tinnitus for a while. Music also helps mask the irritating sound of tinnitus. Avoid anything that can make your tinnitus worse, including smoking, drinking alcohol excessively, and listening to too-loud noise. If you are a construction worker, an airport worker, or a hunter, or if you are regularly exposed to loud noise at home or at work, wear ear plugs or other protective gear (see the box on the previous page) to protect your hearing and prevent your tinnitus from getting worse.

To prevent tinnitus, take the following measures:

- Avoid loud noises. Some forms of hearing loss can cause tinnitus.
- Lower your intake of caffeine, which can reduce blood flow to the ear.
- Don't smoke. Nicotine reduces blood circulation in the ear.
- Exercise regularly. Physical activity makes blood flow better.
- Stay at a healthy weight. Tinnitus develops more frequently in people who are obese.
- Ask your doctor if any medications (including over-the-counter products) you are taking could cause tinnitus.

The nose

Your nose prevents small particles in the air from entering your airways by trapping them in tiny protective hairs that line the nasal passages. The lining cleans, moistens, and warms the air as it travels toward the throat and lungs. Specialized cells in the nose sample the particles and send information to the brain, creating the sense of smell. People who smoke often notice that they cannot smell well, because the smoke damages these cells. Allergies and colds can also temporarily affect the sense of smell. Nosebleeds are the most common preventable nose problem.

Nosebleeds

The nose contains many small and fragile blood vessels that bleed easily. As air passes through the nose, it can dry and irritate the lining of the nose, forming crusts. The crusts can bleed when you rub, pick, or blow your nose. Low humidity compounds the problem, as do colds, allergies, and sinus infections. In rare cases, nosebleeds may signal a bleeding disorder or high blood pressure. Taking blood-thinning medication can cause nosebleeds or make them worse. Nosebleeds are very common, especially in children between the ages of 2 and 10. Although they can be alarming for some children, nosebleeds are rarely serious.

The following factors can cause nosebleeds:

- Very cold or very dry air

- Blowing the nose too hard
- Injury to the nose
- Nose picking
- Allergies
- Repeated sneezing
- Colds or the flu
- Taking blood-thinning medication or large doses of aspirin
- Nasal sprays
- Snorting cocaine

PREVENTION

The following measures can help you prevent nosebleeds:

- Don't blow your nose forcefully.
- Humidify the air in your home.
- During the winter, swab your nostrils with a little petroleum jelly at night.
- Use a saline (saltwater) nose spray if your nose feels dry.
- Don't pick your nose; use a tissue.

The throat

The throat is part of the passageway that leads from the back of the nose and mouth down to the trachea (windpipe) and esophagus. The throat splits into two parts at the opening to the voice box. Breathed air passes through the throat into the trachea, and swallowed food moves down the throat into the esophagus on its way to the stomach.

Obstructive sleep apnea

Obstructive sleep apnea is a serious and potentially life-threatening breathing disorder that affects more than 12 million Americans. In a person who has sleep apnea, breathing stops for short periods during sleep. Each pause in breathing may last 10 to 20 seconds or more, and the pauses can occur 20 to 30 times or more an hour. During the periods when breathing stops, air cannot flow into the lungs. The amount of oxygen in the blood may drop dangerously low. Normal breaths then start again with a loud snort or choking sound. After a few normal breaths, the person falls back asleep and the cycle starts again.

In obstructive sleep apnea, the base of the tongue, the uvula, or the soft palate becomes overly relaxed or sags down too far, obstructing airflow to and from the windpipe. Drinking alcohol or using sleeping pills can worsen the problem by making the tissues more likely to sag.

Sleep apnea interrupts sleep throughout the night, making a person feel very sleepy during the day. In fact, 1 in 25 middle-aged men and 1 in 50 middle-aged women have sleep apnea so severe that it causes them to have daytime sleepiness.

People with obstructive sleep apnea often snore loudly, although not everyone who snores has sleep apnea. People with sleep apnea often don't know they snore, and most people who have sleep apnea don't know they have it. A family member or bed partner may notice the signs of sleep apnea first. Sleep apnea is more common in people who are overweight, but thin people can also have it. Obstructive sleep apnea can also occur in children who snore. If your child snores, you should discuss it with your child's doctor.

Untreated sleep apnea can increase the risk for high blood pressure, heart attack, and stroke, and increase the likelihood of having work-related and driving accidents.

RISK FACTORS

Anyone can have obstructive sleep apnea, but more than half of all people with the disorder are overweight, and most snore heavily. Sleep apnea is more common in blacks, Hispanics, and Pacific Islanders than in non-Hispanic whites. If someone in your family has sleep apnea, you are more likely to develop it than someone who doesn't have a family history of the condition.

The following factors increase a person's risk for sleep apnea:

- Being a loud snorer
- Being overweight
- Having high blood pressure
- Having a structural abnormality in the nose, throat, or mouth
- Having a medical condition that causes congestion in the nose and throat, such as hay fever or other allergies
- Having a family history of sleep apnea
- Being a smoker

PREVENTION

You can reduce your risk for sleep apnea by taking the following steps:

- Lose weight if you are overweight. Sleep apnea can improve with even modest weight loss.
- Stop smoking if you smoke. (Nicotine relaxes the muscles that keep the airways open.)
- Avoid drinking alcohol and using sleeping pills and sedatives before bed. (These substances can slacken the throat muscles and slow breathing.)
- Eat a healthy diet.
- Get regular exercise.
- Sleep on your side. (Sleeping on your back promotes snoring.)
- Raise the head of your bed 4 to 6 inches.

If you have sleep apnea, ask your doctor about a treatment called continuous positive airway pressure (CPAP). In CPAP, you wear a mask over your nose and/or mouth during sleep; pressure from an air blower forces air through your nasal passages, preventing tissue in the throat from sagging, and improving breathing.

Choking

Food or small objects can get caught in the throat and obstruct the airway, preventing oxygen from getting to the lungs and brain. If the brain is deprived of oxygen for more than even a few minutes, the result can be severe brain damage or death. Young children face an especially high risk for choking. Watch for choking hazards, such as toys with small parts, and always supervise your children when they eat.

When someone is choking, you need to act fast to save a life. Learn how to do the Heimlich maneuver and cardiopulmonary resuscitation (CPR). You can find out about CPR classes available in your community by asking your doctor or by contacting a local hospital or fire department. You can also contact the local chapter of the American Heart Association or the American Red Cross.

PREVENTION

Developmentally, young children are at high risk for choking, primarily because putting things in their mouth is one of the ways they explore the world. Anything that fits into the mouth can be a danger. Choking is usually caused by food, toys, and other small objects that can easily lodge in a child's small airway. Pay special attention to the following potential choking hazards.

HEIMLICH MANEUVER

The Heimlich maneuver is an effective first-aid measure for dislodging food or another foreign object in a choking person.

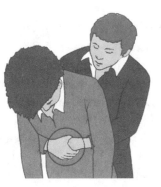

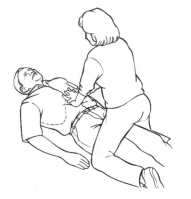

Heimlich maneuver on a conscious adult

If you see someone choking and the person is conscious, stand behind the person and place your fist (with your thumb folded in) slightly above the person's navel and below the ribs and breastbone. Do not touch the breastbone. Wrap your other hand around the fist and give several quick, forceful upward thrusts. Push only on the person's abdomen—do not squeeze the ribs. Repeat until the person coughs up the object. You may have to repeat the maneuver 6 to 10 times.

Heimlich maneuver on an unconscious adult

If a person who is choking is unconscious or becomes unconscious, place the person on his or her back on a hard surface. Straddle the person and place the heel of one hand on the person's abdomen, slightly above the navel and below the ribs (dotted line). Put your other hand on top of the first hand. Keeping your elbows straight, give several quick, forceful thrusts downward and forward (toward the person's head). Do not press on the person's ribs; press on the abdomen only. Repeat until the person coughs up the object.

Food

Don't give a child under age 4 any hard, smooth foods that can partially or completely block the windpipe, including nuts of any type, sunflower seeds, watermelon with seeds, cherries with pits, raw carrots, raw peas, raw celery, popcorn, or hard candy. Some soft foods—including hot dogs, sausages, grapes, and caramels—can also cause choking because they are the right shape for blocking a child's windpipe. Serve these foods only after cutting them into small pieces. Consider chewing gum and spoonfuls of peanut butter to be potential choking hazards. When babies begin eating solids, beware of foods such as raw apples and pears, which may be difficult to chew without teeth (or with just a few teeth).

Encourage children to sit when eating and to chew thoroughly. Teach them to chew and swallow their food before talking or laughing. Never let children run, play sports, or ride in the car with gum, candy, or lollipops in their mouths. Be especially vigilant during adult parties, when nuts and other foods might be easily accessible to small hands. Clean up early and carefully, and check the floor for dropped foods that could cause choking.

Toys

Always follow all manufacturers' age recommendations when buying toys. Some toys have small parts that can cause choking, so read and heed all warnings on a toy's packaging. Never buy vending-machine toys for small children; these toys are not required to meet safety regulations and often contain small parts. Check toys frequently for loose or broken parts, such as a stuffed animal's loose eye or a broken plastic hinge.

Warn older children not to leave loose game parts or toys with small pieces in easy reach of younger siblings. Watch out for toys that contain small magnets that can fall out and be swallowed.

Balloons and other small objects

Never give balloons to a child younger than age 8. A child who is blowing up or chewing on a balloon can choke by inhaling it. Inflated balloons also pose a risk because they can pop without warning and be inhaled. Safely dispose of button-cell batteries. Encourage children not to put pencils, crayons, or erasers in their mouth when coloring or drawing.

Do not reward small children with coins.

18

KEEPING YOUR EYES HEALTHY

THE EYES ARE INTRICATE, delicate structures that process information from light and transmit it to your brain, enabling you to see. The best defense against eye problems is to have regular checkups, because eye diseases don't always produce symptoms. Early detection and treatment can often prevent vision loss. See an ophthalmologist (eye M.D.) right away if you have a sudden change in vision, everything looks dim, or you see flashes of light. Other symptoms that need quick attention are pain, double vision, and prolonged redness. It is also important to protect your eyes from injury during work or recreational activities.

This chapter explains how you can help prevent the common eye disorders cataracts, glaucoma, age-related macular degeneration, and diabetic retinopathy. All of these conditions cause gradual changes in vision. If you have a sudden change in your vision, it is an emergency. Sudden onset of loss of visual fields in parts of one or both eyes, or sudden onset of double vision could be symptoms of a serious problem (such as retinal detachment) or a potentially life-threatening condition (such as stroke; see page 238). If you develop sudden vision symptoms, do not wait to see if they will get better. Get medical help immediately.

Cataracts

A cataract is a clouding of the lens of the eye that can impair vision. The lens is a clear part of the eye that helps to focus light—or an image—on the retina (the light-sensitive tissue at the back of the eye). The lens must be clear for the retina to receive a sharp image. If the lens is cloudy from a cataract, the image seen will be blurred, like looking through a window covered with petroleum jelly.

Most cataracts develop as a result of aging. Cataracts are very common in older people—by age 80, more than half of Americans have a cataract or have had cataract surgery. A cataract can occur in one or both eyes. Cataracts tend to develop slowly, so vision worsens gradually. When a cataract is small, the cloudiness affects only a small part of the lens. Over time, the cloudy area in the lens may enlarge, making it harder to see. Your vision may get duller or blurrier.

Age-related cataracts can develop in two ways. In the first way, clumps of protein reduce the sharpness of the image reaching the retina. The eye's lens consists mostly of water and protein. When protein clumps up, it clouds the lens. The clouding may become severe enough to cause blurred vision. Most age-related cataracts develop from protein clumpings.

The second type of cataract develops when the clear lens slowly changes to a yellowish or brownish color with age, giving a brownish tint to vision. At first, the amount of tinting may be slight and may not make a difference in vision. Over time, increased tinting may make it more difficult to read and to perform other routine activities. This gradual tinting does not affect the sharpness of the image transmitted to the retina, but if the lens discoloration is advanced, the person may not be able to identify blues and purples.

Although most cataracts are related to aging, the following types of cataract can sometimes develop:

- **Secondary cataract** Cataracts can form after surgery for other eye problems such as glaucoma. Cataracts can also develop in people who have certain health problems, such as diabetes. Cataracts have also been linked to the use of steroid medications.

- **Traumatic cataract** Cataracts can form after an eye injury, sometimes years later.

- **Congenital cataract** Some babies are born with cataracts or develop them during childhood, often in both eyes. These cataracts may be so small that they don't affect vision. If they do, the lenses may need to be replaced.

- **Radiation cataract**   Cataracts can develop after exposure to certain types of radiation.

RISK FACTORS

The risk of developing a cataract goes up as you get older. Other factors that raise your risk include the following:

- **Uncontrolled diabetes**   People with diabetes are at increased risk for cataracts.
- **Smoking**   The inhaled chemicals in tobacco smoke directly attack the lens of the eye and lower protective antioxidant levels in the body. Smoking also limits the enzymes that help remove damaged protein from the lens of the eye.
- **Prolonged sun exposure**   Sunshine is a form of radiation, and sun exposure is one of the main causes of cataracts.
- **Long-term use of corticosteroids**   Taking corticosteroids over a long period of time, especially at high doses, is the most common drug-related cause of cataracts.
- **Long-term heavy drinking**   Drinking excessive amounts of alcohol over a long period of time may contribute to the development of cataracts.

PREVENTION

While there is no guaranteed way to prevent cataracts, the following measures can help reduce your risk:

- **Limit your time in the sun.** Whenever you are out in the bright sun, wear sunglasses that block both UVA and UVB rays and wear a large-brimmed hat to protect your eyes from the sun. Never use sunlamps or tanning booths or beds.
- **Quit smoking if you smoke.** Smoking is a major risk factor for cataracts.
- **Control your blood sugar levels.** If you have diabetes, monitor your blood sugar level frequently, according to your doctor's instructions. Consuming a healthy diet, exercising regularly, and keeping your weight down will also help to keep your blood sugar levels in the healthy range.

- **Increase your antioxidant intake.** Eating plenty of antioxidant-rich fruits and vegetables may help protect the eyes.

- **Have regular eye exams.** After age 40, you should have a thorough eye exam by an eye M.D. at least every two years to detect any eye problems at an early stage.

Glaucoma

Glaucoma is an eye disorder caused by elevated pressure inside the eye. Glaucoma can cause gradual loss of vision—often without symptoms. The rise in fluid pressure inside the eyes caused by glaucoma damages the optic nerve. The optic nerve is a bundle of more than 1 million nerve fibers. A healthy optic nerve is necessary for good vision.

- **Open-angle glaucoma**   Open-angle glaucoma is the most common form of glaucoma, which usually develops over several years. A clear, watery liquid (called aqueous fluid) flows in and out of a small space at the front of each eye (the anterior chamber) to bathe and nourish the cornea, iris, and lens and remove wastes. In chronic open-angle glaucoma, the drainage angle (the channel through which aqueous fluid drains from the eyeball) malfunctions and the fluid does not drain properly, causing the normal pressure inside the eye to slowly rise. If not controlled, this abnormally high pressure can permanently damage the optic nerve and other parts of the eye, causing vision loss and, eventually, blindness. Open-angle glaucoma runs in families—your chances of having it are increased if a parent or grandparent had it. African Americans are at especially high risk for this form of glaucoma.

- **Angle-closure glaucoma**   In this form of glaucoma, also called acute glaucoma, the drainage angle suddenly and unexpectedly becomes blocked by part of the iris, which causes a sudden, severe increase in pressure inside the eye. Symptoms usually include severe eye pain on one side with a change in vision, with or without headache or nausea and vomiting. Angle-closure glaucoma is a medical emergency. If not treated immediately, the increased pressure can quickly lead to blindness in the eye. If your doctor is not available, go to the nearest hospital emergency department. Prompt treatment can usually clear the blockage and preserve vision.

- **Low-tension or normal-tension glaucoma**   In low-tension or normal-tension glaucoma, the optic nerve is damaged for no obvious reason in people with normal pressure inside the eye, causing loss of peripheral vision. Doctors do not fully understand this form of glaucoma. Lowering eye pressure at least 30 percent with medication can slow the disease in some people. Glaucoma may worsen in others despite the reduced pressures. Other factors, such as low blood pressure, can contribute to low-tension glaucoma.

- **Secondary glaucoma**   This form of glaucoma develops from an underlying disease or condition such as the eye disorder uveitis (inflammation of the iris), diabetes, a blow to or chemical burn of the eye, and taking drugs such as corticosteroids that can raise the pressure in the eye.

RISK FACTORS

Anyone can develop glaucoma, but some people have a higher risk than others. Following are the major risk factors for chronic open-angle glaucoma, the most common form:

- **Race**   Blacks are at high risk of developing chronic open-angle glaucoma, especially after age 40. Glaucoma is five times more likely to occur in blacks than in whites, and is about four times more likely to cause blindness in blacks than in whites. Hispanics over age 60 also are at high risk.

Acute closed-angle glaucoma

When glaucoma occurs suddenly, without warning, it is acute closed-angle glaucoma, which is a medical emergency. If you suddenly experience any of the following symptoms, call 911 immediately or go directly to the nearest hospital emergency department:

- Blurred vision
- Severe eye pain
- Severe headache
- Seeing rainbows or halos around lights
- Nausea and vomiting

- **Age** The incidence of glaucoma rises with age. Anyone over age 60 has an increased risk.

- **Family history** People with a parent or grandparent with glaucoma are more likely to develop glaucoma than people without a family history.

- **Diabetes** People who have diabetes are nearly twice as likely to develop glaucoma as people without diabetes.

A thorough dilated eye exam can reveal more risk factors, such as high eye pressure, thinness of the cornea, or abnormal optic nerve anatomy. Early detection and treatment to reduce eye pressure is essential to prevent vision loss. In some people with certain combinations of these risk factors, medicated eye drops can cut in half the risk of developing glaucoma.

PREVENTION

The following measures can help prevent the development of chronic open-angle glaucoma:

- **Medications** For many people who have elevated eye pressure, daily glaucoma eye drops can significantly lower eye pressure and decrease the risk of going on to develop glaucoma.

- **Regular screening** The best way to prevent glaucoma and the blindness that can result from it is to have regular eye exams. Eye M.D.s recommend testing for glaucoma as part of the comprehensive adult medical eye evaluation, beginning at age 20. How often to get examined depends on a person's age and other risk factors for glaucoma. If you are at risk for glaucoma, have a dilated eye exam every one or two years by an eye M.D. Encourage at-risk family members to also have dilated eye exams at least once every one or two years. Remember that reducing eye pressure in glaucoma's early stages slows the progression of the disease and helps save vision.

- **Blood sugar control** If you have diabetes, carefully monitor your blood sugar levels to keep them as close to normal as possible.

PROTECT YOUR EYES AND SAVE YOUR VISION

Some of the most common eye problems can be avoided by taking measures to protect your eyes. For example, the risk for two of the most common eye diseases—cataracts (see page 408) and age-related macular degeneration (see below)—is linked to exposure to sunlight. Always wearing sunglasses that block UVA and UVB rays from the sun can significantly reduce your risk for these vision-robbing eye diseases. For extra insurance, wear a hat with a brim that shades your eyes.

More than 2,000 eye injuries occur every day in the United States—half of these in the workplace, mostly from falling or flying objects, or sparks striking the eye. An estimated 90 percent of work-related eye injuries could be prevented by wearing appropriate eye-protection gear. Eyewear must fit properly and must be designed to provide effective protection. Make sure you also wear proper eyewear outside of work when you are doing home repairs or engaging in any other activities that pose a risk for eye injury, including some sports. And don't put yourself in danger by, for example, standing too close to your racquetball opponent or golf partner.

Age-related macular degeneration

Age-related macular degeneration is the leading cause of blindness in Americans over age 60. In age-related macular degeneration, the light-sensitive cells of the macula (the part of the retina that provides sharp focus in the center of the field of vision) deteriorate with age. The retina transforms light into electrical signals that travel along the optic nerve to the brain, which perceives them as visual images. Sharp central vision allows you to see fine details clearly, which is essential for everyday tasks such as reading, driving, and recognizing faces.

In some people, macular degeneration advances so slowly that they notice little change in their vision. In other people, the disease progresses rapidly. Macular degeneration often affects both eyes, one after the other. The condition occurs in two main forms: dry and wet.

- **Dry macular degeneration** Ninety percent of all people with macular degeneration have the dry form, which occurs when the light-sensitive cells in the macula slowly break down, gradually blurring central vision in the affected eye. As dry macular degeneration worsens, you may see a blurred spot in the center of your vision. Over time, as less of the macula functions, central vision gradually diminishes in the affected eye.

- **Wet macular degeneration**   The wet form of macular degeneration occurs when abnormal blood vessels behind the retina start to grow under the macula. These new blood vessels tend to be very fragile and often leak blood and fluid, raising the macula from its normal position at the back of the eye. Damage to the macula is rapid, and the loss of central vision can occur quickly. Wet macular degeneration is also known as advanced macular degeneration. Everyone who has the wet form of macular degeneration had the dry form first.

The dry form of macular degeneration can advance and cause vision loss without turning into the wet form. Or the dry form can suddenly turn into the wet form, even during the early stages. There is no way for doctors to determine if or when the dry form will turn into the wet form.

RISK FACTORS

Late-stage macular degeneration, the most serious form of the disorder with the worst outlook, seems to share risk factors with heart disease, although scientists are not sure what the connection may be. Following are the major risk factors for age-related macular degeneration:

- **Age**   Although macular degeneration can occur in middle age, people over age 60 have the highest risk.
- **Smoking**   Smoking raises the risk for macular degeneration, especially the advanced form, but researchers do not understand why.
- **Obesity**   Obesity has been linked to the progression of early- and intermediate-stage macular degeneration to the advanced form.
- **Race**   Whites are much more likely to lose vision from macular degeneration than are blacks.
- **Family history**   People who have immediate family members with macular degeneration are at increased risk of developing the disease.
- **Being female**   Women appear to be at greater risk for macular degeneration than men.

PREVENTION

Although you can inherit the tendency to develop macular degeneration, it does not mean that you are destined to get the disorder. Your lifestyle can influence how soon you might develop it, or if you develop it at all. The following guidelines may help prevent macular degeneration:

- **Eat a variety of fruits and vegetables.** Consume a variety of colorful fruits and vegetables to get enough of the potentially eye-protecting antioxidants lutein and zeaxanthin. These antioxidants can be found in spinach, corn, peaches, squash, collard greens, kale, honeydew melon, orange juice, red delicious apples, Brussels sprouts, and broccoli.

- **Get your omega-3s.** Eating fatty fish (such as salmon, mackerel, and sardines) that are rich in omega-3 oils may help reduce your risk for macular degeneration. Flaxseeds also contain omega-3s, so consider sprinkling some on your morning cereal. Omega-3 supplements are now widely available.

- **Stop smoking if you smoke.** Add avoiding macular degeneration to your list of reasons to quit.

- **Keep your blood pressure normal.** High blood pressure can cause degenerative changes in the eyes that can lead to macular degeneration.

- **Watch your weight.** Both overall obesity and fat distributed in the abdominal area raise the risk that macular degeneration will progress to the advanced stage.

- **Be more physically active.** Physical activity tends to lower the risk that macular degeneration will reach the advanced stage.

Vision distorted by dry macular degeneration

In dry macular degeneration, the macula—the part of the retina that enables you to see objects in the center of your field of vision in sharp focus—is damaged. An early symptom of the disorder is blurred central vision, which makes it difficult to distinguish fine details on faces or printed pages.

Normal vision

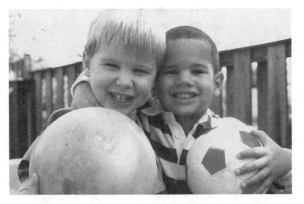

Blurred vision with large central blind spot

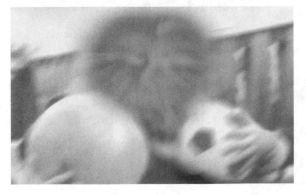

Diabetic retinopathy

Diabetic retinopathy, or diabetic eye disease, is the leading cause of blindness in American adults under age 65. The condition is a complication of diabetes that affects vision by damaging the blood vessels in the retina (the light-sensitive membrane that lines the back of the eye). In some people with diabetic retinopathy, blood vessels in the retina leak fluid. In other people with diabetic retinopathy, abnormal new blood vessels grow on the surface of the retina and may leak blood into the eyeball, preventing light from reaching the retina. The abnormal blood vessels can also produce scar tissue that pulls the retina away from the back of the eye (retinal detachment).

Anyone who has diabetes—either type 1 or type 2—is at risk for diabetic retinopathy. Between 40 and 45 percent of Americans diagnosed with diabetes have some stage of diabetic retinopathy. The longer you have diabetes, the higher your risk. If you have diabetic retinopathy, your eye doctor can recommend treatment to help slow its progression, including careful control of your blood sugar levels and blood pressure.

Some women develop diabetes only during pregnancy, a condition known as gestational diabetes. Every pregnant woman who has gestational diabetes should have a thorough dilated eye exam as soon as possible.

RISK FACTORS

Having diabetes and how long you have had diabetes are the major risk factors for diabetic retinopathy. The following factors also can influence risk:

- **Poor blood sugar control** The higher your blood sugar levels, the higher your risk for diabetic retinopathy.

Vision distorted by diabetic retinopathy

As diabetic retinopathy progresses, vision becomes more and more blurred and specks of blood, which look like spots "floating" in your vision, appear. Left untreated, the disorder can eventually lead to total blindness.

Normal vision

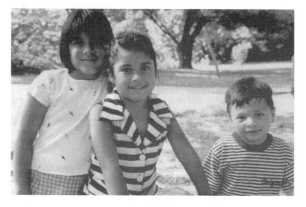

Blurred vision with floating spots

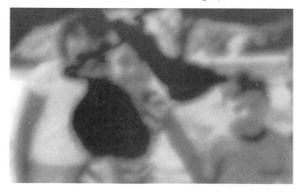

- **High blood pressure** Diabetic retinopathy progresses much more slowly when blood pressure is tightly controlled.

- **High cholesterol levels** Evidence suggests that high cholesterol contributes to the development of diabetic retinopathy by causing deposits of fat and protein to develop inside the retina.

- **Your genes** Some people have a genetic predisposition to developing diabetic retinopathy.

PREVENTION

People with diabetic retinopathy can reduce their risk for blindness by 95 percent by getting early treatment and proper follow-up care. Follow these guidelines:

- **Carefully control your blood sugar levels.** Good control of blood sugar slows the onset and progression of diabetic retinopathy. People with diabetes who keep their blood sugar levels as close to normal as possible also have a much lower risk for other complications of diabetes, including kidney disease and nerve disease. Good control of blood sugar also reduces the need for sight-saving laser surgery.

- **Control your blood pressure.** Have your blood pressure checked once a year; twice a year if you are over age 50. Keep your blood pressure at a healthy level by limiting your intake of salt, keeping your weight down, and improving your response to stress. Take blood pressure medication as prescribed by your doctor.

- **Watch your cholesterol levels.** Controlling abnormal cholesterol levels can help reduce the risk for vision loss. Although diet only partially contributes to abnormal cholesterol, reducing your consumption of saturated and trans fats can help. If your doctor prescribes a cholesterol-lowering medication, take it as directed.

- **Have an eye doctor examine your eyes once a year.** Have regular eye exams even if your vision is fine. The eye doctor will dilate your eyes, which opens the pupils to allow him or her to see inside the back of the eye. Finding eye problems early and getting treatment right away helps prevent more serious problems later on.

19

REDUCING DEMENTIA RISKS

THE TERM "DEMENTIA" describes changes in the normal activity of the brain that can affect memory, speech, personality, and the ability to carry out daily activities. Dementia is not considered a disease but rather a collection of symptoms caused by various disorders that affect the brain. People with dementia have impaired mental functioning that interferes with their normal activities and relationships. They lose their ability to solve problems and maintain emotional control, and they may have personality changes and behavior problems such as agitation, impulsivity, delusions, and hallucinations. While memory loss is a common symptom, it does not by itself mean that a person has dementia. Doctors diagnose dementia only if two or more brain functions—such as memory and language skills—are seriously impaired. Although dementia is common in the very old, dementia is not considered a normal result of aging.

Some conditions that cause dementia or dementia-like symptoms are reversible or partially reversible. Among the most frequent reversible causes are depression, alcohol abuse, certain vitamin deficiencies, and drug interactions. For example, in older people, who often take multiple medications, drug interactions are a common cause of cognitive decline. Depression is a relatively common condition in older people that often goes undiagnosed and untreated. In some cases, the symptoms of depression in older people are mistaken for signs of dementia.

Doctors have identified other conditions that can cause dementia or dementia-like symptoms, including endocrine abnormalities (such as a thyroid problem), nutritional deficiencies (such as vitamin B12 deficiency), infections, brain tumors, and heart and lung problems. The two most common causes of dementia in older people are Alzheimer's disease and vascular dementia (caused by multiple strokes that disrupt the flow of blood to the brain). Less common conditions that cannot be prevented but can cause dementia include Lewy body dementia, Huntington's disease, and Creutzfeldt-Jakob disease.

Alzheimer's disease

Alzheimer's disease is a brain disorder characterized by abnormal clumps and tangled bundles of fibers in the brain that are composed of misplaced proteins. It is the most common form of dementia affecting older people. Alzheimer's disease begins gradually, first affecting the parts of the brain that control thought, memory, and language. People with the disorder may

---

VITAMIN DEFICIENCY AND DEMENTIA

Vitamin deficiency—especially a lack of the B vitamins, including thiamine (vitamin B1), riboflavin (vitamin B2), niacin (vitamin B3), pyrodoxine (vitamin B6), folic acid, and vitamin B12—can cause dementia-like symptoms. Vitamin deficiencies can result from a poor diet or from problems with the body's ability to absorb vitamins from food.

Vitamin deficiencies can be detected through blood tests. The symptoms can often be reversed with measures such as vitamin supplements and an improved diet, or in some cases, treatment of the underlying problem that has caused the poor absorption of vitamins. Because vitamin B12 is especially important in keeping brain cells healthy, researchers are looking into whether taking supplements of vitamin B12 may help protect against dementia.

have trouble remembering things that occurred recently (short-term memory loss) or the names of people they know. As symptoms worsen, affected people may not recognize family members and may have difficulty speaking, reading, or writing. They may forget how to brush their teeth, shave, or comb their hair. Eventually they become anxious or aggressive, may wander away from home, and need total care.

More than 5 million people in the United States have Alzheimer's disease—including one in eight people over age 64 and almost half of all people over age 85. As the number of Americans who live into their 80s and 90s grows, so will the prevalence of Alzheimer's disease. There is no cure for Alzheimer's and no way to slow its progression.

It is not yet known how to prevent Alzheimer's disease because doctors don't fully understand what causes it. Several interacting factors are probably involved, including genes and lifestyle. Scientists have found brain changes in people with Alzheimer's disease that may be responsible for

---

BREAKING NEWS **Physical activity: Good for the brain as well as the body**

Physical exercise doesn't just keep your body healthy—it can also help you stay mentally sharp as you age. People who are physically active are less likely to develop Alzheimer's disease than people who are inactive. Although the reasons for this are not fully understood, the following factors are thought to be involved:

- Exercise may help slow the age-related shrinkage in the frontal cortex, the area of the brain that is important for higher-level thinking skills and memory.

- Exercise increases circulation to the area of the brain involved with short-term memory.

- Exercise triggers the release in the brain of growth factors (proteins that increase the number of connections between brain cells) and stimulates the production of new brain cells in the hippocampus (the region in the brain that is important for memory).

- Exercise may reduce amyloid buildup in the brain, possibly delaying the onset of Alzheimer's disease in people who have mild cognitive impairment, and slowing or stopping the disease from progressing in people who already have it.

impairing thinking and memory—dead nerve cells in areas of the brain that are vital to memory and other mental abilities, disrupted connections between nerve cells, and lower levels of chemicals in the brain that carry messages back and forth between nerve cells.

RISK FACTORS

Alzheimer's disease is a complex disorder that develops over many years. A number of factors may increase or decrease a person's risk of developing the disease. The effect of the following risk factors on an individual depends on the person's genetic makeup and lifestyle:

- **Age**   Getting older is the most important known risk factor for Alzheimer's disease. The disease usually starts after age 60 and the risk of developing it rises with age. The risk of developing Alzheimer's disease doubles every five years after age 65.

- **Family history**   Your risk for Alzheimer's disease is higher if a family member has had it. Doctors believe that genes may play a role in many cases of Alzheimer's disease. A rare form of the disease that usually occurs between the ages of 30 and 60 (called early-onset familial Alzheimer's disease) is inherited. The more common form (which is known as late-onset Alzheimer's disease) occurs later in life, and has no obvious inheritance pattern. But one group of risk-factor genes has been identified so far for late-onset Alzheimer's, and it is likely that other genes will be found that may increase the risk for Alzheimer's disease or protect against it.

Although no firm evidence yet exists, researchers are looking into possible links between Alzheimer's disease and some other conditions or disorders that can affect the health of the brain—including abnormal cholesterol

ALCOHOL ABUSE AND DEMENTIA

Two overlapping forms of reversible dementia-like symptoms—called Korsakoff syndrome and alcoholic dementia—can result from long-term heavy drinking. In Korsakoff syndrome, heavy drinking causes a deficiency of the B vitamin thiamine, which is important for brain function. The vitamin deficiency may result from a combination of a poor diet and the harmful effects of alcohol on the body's ability to absorb nutrients from food. Korsakoff syndrome, whose major symptom is loss of short-term memory, is not considered a true dementia because the brain damage is confined to small areas of the brain and it can be reversed by stopping drinking and eating a healthy diet.

Alcoholic dementia is thought to result from the direct effect of alcohol on nerve cells in the outer layer of the brain, influencing a wide range of skills and abilities. People with this form of dementia may recover some, but usually not all, of their function by abstaining from alcohol.

levels, high blood pressure, uncontrolled blood glucose in diabetes, and lack of physical activity.

PREVENTION

There is no known way to prevent Alzheimer's disease, but some promising research is being done to determine if there are some steps people can take to reduce their risk:

- **Being physically active** Physical exercise has been shown to maintain and improve brain health, and is strongly linked to a reduced risk of developing dementia late in life. People who exercise regularly in middle age are one third as likely to develop Alzheimer's disease in their 70s as people who are not physically active. Even if you don't start exercising until your 60s, you can significantly cut your risk for dementia. As little as 30 to 60 minutes of fast walking several times a week has been shown to improve brain function in people in their 70s.

HOW TO SPOT MEMORY PROBLEMS

Do you or does someone in your family have increasing difficulty with any of the activities listed below? If so, the person needs to see a doctor for screening for the possibility of dementia.

- **Learning and retaining new information** Repeats questions and statements; has more trouble remembering recent conversations, events, and appointments; frequently misplaces objects.

- **Handling complex tasks** Has more trouble following a complex train of thought or performing tasks that require many steps, such as balancing a checkbook or cooking a meal.

- **Reasoning ability** Cannot respond to problems at work or at home with a reasonable plan, such as knowing what to do if the bathroom floods; shows uncharacteristic disregard for the rules of social conduct.

- **Spatial ability and orientation** Has trouble driving, organizing things around the house, or finding his or her way around familiar places.

- **Language** Has increasing trouble finding the words to express what he or she wants to say, and following conversations.

- **Behavior** Appears more passive and less responsive than usual; is more irritable and suspicious than usual; misinterprets things seen or heard; has a disheveled appearance.

- **Having a social network**   Studies have suggested a link between social engagement and increased mental abilities. Having lots of friends and participating in many social activities seems to reduce mental decline and lower the risk for Alzheimer's disease in older adults.

- **Staying mentally active**   Activities that require intense information processing, such as listening to the radio, reading newspapers, working puzzles, playing games, and going to museums, may help prevent mental decline. Other research has found that the more formal education a person has, the sharper his or her memory and learning abilities are likely to remain as he or she ages. Engaging in mentally stimulating activities during early and middle adulthood may help provide a buffer against Alzheimer's disease later in life.

  - Mental stimulation may protect the brain by establishing a "thinking reserve."

  - Mentally stimulating activities may help the brain become more adaptable and flexible, enabling it to compensate for declines in other areas.

  - People who engage in these activities might have other lifestyle factors that protect them against Alzheimer's disease.

- **Taking NSAIDs**   Some studies have suggested a link between a reduced risk for Alzheimer's disease and the commonly used painkillers nonsteroidal anti-inflammatories (NSAIDs) such as aspirin, ibuprofen, naproxen, and indomethacin. The link between NSAIDs and a lower Alzheimer's risk was made when researchers observed that people who take NSAIDs for chronic conditions such as arthritis or other immune disorders have lower rates of Alzheimer's disease. More studies are needed to confirm or refute this finding.

- **Taking cholesterol-lowering medications**   Drugs called statins, which are used to improve cholesterol in the blood, may also provide some protection against Alzheimer's disease. Cholesterol in the brain contributes to the formation of waxy buildups called amyloid plaques, which are linked to Alzheimer's disease.

Even though no treatments, drugs, or pills have yet been proven to prevent Alzheimer's disease or delay its development, the following steps might

SAFETY CHECKS FOR PEOPLE WITH ALZHEIMER'S DISEASE

A safe home can be a less stressful home for a person with Alzheimer's disease and his or her caregivers and family members. You don't have to make these changes alone. Enlist the help of a friend, a professional, or a community service agency such as the local Alzheimer's Association. The following tips can make life easier for everyone in the household:

- If the person can't answer phone calls, use an answering machine and set it to turn on after the fewest number of rings. Turn ringers on low to avoid distraction and confusion. Put all portable and cell phones and equipment in a safe place so they won't get lost.

- Hide a spare house key outside in case the person locks you out of the house.

- Anticipate the reasons a person with Alzheimer's disease might get out of bed, and try to meet those needs by, for example, offering food and water and scheduling ample time to use the bathroom before bed.

- Cover unused outlets with childproof plugs.

- Place red tape around floor vents, radiators, and other heating devices to deter the person from standing on or touching a hot surface.

- Keep all medications (prescription and over the counter) locked. Ask the pharmacist for child-resistant caps.

- Keep all alcohol in a locked cabinet or out of reach. Drinking alcohol can increase confusion in a person with Alzheimer's disease.

- If smoking is allowed, monitor the person while he or she is smoking. Remove matches, lighters, ashtrays, cigarettes, and other smoking materials from view to reduce potential fire hazards. These measures may also reduce the person's desire to smoke.

- Keep plastic bags out of reach to prevent choking or suffocation.

- Remove all guns or other weapons from the home, or safety-proof them by installing safety locks or by removing ammunition and firing pins.

- Lock all power tools and machinery in the garage, workroom, or basement.

- Keep all computer equipment and accessories, including electrical cords, out of the way. If valuable documents or materials are stored on a home computer, protect the files with passwords.

- Keep fish tanks out of reach. The combination of glass, water, electrical pumps, and potentially poisonous aquatic life could be harmful to a curious person with Alzheimer's.

- Restrict access to a swimming pool by fencing it off with a locked gate, covering it, and keeping it closely supervised when in use.

- In the patio area, remove the fuel source and fire starters from grills when not in use.

- Install childproof door latches on storage cabinets and drawers. Lock away all household cleaning products, matches, knives, scissors, blades, small appliances, and

(continued)

help reduce your risk. Even if they aren't effective against Alzheimer's disease, they are beneficial in other ways, by maintaining and improving overall health and lowering the risk for other diseases.

- Improve your cholesterol profile.

- Control your blood pressure.

- Control your diabetes through diet, exercise, and, if prescribed, medication.

Vascular dementia

Vascular dementia, also known as multi-infarct dementia, accounts for 10 to 20 percent of all cases of gradually worsening dementia. It usually affects people over the age of 60, and is more likely to occur in men than in women. Vascular dementia results from accumulated brain injury caused by repeated small strokes (TIAs; see page 241). Some of these small strokes do not produce any symptoms and are sometimes referred to as "silent" strokes. A person can have a number of small strokes before having noticeable changes in memory.

Following are some of the factors that cause strokes that produce vascular dementia:

- Untreated high blood pressure
- Uncontrolled blood sugar in diabetes
- Unfavorable cholesterol profile
- Heart disease

Of these, high blood pressure is the most important risk factor for vascular dementia. People with vascular dementia can appear to improve for short periods of time, and then decline again after having more strokes. Eventually death can occur from stroke, heart disease, or pneumonia or another infection.

RISK FACTORS

Advancing age is one of the principal risk factors for vascular dementia, which seldom appears before age 65. The older you are, the higher your risk. Additional risk factors include the following:

- **Having a stroke**   The brain damage that can result from a stroke raises the risk of developing dementia.
- **Having high blood pressure**   Increased blood pressure puts additional pressure on the blood vessels throughout the body, including those leading to the brain.
- **Having diabetes**   High blood sugar levels damage blood vessels, boosting the risk for stroke.

PREVENTION

The most important step you can take to prevent vascular dementia is to keep your blood pressure within the healthy range (below 120/80). Improving cholesterol levels and keeping blood sugar controlled in diabetes are also important. To prevent strokes, your doctor may prescribe medications to control your high blood pressure and improve your cholesterol, heart disease, or diabetes. He or she will also recommend that you be more physically active, stop smoking if you smoke, restrict your intake of alcohol, and eat a heart-healthy diet low in saturated and trans fats.

To reduce symptoms in someone who already has vascular dementia, doctors may change or stop medications that can cause confusion, such as sedatives, antihistamines, and strong painkillers. Some people may also need to be treated for medical conditions that can increase confusion, such as heart failure (see page 230), thyroid disorders, anemia, or infections. Doctors sometimes prescribe aspirin, warfarin, or other drugs to prevent clots from forming in small blood vessels. Medications also can be prescribed to relieve restlessness or depression or to help improve sleep.

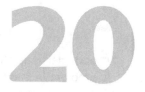

20

KEEPING YOUR MOUTH, TEETH, AND GUMS HEALTHY

TEETH ARE LIVING TISSUE. The pulp that makes up the center of each tooth contains blood vessels that nourish the tooth, along with nerves that sense heat, cold, pressure, and pain. A tough, durable substance called dentin surrounds the pulp, and a hard material called enamel covers the dentin. Each tooth has one to three roots. Healthy gum tissue fits snugly around each tooth, and the roots reach deep into sockets in the jawbone.

Although tooth enamel is the hardest substance in the body, acids formed during the breakdown of simple carbohydrates such as sugar in food can erode the enamel and cause tooth decay. Failing to brush and floss your teeth every day promotes tooth decay and can lead to gum disease, which can cause pockets to form between the gums and teeth, where infectious material can collect. Left untreated, gum disease ultimately leads to tooth loss.

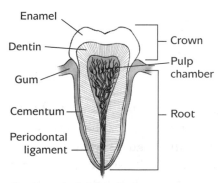

Structure of a tooth

Your teeth start the digestive process by helping you bite and chew food, but they also give shape to your face and play an important part in speech. This cross section of a premolar shows the many parts that make up a tooth.

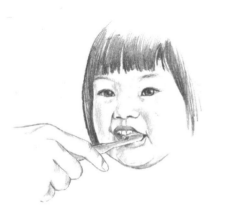
Gum disease

If you have been told that you have periodontitis, commonly known as gum disease, you are not alone. About 80 percent of American adults have some form of gum disease, which can range from simple gum inflammation to serious disease that results in major damage to the soft tissue and bone that support the teeth. In severe cases, teeth are lost. People usually don't show signs of gum disease until they are in their 30s or 40s. Men are more likely to have gum disease than women. Although teenagers rarely develop periodontitis, they can develop gingivitis, the milder form of gum disease.

Your mouth is full of bacteria. These bacteria, along with mucus and other particles, constantly form a sticky, colorless substance called plaque on the teeth. Brushing and flossing help to eliminate plaque. Plaque that is not removed can harden and form bacteria-harboring tartar that brushing cannot clean away. Only a professional cleaning by a dentist or dental hygienist can remove tartar.

The longer plaque and tartar stay on the teeth, the more harmful they become. The bacteria cause inflammation of the gums (gingivitis). The gums become red and swollen, and can bleed easily. If your gums bleed when you brush your teeth, you probably have gingivitis. Gingivitis can usually be reversed with daily brushing and flossing and regular dental checkups and cleanings. This form of gum disease does not cause any loss of the bone or tissue that holds teeth in place.

But when it goes untreated, gingivitis can advance to periodontitis (which is inflammation around the teeth). Periodontitis causes the gums to pull away from the teeth and form pockets of infectious material. The immune system fights the bacteria as the plaque spreads and grows below the gum line. Toxins formed by the bacteria, combined with enzymes produced by the body to fight the infection, start to break down the bone and connective tissue that hold the teeth in place. If periodontitis is not treated, the bones, gums, and connective tissue that support the teeth can be destroyed. The teeth eventually become loose and fall out or need to be removed.

Researchers have uncovered some possible health effects of gum disease that go beyond the mouth and may raise the risk for heart disease and stroke. Inflammation seems to be the cause. Here are some possible connections:

- **Heart disease and stroke**   A number of studies have suggested that people with gum disease are at increased risk for heart and vascular disease. Whether the gum disease may directly cause or promote the atherosclerosis (see page 218) that underlies heart and vascular disease remains unclear. It could be that people with poorer oral hygiene also tend to have poorer health habits in general. However, there are possible links through the activation of inflammation from gum disease that could help to damage arteries.

- **Poor blood sugar control in diabetes**   Having an infection, including gum disease, can impair the body's ability to process and use insulin. Researchers speculate that if the infection is controlled, it might be easier to control blood sugar. Researchers are looking at people with diabetes who have difficulty controlling their blood sugar and

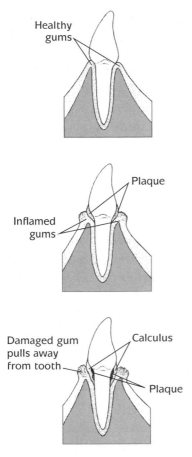

Healthy gums

Plaque

Inflamed gums

Damaged gum pulls away from tooth

Calculus

Plaque

Gum disease caused by neglect

Inadequate brushing and flossing allow plaque to build up, which promotes gum disease. Left untreated, the disease worsens over time and can eventually lead to tooth loss. Healthy gums (top) fit firmly around the necks of the teeth and don't bleed easily. Plaque that accumulates between the teeth and gums can cause pain and inflammation (center). Unremoved plaque can harden to form a substance called calculus, which can make the gums recede (bottom). The bacteria in the calculus can cause severe damage to the teeth, gums, and jawbone.

who also have gum disease. They are treating the gum disease to see if it improves their blood sugar. The research is still ongoing, but the link between diabetes and gum disease is strong enough to stress to people with diabetes the importance of daily brushing and flossing and regular dental checkups to perhaps help them control their diabetes.

RISK FACTORS

Researchers have identified the following risk factors for gum disease:

- **Smoking** Smoking is one of the most important risk factors for the development of gum disease. Smoking can also lower the effectiveness of some treatments for gum disease.

- **Use of smokeless tobacco** Using snuff and chewing tobacco can raise the chances of developing gum disease. The sugar and other harmful substances in tobacco can cause irritation and make the gums pull away from the teeth, making it easier for bacteria to invade.

- **Hormonal changes** A woman's changing hormone levels during puberty, the menstrual cycle, pregnancy, and menopause can cause changes in the mouth. These hormone changes can make the gums more sensitive and more susceptible to gingivitis.

- **Diabetes** Diabetes makes you more susceptible to infections, including gum disease. And there is evidence that people with diabetes tend to have more gum disease. The more poorly controlled the diabetes, the more severe the gum disease is likely to be.

- **Stress** Stress can make it harder for the body to fight infection, including gum disease. When you are chronically stressed, the brain pumps out stress hormones that can reduce the immune system's ability to fight invaders like bacteria or viruses.

KEEPING YOUR TEETH AND GUMS HEALTHY

Even if you brush your teeth twice a day, you can develop gum disease if you don't floss your teeth daily and see your dentist for a professional cleaning twice a year. You can keep gum disease at bay by taking the time to do the following simple steps every day. Make them a regular part of your daily routine, like showering and shaving.

- **Brush your teeth thoroughly for at least two minutes, at least twice a day, every day.** Squeeze some toothpaste onto your brush, place your toothbrush at an angle, and gently move the brush back and forth, away from the gum line. Use only a soft-bristled brush to prevent damage to your gums that could cause them to recede. Electric toothbrushes are especially effective, and many models have a two-minute timer. Finish by brushing your tongue to remove bacteria and freshen your breath.

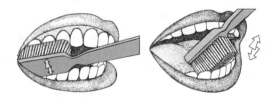

Brushing your teeth

When you brush your teeth, the action of the bristles on your toothbrush gently massages your gums, stimulating blood circulation and keeping the gums healthy. Replace your toothbrush at least every three months.

- **Floss your teeth every day.** Using dental floss helps to remove plaque buildup and dislodge food particles from between the teeth. For best results, floss before you brush your teeth, at least once a day, preferably before bedtime.

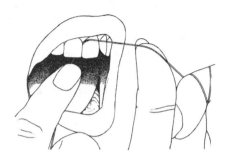

Flossing your teeth

To floss your teeth properly, take about 18 inches of floss and wind some around the middle fingers of each hand. Hold about an inch of floss between both index fingers, or between the thumb of one hand and the index finger of the other—whatever way works best for you. Slide the floss between your teeth and gently rub the sides of each tooth with an up-and-down motion. Use a clean section of floss for each tooth.

- **Cut back on sweets, avoid snacking between meals, and eat a healthy diet.** Munching candy and other sugary foods or refined carbohydrates (such as cookies) between meals harms your teeth because the bacteria in the mouth that break down such foods produce acid that can dissolve tooth enamel. The next thing you know, you may have a cavity. Don't give your kids fruit roll-ups or gummy candy that sticks to the teeth. If you must give your children candy, make it sugar-free gum or small amounts of chocolate (because chocolate quickly dissolves in the mouth).

(continued)

- **Medications**   Certain drugs, such as antidepressants and some heart medicines, can adversely affect oral health by reducing the flow of saliva, which protects the teeth and gums.

- **A weakened immune system**   Diseases such as cancer or HIV/AIDS and their treatments, which weaken the immune system, can affect the health of the gums.

- **Genetic susceptibility**   Some people are more prone to developing severe gum disease than others, especially if they have close relatives who have had it.

PREVENTION

Gum disease is relatively easy to prevent if you are willing to spend some time cleaning your teeth well every day. Being vigilant about brushing and flossing daily can make a huge difference in the health of your teeth and gums. Dental hygiene involves the following daily steps:

- Brush your teeth at least twice a day.

- Floss your teeth at least once a day.

- Visit your dentist at least twice a year for a checkup and professional cleaning.

- Eat a well-balanced diet.

- Don't smoke, and don't use smokeless tobacco products (such as chewing tobacco or snuff).

PART THREE

Prevention and Wellness Throughout Life

21

KEEPING YOUR CHILDREN HEALTHY

THIS CHAPTER GIVES YOU USEFUL information about ways to keep your children healthy, especially by helping them adopt healthy habits from a young age. You will learn some basics about healthy eating, the importance of being physically active, and why sleep is essential for health. You will also learn how to help your children resist using alcohol, tobacco, and other drugs, and to help them make good choices to keep themselves healthy and safe.

The health of America's children has improved enormously over the past century. Infant and early childhood death has fallen dramatically, thanks mostly to widespread childhood immunization against common life-threatening childhood infectious diseases and the development of antibiotics to fight bacterial infections. But now we are witnessing the rise of a different public health threat—the alarming increase in childhood obesity, which doctors now consider the most serious health problem facing American children.

Instill healthy eating habits

The typical Western diet contains too much fat, sugar, and salt, and not enough fruits and vegetables, whole grains, and fiber. This diet (along with an increasingly inactive lifestyle) is one of the major factors that doctors say are causing more and more American children to become overweight and therefore susceptible to weight-related health problems at younger ages. The best way to teach children the basics of good nutrition is for parents to be good role models and eat as many meals together as possible. When kids are offered nutritious foods from a young age, they acquire a taste for them and are less likely to become overweight—and they learn to make healthy food choices on their own.

The Dietary Guidelines for Americans (see page 23) are scientific recommendations produced jointly by the U.S. Department of Health and Human Services and the U.S. Department of Agriculture every five years. The guidelines promote a diet that emphasizes fruits, vegetables, whole-grain foods, and fat-free or low-fat dairy products. For a complete discussion of nutrition and healthy eating, see chapter 1.

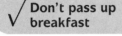

Don't pass up breakfast

Make sure your child eats a healthy breakfast so he or she can get the energy needed to learn and perform well in school.

MyPyramid for kids

The U.S. Department of Agriculture's food guidelines for children, called MyPyramid for Kids (www.mypyramid.gov/kids), shows how you can use the Dietary Guidelines when planning meals for your children. It also stresses the importance of getting 60 minutes of exercise every day. The Web site has many appealing and fun tools to help kids learn the basics of the guidelines and see how their food choices fit into MyPyramid.

Watch for added sugars

Sugars are added to a wide variety of calorie-dense foods and beverages ranging from soft drinks and fruit-flavored drinks to cookies, energy bars, jams, jellies, and baked goods. Fifty years ago, the major sweetener added to foods was sucrose, which we know as table sugar. Today, the major sugar added to foods is high-fructose corn syrup. And that may be a problem.

Some studies have suggested that high-fructose corn syrup is absorbed and used differently by the body than other sugars, acting in the body more

> **BREAKING NEWS** **Some food additives may increase hyperactivity**
>
> A scientific study has found a link between some food additives found in many children's foods and drinks—a variety of food colorings and the common preservative sodium benzoate—and increased hyperactivity behavior and decreased attention span in children. The most surprising result was that the effect was found not just in children who had been diagnosed with attention deficit hyperactivity disorder, but in a wide range of children.
>
> Some children are more sensitive to these effects than others. As a parent, you might want to monitor your children's activity and behavior. If you notice a marked change after your child eats or drinks something containing food additives, try eliminating foods containing additives from his or her diet to see if it makes a difference.

like fat than other sugars. As a result, consuming a lot of fructose may contribute to weight gain, elevate the blood level of triglycerides (linked to an increased risk for heart disease), alter the balance of the bone-strengthening mineral magnesium (leading to bone loss), increase the risk for type 2 diabetes, and raise blood pressure.

The National Academy of Sciences has suggested that added sugars should not exceed 25 percent of daily calories. For a 2,000-calorie daily diet, the 10-percent limit equals 200 calories—the amount in one 16.9-ounce sugary soft drink. The 25-percent limit equals 500 calories—the amount in two and a half 16.9-ounce sugary soft drinks. Check food labels for added sugars and look at the ingredient list to see if the product has high-fructose corn syrup.

Most experts add that while it's a good idea to limit added sugar it takes more than just eliminating one food ingredient from the diet to lose weight or avoid weight gain and stay healthy. Children also need to increase their physical activity to at least an hour a day.

Physical activity: Essential for health

You may have fond memories of running down the block to your friend's house to play ball, or of riding your bike for miles, but your children's memories of childhood may be very different. Your kids are more likely to be spending time in front of a computer screen or a TV—the sedentary

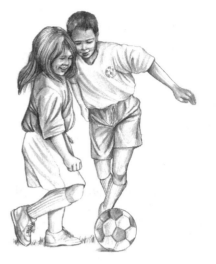

Kids need to exercise vigorously and often

New guidelines suggest that kids need to exercise at least an hour every day—90 minutes is optimal. Exercise makes the heart pump more efficiently, improves the strength and endurance of the muscles, makes bones stronger, increases flexibility, helps burn excess calories, and lowers stress.

activities that doctors warn are promoting weight gain among children. Doctors advise parents to limit their children to no more than two hours per day of screen time—including both TV time and computer time. Most American children spend four to six hours or more each day on these activities. Be firm in setting limits on your child's TV and computer time, and don't put a TV or computer in your child's bedroom. Put the computer in a central place in the home, such as the family room, so you can monitor what your child sees and does online.

Here are some steps you can take to make your child more physically active:

- Talk to your child's school about scheduling gym time every day.
- Sign your child up for exercise programs at the local park district, YMCA, or other recreation center.
- Assign active chores such as yard work, washing the car, vacuuming, and walking the dog.
- Allow older children to work delivering papers on a bike, raking leaves or shoveling snow for neighbors, or working for the local park district.
- Celebrate a special occasion with a hike or a softball game.
- Take your children to the playground frequently.

BREAKING NEWS **Kids' daily exercise levels may be too low**

Doctors recommend that children get at least one hour of physical activity on most days of the week. But a new report suggests that kids may need 90 minutes of daily exercise to help avoid heart disease risk factors. Kids' physical activity doesn't need to be extreme. Walking and playing will do, as long as children are moving. These recommendations are not just for overweight kids; fitness is the goal for all children. Getting into the habit of being active for 90 minutes a day will help kids stay physically active into adulthood, further reducing their risk for heart disease.

Preventing exercise-related injuries

More than 30 million children participate in organized sports in the United States. Even more children engage in less-formal recreational activities. While exercise provides numerous physical and social benefits, it also poses a risk for injuries. Nearly 2 million children under the age of 15 are treated in emergency departments every year for sports-related injuries. It's important to encourage your children to be physically active, but it's also important to match your children to the sport, and not push them too hard into an activity they may not like or be capable of doing. Teach your children to follow the rules and to play it safe when they get involved in sports. Here are some tips to help reduce your child's chances of injury:

- Enroll your child in organized sports through schools, community clubs, and park districts that are properly maintained. Coaches should be trained in first aid and CPR and should enforce rules on equipment use.
- Look for adults on staff who are Certified Athletic Trainers. These are people who are trained to prevent, recognize, and provide immediate care for athletic injuries.
- Make sure your child has the proper protective gear for a sport and that he or she uses it every time.
- Make warm-ups and cool-downs part of your child's routine before and after exercise or sports participation.
- Make sure your child has enough water to drink while playing. Encourage him or her to drink frequently before, during, and after exercise.
- Provide sunscreen and a hat to reduce the chance of sunburn. Sun protection also lowers the risk for skin cancer.
- Encourage your child to do strength-training exercises for the arms, shoulders, and legs to strengthen and condition the muscles.

Limiting screen time

An excellent way of getting your child to be more active is to limit his or her screen time—the total time spent inactive in front of a TV, computer, or video-game screen. Not only will your child have more time for active play and sports—he or she will also be less exposed to commercial interests that are promoting unhealthy food, expensive toys, alcohol, violence, and sexual content. Doctors recommend no more than one to two hours of quality screen time a day for older children and no screen time at all for children under the age of 2.

Getting enough sleep

Sleep has been linked to our ability to learn, create memories, and solve problems—and even to our moods. Insufficient sleep can cause fatigue, irritability, easy frustration, and difficulty regulating emotions. Daytime sleepiness can interfere with a child's ability to learn and perform well in school. Children with chronic sleep deprivation can appear to be overactive, causing some to be mistakenly diagnosed with attention deficit disorder or learning disabilities. Even more troubling is the mounting evidence that links a chronic lack of sleep with an increased risk of developing obesity, diabetes, and heart disease.

Help your child get a good night's sleep

Many young children fight going to sleep at night and end up being drowsy and irritable the following day. Here are some ways you can cope with bedtime resistance and make sure your child gets a full night of sleep:

- Set a regular time for sleep and stick to it.
- Avoid active play right before bedtime
- Establish a relaxing bedtime routine, such as giving your child a warm bath or reading a story.
- Don't give your child a big meal near bedtime.
- Avoid giving your child drinks that contain caffeine.
- Set the bedroom thermostat so that it's not too warm or too cold.
- Make sure the bedroom is dark. Provide a small nightlight if your child needs it for comfort.
- Keep the noise level low.
- Don't put a TV, computer, or other electronic media in your child's bedroom.

Preventing common childhood infections

A child's immune system constantly encounters, fights, and develops resistance to microorganisms that cause disease. By adulthood, the immune system has built up a defense against a wide range of infections. Most childhood infections are caused by viruses and bacteria that infect the airways or the digestive system.

Childhood immunizations

Many once-common childhood infections can now be prevented by routine vaccinations. A vaccination is usually a shot that helps prevent the development of a specific disease. Some vaccinations require a single shot; others require a series of injections over time. Your child's doctor can suggest the

---

HUMAN PAPILLOMAVIRUS VACCINATION

A vaccine is available that may protect against the human papillomavirus virus (HPV; see page 170), the virus that causes cervical cancer (see page 287) in women. HPV is the leading cause of cervical cancer. About 11,150 women are diagnosed with cervical cancer each year in the United States and nearly 3,700 women die from the cancer each year. Approximately 20 million people are currently infected with HPV. At least half of sexually active men and women acquire HPV at some point in their lives. More than 6 million new cases of HPV occur each year in the United States.

The HPV vaccine is given in three doses and, because it is intended for use before a girl becomes sexually active and can be exposed to the virus, girls can receive it when they are 11 or 12 years old. Girls and women ages 13 to 26 years may also benefit from the vaccine. Those who are sexually active should still be vaccinated, to possibly prevent cervical cancer, precancerous tissue changes, and genital warts from HPV.

The vaccination protects against four types of the HPV virus, including two that cause about 70 percent of cases of cervical cancer. Girls who have not acquired HPV would get the full benefits of the vaccine. The vaccination is an important medical breakthrough, but you should talk to your daughter's doctor and thoroughly evaluate the benefits and risks before allowing your daughter to have the vaccination. The vaccination's long-term risks are not yet fully understood, especially in the age group—11- and 12-year-old girls—for whom it has been designed. The vaccine is less effective in girls who have already been exposed to one of the HPV types covered by the vaccine, and the vaccine does not treat existing HPV infections, genital warts, precancers, or cervical cancer. And keep in mind that the HPV vaccine is not intended to replace other preventive measures, such as having regular Pap smears (see page 188) or using a condom and practicing other safe sex measures (see page 175).

exact timing that is best for each vaccination. The schedule will vary for children who have not had the vaccinations as recommended or who have a serious illness such as cancer.

Recommended Schedule of Childhood Immunizations

Child's age	Vaccination
Birth to 2 months	HepB (1st dose)
2 to 4 months	IPV
2 to 6 months	Rotavirus, DTaP, Hib, PCV
6 months—begin yearly vaccination	Influenza vaccine
6 to 18 months	HepB (2nd and 3rd doses)
12 to 15 months	MMR, Varicella (1st dose)
12 to 23 months	HepA (2 doses)
4 to 6 years	MMR, Varicella (2nd dose)
11 to 12 years	DTaP, HPV (3 doses), MCV4
13 to 18 years	MCV4 (if not given at 11 to 12)

Key

DTaP	=	Diphtheria, Tetanus, Pertussis
HepA	=	Hepatitis A (2 doses)
HepB	=	Hepatitis B
Hib	=	Haemophilus influenzae, type b
HPV	=	Human Papillomavirus
IPV	=	Inactivated Poliovirus
MCV4	=	Meningococcus
MMR	=	Measles, Mumps, Rubella
PCV	=	Pneumococcus
Varicella =		Chicken pox

Preventing common infections

The common cold and the flu (influenza) are respiratory disorders that are caused by different viruses. Because the two types of illnesses have similar symptoms, it can be difficult to tell the difference between them based on symptoms alone. In general, the flu is worse than the common cold, with more severe symptoms such as a high fever, severe body aches, extreme

Antibiotics: Not for treating colds or the flu

If your child has a cold or the flu, antibiotics will not be helpful. In fact, they could be harmful. Colds and the flu are caused by viruses; antibiotics work only against infections caused by bacteria. When antibiotics are taken incorrectly or for illnesses other than bacterial infections, they can lead to bacteria that have developed resistance to antibiotics, and bacterial infections that cannot be treated effectively with available antibiotics. An example of this is MRSA (methicillin-resistant Staphylococcus aureus; see page 301), which can cause serious infections and is much more difficult to treat because of its resistance. For information about antibiotics and how to take them correctly, see page 303.

fatigue, and a dry cough that can last two weeks or longer. Colds tend to be milder than the flu, often with no symptoms other than a runny or stuffy nose, mild sore throat, and low (or no) fever; and they usually last only a few days to a week.

The primary way in which the viruses that cause colds and the flu are spread is in airborne droplets from an infected person's coughs or sneezes. These droplets can spray up to 3 feet through the air and deposit themselves on the mouth or nose of a person nearby. The viruses also can be spread when a person touches droplets that have landed on another person or on an object and then touches his or her mouth or nose (or someone else's mouth or nose) before washing his or her hands. Some viruses and bacteria can live from 20 minutes to two hours or more on inanimate surfaces such as cafeteria tables, doorknobs, and desks.

When your children are sick, keep them home from school to avoid spreading the infection. To help reduce your children's risk of getting a cold or the flu, teach them the following precautions that should become lifelong habits:

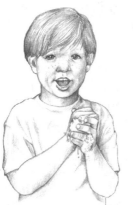

- **Cover your nose and mouth** with a tissue when you cough or sneeze. Throw the tissue away after you use it. If no tissue is available, sneeze into the inside bend of your elbow.

- **Wash your hands often with soap and water,** especially after you cough or sneeze. If water is not available, use an alcohol-based hand cleanser.

- **Avoid touching your eyes, nose, or mouth.** Don't chew on pens and pencils; germs are often spread in this way.

- **Avoid close contact with people who are sick.** When kids are sick, tell other people to keep their distance to avoid getting sick.

Children also need to get plenty of sleep and regular physical activity, drink lots of water, and eat nutritious foods to help them stay healthy.

Preventing lead poisoning

Lead is no longer added to gasoline, or used to solder plumbing pipes or seal the seams of food cans. For this reason, levels of lead in food and water are lower than in the past, but children can still be exposed to lead in a number of ways. The body easily absorbs lead into the bloodstream, and children take in proportionally more lead than adults because of their smaller size. Also, children, especially those under age 6, are more exposed to lead than older people because they tend to put their hands and other objects into their mouth more frequently. When large amounts of lead are absorbed daily, the mineral can get deposited into vital organs such as the brain, bones, and kidneys, where it can cause damage. Lead poisoning can cause learning disabilities, behavior problems, and at very high levels, seizures, coma, and death.

Lead poisoning usually has no obvious symptoms, and for this reason, it frequently goes undiagnosed. The top source of lead exposure in American children is lead-based paint and lead-contaminated dust found in older buildings. Lead-based paints were banned for use in housing in 1978, but millions of homes in the United States still contain layers of leaded paint and high levels of lead-contaminated house dust.

You can prevent much of your child's exposure to lead by taking the following simple measures:

- **Run the cold tap water for a few minutes every morning.** Running the cold water flushes out the lead that has accumulated in the pipes overnight.

- **Use only cold tap water for cooking or drinking.** Babies have been poisoned when hot tap water was boiled and used to make baby formula. Boiling the water concentrates the lead.

- **Never store food in lead-containing glassware or ceramics.** Store food only in glass, stainless steel, or plastic containers. If you use ceramic food containers to store food, make sure they are made with lead-free glazes. Never put food or drinks—especially baby formula or juices—in leaded crystal.

- **Provide foods containing iron and calcium.** Children who get enough of the minerals iron and calcium absorb less lead. Iron-rich foods include lean red meat, dried beans, fortified breakfast cereals, and eggs. Foods high in calcium include dairy products, calcium-fortified orange juice, canned fish with bones, nuts, fruits, and dried beans.

- **Limit exposure to lead outdoors.** Always wash your child's hands after playing outside to prevent intake of lead from the soil or sandboxes.

- **Before growing vegetables in an urban garden, have the soil tested for lead.** The soil could have an elevated lead content if exterior renovations, including the scraping of old paint, have ever occurred, or if you live near a highway or expressway, because lead from leaded gas can still be in the soil.

- **Find out the sources of food supplements.** Dietary supplements from "natural" sources, such as calcium supplements derived from animal bone, can be contaminated with lead.

- **Never burn lead-painted wood in home fireplaces or stoves.** You'll generate lead fumes, and the ashes may be deposited in the backyard, contaminating the soil.

- **If you work in an industry that uses lead, don't launder your clothes at home.** Take-home exposures can occur when workers wear their work clothes home, launder them with the family laundry, or bring scrap or waste material home from work.

- **Avoid using home remedies that contain lead.** Examples to avoid include azarcon, greta, pay-loo-ah, and cosmetics such as kohl and alkohl.

- **Remove lead hazards from your child's environment.** If you live in a house that was built before 1978 and has layers of lead-based paint, contact a certified lead-abatement contractor. Lead abatement involves treating or removing lead-based paint and lead-based paint hazards from a home to make the property lead-safe for young children and other occupants.

To further reduce lead exposure, frequently damp-mop your floors, damp-wipe all furniture and windowsills, and wash your child's hands, pacifiers, and toys to reduce the exposure to lead.

Obesity in children: An alarming trend

Obesity-driven conditions such as high blood pressure, unfavorable cholesterol levels, and type 2 diabetes, once seen primarily in older adults, are now appearing with increasing frequency in children as young as age 5. These health problems can lead to serious complications, including blood vessel damage, organ damage, nerve problems, vision loss, and kidney failure, increasing the risk for disability and premature death.

A child who consumes about the number of calories needed to grow and be active is likely to stay at a healthy weight throughout childhood and has a better chance of maintaining a healthy weight throughout life. But keep in mind that normal weight lies within a fairly wide range. How do you know if your child's weight is normal or too high?

Your child's doctor is the best person to determine if your child's weight is healthy. Doctors use a standard growth chart to measure a child's height and weight against those of other children of the same age and gender. In general, doctors consider a child to be overweight if he or she is heavier than 85 percent of children of the same age and gender. A child who is at or above the 95th percentile is considered obese.

Using the information from the growth charts, doctors calculate a child's body mass index (BMI), which measures the ratio of weight to height. The BMI is the tool used most widely to judge whether a child is at a normal weight, overweight, or obese. You can get a rough idea of whether or not your child is overweight by using one of the many BMI calculators available on the Internet.

From 1980 to 2000, the prevalence of obesity more than doubled for preschoolers and teenagers, and more than tripled for children ages 6 to 11. Many factors have played a role. Technology has become more labor-saving, and daily life less physically active. At the same time, kids learn unhealthy patterns of eating from their parents and friends. Fast food tends to be relatively inexpensive and readily available. Much of the food advertising in the media—especially for high-sugar, high-calorie, high-fat, and high-sodium packaged foods—directly targets young children. Many schools still make high-fat, calorie-dense snacks and sugary soft drinks available to kids in vending machines.

Obesity's health consequences

The soaring prevalence of overweight and obesity in children has brought a corresponding increase in serious health problems, including high blood pressure, unfavorable cholesterol levels, heart disease, type 2 diabetes, arthritis, and respiratory disorders such as sleep apnea. These disorders, which used to occur primarily in adults over age 40, are now appearing in children and young adults with increasing frequency.

HIGH BLOOD PRESSURE

The average blood pressure measurement in American children has risen in recent decades, putting them at risk of developing early heart disease. As many as 1 to 3 percent of children and adolescents may have hypertension or prehypertension (see the box below). High blood pressure, the leading cause of stroke, is called a silent killer because it causes no symptoms in the early stages, even as it is damaging blood vessels and organs.

The increase in the number of overweight American children is the major cause of the increase in blood pressure among children. African American and Hispanic American children usually have higher blood pressure measurements than non-Hispanic white children. Doctors think this difference may result from the higher average weights of children in these groups. However, many of these children may also have inherited a genetic susceptibility to developing high blood pressure that is triggered when they become overweight.

Pediatricians measure the blood pressure of all children ages 3 and older at each well-child office visit. Make sure that your child's blood pressure is checked at every doctor visit, especially if your child is significantly overweight or if other members of your family have high blood pressure. If your child has high blood pressure, his or her doctor may recommend an echocardiogram (an ultrasound imaging test of the heart) to check for enlargement of the left ventricle (the heart's main pumping chamber). Enlargement of the left ventricle is the most obvious sign of heart damage from high blood pressure in children and adolescents.

The first treatment that doctors recommend for high blood pressure in children is

---

CLASSIFYING BLOOD PRESSURE IN CHILDREN AND TEENS

Normal blood pressure readings vary, depending on a child's gender, age, and height. For this reason, blood pressure readings are given in average percentiles so that children aren't mistakenly diagnosed with high blood pressure if they are taller or shorter than average for their age. Also, normal blood pressure is significantly lower in children and adolescents than it is in adults, so readings that doctors regard as elevated in teenagers can be significantly less than readings considered high in adults.

In children younger than 18, hypertension is defined as blood pressure above the 95th percentile (which means that 95 percent of children of the same gender, age, and height have lower blood pressure). Prehypertension is defined as blood pressure between the 90th and 95th percentiles. In adolescents and adults, prehypertension is defined as blood pressure between 120 and 139 on the top (systolic) and 80 to 89 on the bottom (diastolic).

weight loss and exercise. Depending on the degree of hypertension, some doctors may also prescribe an antihypertensive medication. It's essential to work closely with the doctor to bring your child's blood pressure down to normal to prevent the potential long-term harmful effects of high blood pressure, especially on the blood vessels, heart, and kidneys. Children and teenagers with high blood pressure should never start smoking, because smoking can worsen these long-term health risks.

UNFAVORABLE CHOLESTEROL LEVELS

Doctors are finding that childhood obesity can lead to unfavorable blood cholesterol levels. Having unfavorable cholesterol levels, even early in life, may cause fatty deposits to develop in artery walls (atherosclerosis; see page 218). These fatty deposits in arteries that begin in childhood can build up over time, eventually leading to heart disease.

If your child's cholesterol profile is unfavorable, limit his or her intake of foods such as full-fat dairy products (including whole milk, cheeses, and ice cream) and fatty meats (which are high in saturated fats), processed baked foods and snacks such as chips that are often made with trans fats, and cholesterol-rich foods such as egg yolks. Diet isn't the only factor that affects blood cholesterol levels and heart disease risk. Regular exercise also helps to keep cholesterol levels in the healthy range.

CHOLESTEROL: WHAT THE NUMBERS MEAN

The following table shows desirable, borderline, and high cholesterol ranges for children. (Readings are measured in milligrams per deciliter of blood.) Blood cholesterol levels are important determiners of long-term risks for heart disease, so it is never too early to pay attention to them. In general, the lower the level of bad LDL cholesterol, the better. HDL (the good cholesterol) levels should be higher than or equal to 35.

LDL cholesterol	Total cholesterol	What it means
Less than 110	Less than 170	Desirable
110 to 129	170 to 199	Borderline high
130 or higher	200 or higher	High

TYPE 2 DIABETES

When diabetes appears during childhood, doctors usually assume it is type 1 diabetes, which used to be called juvenile diabetes. Over the past few decades, however, type 2 diabetes (formerly known as adult-onset diabetes) has been diagnosed in increasing numbers of American adolescents and young adults, and the problem seems to be occurring worldwide. Type 2 diabetes develops when the body's cells become resistant to the effects of the hormone insulin, which is needed to process glucose, a simple sugar that is the body's main source of fuel. Insulin resistance is the first step toward type 2 diabetes.

Young people with type 2 diabetes represent all ethnic groups, but larger percentages come from Native American, Hispanic, and African American backgrounds. In fact, Native Americans have the highest prevalence of type 2 diabetes in the United States. However, although people in these ethnic groups are at increased risk for type 2 diabetes, people from any racial or ethnic background can develop the disorder, especially if they are significantly overweight and physically inactive.

The major risk factors for type 2 diabetes in young people include the following:

- Being overweight
- Having a history of type 2 diabetes
- Being Native American, Hispanic American, African American, or Asian American
- Eating too much
- Being physically inactive
- Having a mother who developed diabetes during pregnancy
- Having a low birth weight

You may not be able to tell that your child has type 2 diabetes because the disease may not produce any symptoms. For this reason, the disease can go undiagnosed for some time. The only way for a doctor to make an accurate diagnosis is with a blood test. If your child is overweight and inactive, talk to your doctor about your child's risk of developing diabetes.

PUBERTY AND TYPE 2 DIABETES RISK

Some at-risk children develop type 2 diabetes when they reach puberty. In all children, the changes in hormone levels during puberty make the cells less sensitive to insulin, a condition called insulin resistance. Most children do not go on to develop diabetes, but this extra insulin resistance triggered by puberty can bring on type 2 diabetes in children who are already insulin resistant because they are overweight and inactive.

Helping your child reach a healthy weight

The alarming increase in weight among American children is compelling more and more doctors and parents to take action. Many school systems and local and state governments—even the federal government—are enacting legislation aimed at helping children reach and maintain a healthy weight. As a parent, you can have a great influence in helping your child reach a healthy weight by taking some simple—but not always easy—steps. For example, you can learn the basics of nutrition and teach them to your child, be a good role model by eating a nutritious diet and providing healthy meals for your family, and get the whole family (including you, of course) more active. See chapters 1, 2, and 3 to learn the basics of nutrition, exercise, and healthy weight.

Preventing risky behaviors

Risky behaviors are those that have the potential to cause harm. In childhood, risky behaviors usually include experimenting with smoking or using alcohol or other drugs. About 15 percent of boys and 12 percent of girls admit to using drugs before age 13. Because of the delayed effects many of these behaviors can have on health, children often ignore or deny the risks involved.

Keeping kids from smoking

Most adults who smoke started and became addicted when they were teenagers. But even some preteens are taking up smoking. For this reason, it's never too soon to start talking to your children about the dangers of smoking. Firmly root the anti-smoking message in their mind at a young age. The younger your children are when they learn about the harmful effects of smoking, the more likely they are to resist the temptation or pressure from friends to smoke. Many kids who smoke do so because their parents smoke. Here are some things you can do to help your children avoid becoming smokers:

- **Talk with your children about the health effects of smoking.** Give examples of family members or friends who have suffered or died from smoking-related illnesses to make the effects of smoking real. Children seem to respond more strongly to anti-smoking information that focuses on the severely damaging health effects of smoking (such as lung cancer and emphysema) than on the cosmetic effects (such as yellow teeth and bad breath).

- **Teach your children how to resist pressure to smoke.** Know if your kids' friends use tobacco. Talk with your children about ways to tell their friends that they don't want to smoke. A simple "no thanks" is sometimes not enough to get smokers to stop pressuring their friends to smoke.

- **Be a good role model—don't smoke.** If you smoke, quit now (see page 135). (Or at least refrain from smoking in the house.) Teens whose parents smoke are more likely to also smoke. What you do affects your children more than you think.

- **Set rules and stick by them.** Make sure your children know that smoking is not allowed. Frequently remind them of the rules and the consequences of breaking them. This helps children handle peer pressure to smoke by allowing them to use these consequences (such as being grounded for a month) as their reason for not smoking.

- **Talk to your children about smoking in the media.** Smoking may look cool in movies and ads, but the media don't show the damaging health problems and wrinkled skin caused by smoking.

- **Ask teachers and coaches not to use tobacco around teens.** People who are in responsible positions with children should recognize their influence on them.

Helping kids avoid alcohol and other drugs

When it comes to alcohol and other drugs, communicating with your children is the key to prevention. Here's what you can do:

- Talk early and often about drugs with your children. Tell your children what you expect from them if they are offered alcohol or drugs at any time, anywhere.

- Learn the warning signs of drug use.

- Find out how alcohol and drug use can harm a child's mind, body, and emotional health.

- Be aware of all of your children's activities. Encourage them to participate only in supervised groups, clubs, and events that are alcohol-free.

- Be a good role model. Don't abuse alcohol or use drugs yourself.
- Tell your kids to use you as their reason for resisting negative peer pressure. Remind them of your rules and the consequences of breaking those rules each time they leave the house with friends. Kids whose parents establish rules and are consistent in enforcing them are more likely to make good choices.
- Teach your kids the importance of choosing friends wisely and forming positive relationships.
- Set this rule in stone: No riding in a vehicle with anyone who has been drinking. Tell your children to call you if they find themselves in such a situation, and assure them you will come and get them or find a way for them to get home safely.

Remember, the earlier you start talking to your children about drinking and drugs, the more influence you have on their values and decisions—and the more confident your children will be in those values and decisions. Short, frequent conversations are better than one long lecture. See pages 466 to 475 for a more complete discussion of underage drinking and drug use.

Preventing inhalant use

To get high, more and more preteens are inhaling chemicals found in common household products. The list of these products is long and includes model airplane glue, rubber cement, gasoline, propane gas, correction fluid, household cleaners, nail polish remover, marking pens, paint thinner, spray paint, butane lighter fluid, cooking sprays, deodorant, fabric protec-

WARNING

Could your child be using inhalants?

The telltale signs of inhalant use include the following: an unusual breath odor, chemical odors on clothing, slurred speech, disorientation, intoxicated or dazed appearance, red eyes, runny nose, sores around the mouth, or loss of appetite. Some children put chemicals on their sleeves and frequently inhale them, hide rags or empty chemical containers, or have paint stain marks on their faces. If you notice any of these signs, get help immediately. If your child is in imminent danger, call 911 or your local emergency number. Otherwise, talk to your child's doctor right away. Your child's life could depend on it.

tors, and air-conditioning coolant (freon). These chemicals are attractive to kids because they produce a quick high, cost little, are easy to get, and are legal.

Using inhalants—even once—can be life-threatening. Inhalants can cause what is referred to as sudden sniffing death, in which the heart beats rapidly but unevenly and triggers cardiac arrest. Inhaling these chemicals can also cause hallucinations, severe mood swings, numbness and tingling, heart palpitations, breathing difficulty, dizziness, and headaches. Prolonged use can cause short-term memory loss, muscle spasm, an irregular heartbeat, liver and kidney failure, and permanent brain damage.

To prevent inhalant use, lock up all household cleaners, chemicals, paints and paint thinner, gasoline, and even nail polish remover, and keep these products out of the reach of children—your own kids and their friends. Even if you trust your kids and their friends not to do something stupid or dangerous, you could be tempting them by not taking proper precautions. It's better to be safe and lock all potentially dangerous chemicals away in a secure cabinet. Teach your children, starting at a young age, about the dangers of inhaling chemicals—especially that it can kill them instantly, even the first time. Elementary-school age is when many children begin experimenting with inhalants.

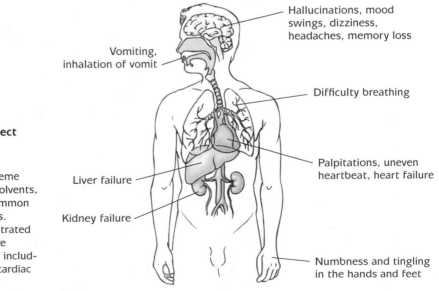

How inhalants affect the body

Children are usually unaware of the extreme danger of inhaling solvents, gases, and other common household chemicals. Chemicals in concentrated form can have severe effects on the body, including organ damage, cardiac arrest, and death.

Hallucinations, mood swings, dizziness, headaches, memory loss

Vomiting, inhalation of vomit

Difficulty breathing

Liver failure

Kidney failure

Palpitations, uneven heartbeat, heart failure

Numbness and tingling in the hands and feet

22

ADOLESCENTS AND WELLNESS

ADOLESCENCE IS A TIME OF RAPID CHANGE. Not only is the body changing physically, but changes are also occurring in a child's intellect and feelings. The teen years can often be a time of stress because kids are coping with their body changes at the same time that they feel pressure to conform to social trends as well as higher expectations from parents and teachers. This chapter discusses the emotional, physical, and behavior issues that can occur during the teen years. While your child is an adolescent, keep in mind that parents and family remain the most important influences for most teenagers. If you educate yourself about the issues facing teens, you will be able to help your child avoid them and know what signs of potential problems to watch for. If problems arise, it's best to take action early, when problems are generally easiest to solve.

Mental and emotional well-being

Adolescence is a developmental period that encompasses many changes for young people—in their body, at school, and in their social life. For some, parental divorce, being part of a new family with stepparents and stepsiblings, or moving to a new community can be an added source of stress. Teens are often exposed to new situations, new people, and new opportunities—both good and bad. For example, driving can be an exciting challenge that promises newfound independence, while smoking and drug and alcohol use are harmful behaviors that can promote lifelong unhealthy habits.

Adolescents can experience intense feelings of anxiety, confusion, self-doubt, pressure to conform, and demands to succeed. This section describes how you can help your adolescent navigate this exciting but challenging stage of life to become a physically and emotionally healthy adult.

Managing stress and anxiety

Teens face many situations that can cause high levels of stress and anxiety, including school demands, problems with friends, lots of activities, the separation or divorce of their parents, moving or changing schools, or breaking up with a boyfriend or a girlfriend. You can help your adolescent children manage stress by helping them organize their schedules, promoting activities that benefit others as well as themselves, allowing unscheduled time to have fun, and keeping your lines of communication open. Here are some tips:

- **Establish a family routine.** Studies suggest that successful students have a flexible family routine that includes eating meals with the family, having a regular time for homework, and going to bed at a set time.

- **Set boundaries.** Children feel reassured and protected when parental guidelines are firm. But keep in mind that saying no with a tone of care and concern is more likely to get a cooperative response. Learn new ways to say no, such as "Yes, after your homework is done." Help children learn how to say no to peer pressure when they need to—and mean it. This skill will be useful when difficult and stressful choices have to be made now, and throughout their life.

- **Listen and be encouraging.** Listen to your children and encourage them to express their feelings, especially if you sense that they may be overwhelmed or experiencing stress. Respect their feelings and reassure them that everyone experiences nervousness, fear, and anxiety, and that it's okay to feel this way.

- **Provide safety valves for stress.** Every teen needs a collection of stress safety valves—ways to relax or enjoy some downtime. Some effective safety valves include listening to music, reading a book, taking a walk, dancing, jogging, talking with a friend, doing yoga, playing sports, or drawing pictures.

Healthy behaviors also help to relieve stress. Encourage your kids to adopt the following healthy lifestyle habits:

- Exercise regularly.
- Eat a healthy diet.
- Avoid skipping meals.
- Eat breakfast every day.
- Avoid excessive caffeine intake because it can increase anxiety and agitation.
- Resist using alcohol, tobacco, and illegal drugs.

CAFFEINE-RICH ENERGY DRINKS: NOT A GOOD WAY TO HANDLE STRESS

Busy teenagers often don't get the sleep they need, leaving them more likely to reach for a caffeine jolt. Caffeine stimulates the central nervous system and provides an energy lift, but the high levels of caffeine in energy drinks can cause health problems. Because caffeine promotes water loss from the body, it can cause dehydration. Dehydration is even more likely if you are also sweating a lot from exercise.

Excess caffeine can also increase heart rate and raise blood pressure. For this reason, energy drinks are not good for children or adolescents. Caffeine can cause children to become agitated, irritable, and nervous. How much caffeine is too much? It depends. The effects of caffeine vary from one person to another depending on age, size, and health. For most people, three 8-ounce cups of coffee a day is considered a moderate amount of caffeine. But some other ingredients in energy drinks, including guarana and taurine, add to the potential problems. Guarana, or guarine, is a caffeine-like substance. Taurine is an amino acid that the body produces naturally, but exactly how it works or how much is too much is not known. Also, energy drinks contain carbohydrates—more than most people need. The result—excess calories—can contribute to weight gain.

Mixing energy drinks with alcohol poses an added risk. The stimulation from a caffeine-heavy energy drink can make a person feel less intoxicated than he or she is. An adolescent may keep drinking or drive a car without understanding the danger. Also, because caffeine can promote dehydration, alcohol becomes harder to absorb, making its toxic effects more damaging to the body.

Remember that your children look to you as an example, so use good stress-management techniques yourself to help them learn to handle stress in positive ways.

Why teens need their sleep

Teenagers are especially susceptible to sleep loss. Teenage sleep patterns are different from those of adults and younger children. During adolescence, a teenager's circadian rhythm, or internal biological clock, becomes reset, telling him or her to fall asleep later at night and wake up later in the morning. This change occurs because the adolescent brain produces the hormone melatonin (which controls sleep and wake cycles) later at night than do the brains of children and adults, making it more difficult for teens to fall asleep at what parents might consider a more reasonable hour.

This biological readjustment occurs when most teens' lives are busier than ever. Activities that can include school, homework, sports, a part-time job, and a busy social life place competing demands on an adolescent's time. But most schools start early in the morning, and as a result, many young people are getting only six or seven hours of sleep a night. Research has shown that kids ages 12 to 17 need eight and a half to nine and a half hours of sleep every night. An hour or two of missed sleep can cause daytime drowsiness that can affect concentration, learning, and performance at school. Sleep-deprived teens may forget what they were taught because memory is formed partly during sleep. In response to parental pressure, some high school districts in the United States are changing school hours to start later.

Sleep deprivation can also have a harmful effect on a teen's physical and emotional health. Lack of sleep may reduce the body's ability to fight infection, and in some teens, may bring on feelings of stress, anger, or sadness. According to the National Sleep Foundation, lack of sleep increases a teen's already elevated risk of being in a car collision. Drowsiness and fatigue play a role in 100,000 traffic accidents a year, and drivers 25 and under are responsible for more than half of these. Here are some things parents can do to help their teen get a good night's sleep:

- Educate your kids about the need for sleep.
- Establish a regular sleep-wake schedule, with a routine bedtime on school nights and staying up no more than one hour later on weekends.

- Monitor late-night activities; limit the amount of time spent on TV, the Internet, and the phone on school nights.

- Limit caffeine intake: no more than two caffeinated drinks during the day and none after 5 p.m.

- Set a good example for your children by having a healthy sleep routine yourself.

- Get involved with other parents to encourage school administrators to institute a later start time at your teen's school.

Teen suicide

Some teenagers experience adolescence as stressful and anxious, and severely stressed-out kids can slip into feelings of helplessness and hopelessness—feelings that could lead to thoughts of suicide. Suicide is the third leading cause of death among adolescents, after car crashes and homicide. In 2004, 4,599 young people between ages 10 and 24 committed suicide, and many more attempted suicide. Between 1990 and 2003, the suicide rate for this age group fell by more than 28 percent, but from 2003 to 2004, the Centers for Disease Control and Prevention (CDC) reports, the rate jumped 8 percent, the biggest single-year increase in 15 years. The largest increase—67 percent—was among girls ages 10 to 14.

The method of suicide also changed during this time, especially among females. In 1990, guns accounted for more than half of all suicides among young females. By 2004, however, death by suffocation from hanging became the most common method, accounting for 71 percent of suicides among girls ages 10 to 14, about half among girls ages 15 to 19, and 34 percent among young women between ages 20 and 24.

A 2007 survey of high-school students found that almost one in five had seriously considered suicide, and more than one in twelve had made a suicide attempt in the past year. In all racial and ethnic groups, female students are more likely than male students to feel sad or hopeless, but boys are more likely to succeed when they attempt suicide.

√ **Suicide risk: Take action**

If you think your child, or one of his or her friends, could be suicidal, remove from your home or lock away all ropes, guns, pills, kitchen knives, and household chemicals. These are the items that teens use most often to kill themselves.

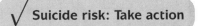

Suicide warning signs

If your child ever talks about suicide, even in a joking way, take him or her seriously and get help immediately. Any adolescent who talks about suicide needs to be taken seriously and immediate action needs to be taken. An adolescent who displays any of the following signs listed below may be thinking about suicide. However, you should know that the signs of depression and risk of suicide can be subtle, and a teen who may be at risk may not have any of the signs listed below. If you have any questions, concerns, or instincts about your child that something could be wrong, seek help immediately. You could be saving your child's life.

- Feeling sad and hopeless for no reason, and these feelings don't go away
- Feeling very angry most of the time
- Crying a lot or overreacting to things
- Feeling worthless or guilty often
- Feeling anxious or worried often
- Being unable to get over a loss or the death of someone important
- Performing less well in school
- Losing interest in things he or she once enjoyed
- Experiencing unexplained changes in sleeping or eating patterns
- Avoiding friends or family and wanting to be alone all the time
- Feeling life is too hard to handle.

PREVENTION

If you think your child, or the child of a friend or family member, might be considering suicide, get help immediately. Call your child's doctor or a local hospital emergency department, where a suicide crisis worker should be available 24 hours a day to evaluate the situation and intervene. If not, look for suicide hotline and crisis center phone numbers in your local phone book or call 1-800-273-TALK (8255). This 24-hour toll-free number is for the National Suicide Prevention Lifeline, which will route you to the nearest crisis center in your area. (All calls are confidential.) If you think your child is in imminent danger, call 911 or your local emergency number.

Listen carefully to your child and tell him or her that you care about what happens to him or her and that help is available, no matter how overwhelming the problems seem. Find a doctor, community health center, counselor, psychologist, social worker, youth worker, or clergy member to work with your child. Most cases of depression can be successfully treated.

Teen self-injury

Self-injury—also called self-mutilation or "cutting"—is the intentional harming of the body, usually by cutting, to cope with overpowering emotions. Although only about 3 percent of the population engages in self-injury, it is on the rise among adolescents. Adolescents who self-mutilate typically make cuts or scratches with a sharp object on their arms, legs, or torso. Other types of self-injury include burning, scratching, carving words or symbols on the skin, breaking bones, banging the head, pulling out hair, biting themselves, or overdosing on drugs.

The practice can be an impulsive act done in response to an emotionally upsetting event. Or a teen might engage in self-injury in a controlled, systematic way, planning ahead for it and being careful not to be discovered. The emotional relief that people say they get from self-injury is always only temporary because the painful underlying emotions and problems quickly return, often leading to a repeating cycle of self-abuse. Self-mutilation may be related to depression or borderline personality disorder (which is characterized by impulsive behavior). The practice is more common in people who have been sexually abused and is more prevalent among girls and women than boys and men.

Teens who hurt themselves usually try to keep their behavior hidden, so it can be hard to recognize the signs of self-injury, which include having unexplained scars, cuts or other wounds, bruises, or broken bones, and repeatedly pretending to have accidents or making up accidents to explain their injuries.

PREVENTION

To prevent self-injury, it's important to identify the adolescents who are most at risk, and try to teach them more positive ways of coping with their strong emotions. If you think your child could be at risk for self-injury, help him or her learn to deal with emotional stress in the following healthier ways:

- **Accept what cannot be changed.** If life hands your child a setback, let him or her know that it's okay to grieve for a time, but then it's important to move on.

- **Find someone to talk to.** Urge your child to open up to a trusted friend, adult, or trained professional, who can help him or her see problems in a new light and learn positive ways to deal with them.
- **Learn how to relax.** Find activities to enjoy—such as a yoga class or meditation (see page 121)—that can help take the mind off troubles.
- **Exercise.** Work off tensions through a physical activity such as walking, jogging, playing a sport, or taking an exercise class.

Preventing acne

Acne is a common skin condition that results from inflammation of the hair follicles and sebaceous glands, which produce an oily substance called sebum that lubricates the skin. Acne is most common during puberty and adolescence because the level of male hormones rises in both males and females at this time, stimulating the sebaceous glands to increase sebum production. About 85 percent of all teenagers develop acne. Acne usually clears up in the late teens or early 20s. Although acne is not a serious health threat, it can be a source of emotional distress during the teen years, and severe acne can lead to permanent scarring. The tendency to develop acne can be inherited.

Acne tends to occur in flare-ups. Chocolate and greasy foods are often blamed for acne flare-ups, but no evidence has shown that foods have much effect on the development of acne. Common factors that can cause a flare-up include changing hormone levels that can occur in the days before a menstrual period; oil from moisturizers or cosmetics, or from unwashed hair that hangs over the face; pressure from sports helmets or equipment, backpacks, tight collars, or tight sports uniforms; pollution or high humidity; squeezing or picking at blemishes; or scrubbing the skin too hard.

Here are some guidelines for keeping acne outbreaks in check:

- Gently wash your face with a mild soap in the morning and evening. Don't forget to also wash your face after exercising.
- Never use strong soaps or rough scrub pads. Rubbing acne can make the problem worse.
- Keep your hair off your face. Hair contains oil that could trigger acne breakouts.
- Shampoo your hair regularly. If you have oily hair, wash it every day.

- Avoid rubbing and touching skin blemishes. Squeezing, pinching, or picking blemishes can cause scarring.

- Don't wear makeup. Foundation and blusher create a barrier over clogged pores, preventing them from healing.

- Change your pillowcase every other day. Oil and dirt from your face build up on your pillowcase and go back onto your skin when you lie down.

- Eat a healthy, balanced diet. Your body needs proper nutrition to heal your skin and fight bacteria.

Reducing osteoporosis risk

Osteoporosis (see page 325), weak bones from the loss of bone density, is not a disorder of adolescence. However, because bones grow and incorporate calcium most rapidly during the teen years, adolescence is the time to build strong bones that can withstand the normal bone loss that occurs with age. About 90 percent of adult bone mass is established by age 17. By age 21 or soon after, peak bone density is reached; a few years later, a steady loss of calcium from the bones begins that continues throughout life. You can help your teen avoid the devastating consequences of osteoporosis later in life by teaching him or her the importance of building strong bones now. Think of it as putting money in the bank for later. Here are the most important things that teens can do to build strong bones now to reduce their risk for fractures later in life:

- **Get enough calcium.** Consuming calcium-rich foods, such as low-fat dairy products and nondairy calcium-rich foods, during adolescence helps build strong bones. But 8 out of 10 teen girls and 6 out of 10 teen boys do not get enough calcium in their diet. Most teens get only about 800 milligrams out of the 1,300 milligrams they need each day. They should try to increase their consumption of dairy products and calcium-fortified juices and breakfast cereals. If your teen is not getting sufficient calcium from the diet, make calcium supplements available and make sure he or she takes them regularly to reach the 1,300 milligram daily requirement.

- **Get enough vitamin D.** Vitamin D strengthens bones by helping the body absorb bone-building calcium. Adolescents need at least 5 micrograms (200 IU) of vitamin D from food every day. Another good way to get vitamin D is to be outside in the sun so the skin can make vitamin D from sun exposure. Ten or 15 minutes a day in the sun is all you need; more than that can cause sunburn and skin changes that could lead to skin cancer.

- **Exercise regularly.** Weight-bearing exercise that forces you to work against gravity stimulates the growth of bone. Bones respond to exercise by becoming bigger and stronger; without use, they weaken and shrink. Exercise also boosts blood flow to the bones, transporting needed bone-building nutrients. Strength-training exercises (see page 52) are especially good for building bone.

- **Avoid excessive weight loss and excessive exercise.** Eating too little and exercising too much can make you lose bone mass because you don't get enough nutrients to maintain health. In girls, the stop of periods is a key warning sign. Increasing numbers of young women with eating disorders are developing osteoporosis.

Avoiding bacterial meningitis

If they have not done so already, college students may want to be vaccinated against meningitis (inflammation of the tissues that cover the brain and spinal cord). Once rare, outbreaks of bacterial meningitis began to occur more frequently in the 1990s, especially among college students who live in dormitories or residence halls. Bacterial meningitis can cause disability or death if not treated promptly.

The meningococcal vaccination (see page 444) is recommended for all children at ages 11 to 12, and at age 15 for kids who did not receive the vaccination earlier. If your child has not had the meningococcal vaccination and is about to enter college, talk to the doctor about having your child vaccinated, especially if your child will be living in a dorm or residence hall. While the vaccination significantly reduces the risk for meningitis, it does not completely eliminate the risk. It protects against only certain strains of the bacteria, and the vaccine is not 100 percent effective.

Recognizing drug and alcohol use and abuse

Every day, children make choices that are good or bad for their health. Sometimes they face choices about potentially dangerous behaviors, including drug and alcohol use—often while under pressure from their peers. Alcohol is the drug most commonly used and abused by adolescents. It can cause many problems for teenagers, including motor vehicle crashes, injuries, and death; school problems; fighting; and crime. Nearly half of all teens have tried marijuana by the time they leave high school, but only a small percentage goes on to use stronger drugs such as cocaine. Prescription drug use is growing among teens because of their easy availability and the false perception that they are safer than illegal drugs. This section shows you how to help adolescents understand the impact that drug and alcohol use can have on their future, and how to give them the tools they need to be able to resist the peer pressure to use these dangerous substances. For more thorough discussions about the use and abuse of alcohol and other drugs, see pages 140 to 165.

Alcohol

By the time they are seniors in high school, most American teens have used alcohol or been drunk (see the chart on the next page). Drinking can have especially harmful effects on an adolescent's still-developing brain and body. Alcohol use can cause learning problems and lead to alcohol abuse and dependence in adulthood. In fact, people who begin drinking by age 15 are five times more likely to abuse or become dependent on alcohol than those who begin drinking after age 20.

Alcohol affects girls more strongly than boys, because girls tend to be smaller than boys and the female body lacks certain digestive enzymes that help break down alcohol before it enters the bloodstream. For this reason, girls can become dependent on alcohol more quickly than boys and are more vulnerable to liver damage and other health problems that result from long-term alcohol use.

Alcohol most noticeably affects the central nervous system. Just one or two drinks can slow reaction time, distort vision, block memory, and impair judgment. Teenage alcohol use has been linked to poor academic performance, date rape, blackouts, unplanned pregnancy, suicide, and murder. Driving and drinking can be especially dangerous, particularly for inexperienced teen drivers.

Binge drinking—having five or more drinks in a row in one session—is a particularly dangerous but common feature of adolescent drinking. Drinking large amounts of alcohol at one time or very rapidly can cause

Alcohol use by American teens

The 2006 Monitoring the Future Survey found the percentages shown on the chart of American students who reported that they had used alcohol or had been drunk at some time in their life. The numbers have declined steadily since 1991, when 70 percent of eighth graders, 84 percent of tenth graders, and 88 percent of twelfth graders reported that they had ever used alcohol.

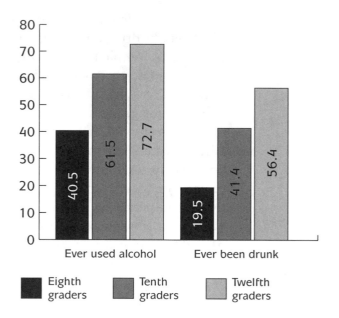

	Ever used alcohol	Ever been drunk
Eighth graders	40.5	19.5
Tenth graders	61.5	41.4
Twelfth graders	72.7	56.4

alcohol poisoning, which can lead to coma or even death. Alcohol poisoning is more common among preteens and teens than any other age group; having more than one drink in an hour increases the risk. Binge drinking and heavy drinking can also lead to bone loss, increasing the risk for osteoporosis (see page 325) later in life.

Alcohol can be harmful even to teens who are not drinking. If your teenager is around people who are drinking, he or she has an increased risk of being seriously injured, involved in a vehicle collision, or affected by violence.

Remind your child that most teens don't drink alcohol, and that he or she will be in the majority by declining to drink. Tell your child to simply say, "No thanks," or, "I don't drink," or, "I don't feel like it." Tell your child to use you as the excuse: "My parents will ground me for a month if I drink. It's not worth it." (For a complete discussion about the harmful effects of alcohol, including what to do about alcohol abuse, see pages 140 to 153.)

Marijuana

After alcohol, marijuana (also known as cannabis) is a major drug of choice of adolescents. Long-term marijuana use can damage the airways and lungs and lead to chronic bronchitis or emphysema. Marijuana smoke contains cancer-causing agents that can increase the risk for lung cancer. Although marijuana is not thought to be physically addictive, heavy, chronic use can cause psychological dependence that could lead to a loss of energy, ambition, and drive. For more about marijuana, see page 155.

Your child could be using marijuana if you find any paraphernalia designed for marijuana use in your child's room or backpack. These items might include rolling papers, clips, pipes, or bent paper clips (used for cleaning out pipes). Other telltale signs of marijuana use include the distinctive odor on your child's clothing, the use of incense or other room deodorizers to hide the odor, and wearing clothing or jewelry that promotes marijuana use.

Prescription drugs

Teens are increasingly using prescription drugs to get high. Studies have shown that the intentional abuse of prescription drugs—including pain relievers, tranquilizers, stimulants, and sedatives—is growing. Prescription-drug abuse is an increasing problem among American teens between ages 12 and 17.

Teens abuse prescription drugs because they believe the myth that the drugs provide a medically safe high. They often characterize their use of the drugs as "responsible," "controlled," or "safe," because of the perception that prescription drugs are safer than street drugs. Young people also admit to abusing prescription medicine for reasons other than getting high, including to relieve pain or anxiety, to sleep better, to help with concentration, or to increase alertness. Many kids have no idea that these drugs can be addictive.

Teens who use prescription drugs to get high obtain the drugs easily, often from friends or relatives. Nearly half of adolescent prescription-drug users get them from their friends for free. And parents, take note: more than three in five teens say prescription pain relievers are easy to get from their parents' medicine cabinet. Girls are more likely than boys to intentionally abuse prescription drugs to get high. Pain relievers such as oxycodone and hydrocodone/acetaminophen are the prescription drugs most commonly abused by teens, followed by stimulants and tranquilizers. Adolescents are more likely than young adults to become dependent on prescription drugs.

Anabolic steroids

Anabolic steroids are synthetic forms of the male sex hormone testosterone, which some teenagers use to increase their strength, get a hard-bodied appearance, and improve their athletic performance. Although this practice is most common among boys who play varsity football and wrestling, anabolic steroid use has also been rising among girls. Young people can take these drugs in pills, by injection (which boosts their risk for HIV or hepatitis infection if they share needles), or by rubbing them onto their skin.

Use of anabolic steroids can have numerous harmful physical effects, mainly on the liver, heart, and reproductive system, as well as psychological effects. In males, steroids can cause the testicles to shrink and breasts to develop, and can raise the risk for male infertility, erection problems, and baldness. In females, the drugs can stimulate the development of irreversible masculine traits, including facial hair, breast reduction, and deepening of the voice. Irregular menstrual periods and infertility are also risks in females. In both sexes, the drugs can induce extremely aggressive behavior, commonly known as 'roid rage, as well as depression. Steroid use also increases the future risk for heart attacks and stroke.

Signs of anabolic steroid use include a rapid increase in weight and muscle bulk, aggressiveness, hostility, moodiness, severe acne, baldness, and yellowing of the skin and whites of the eyes (jaundice). Some children begin using steroids as early as junior high. If you suspect that your child might be using anabolic steroids, talk to his or her doctor and coach. Ask them to counsel your child against the drugs and to recommend safe ways to build muscle and strength without them. Remind your children that steroid use in sports is illegal and that athletes are tested for steroid use to prevent them from gaining an unfair advantage.

How to prevent drug and alcohol use and abuse

The key risk periods for drug abuse in adolescence are during major transitions in children's lives. These transitions can include puberty and family milestones, such as moving or parents divorcing. When they enter high school, young people face social, emotional, and educational challenges. At the same time, they may be exposed to greater availability of drugs, drug abusers, and social situations involving alcohol, tobacco, and other drugs.

Some children are abusing drugs by age 12 or 13, and some begin even earlier. Early abuse usually includes such drugs as tobacco, alcohol, inhalants, marijuana, and prescription drugs. If drug abuse persists into later adolescence, teens often become more heavily involved with marijuana and advance to other illegal drugs, while continuing to use tobacco and alcohol.

Building a strong and protective relationship with your children from infancy will help reduce their risk of abusing drugs. As a parent, you can take a number of steps to prevent your children from using and abusing alcohol and other drugs. Here are some strategies that have been shown to work:

- Be involved in your children's lives, at home and at school.
- Provide emotional, intellectual, and financial support.
- Keep tabs on who your children choose as friends, and know your children's friends. Most teens get their first exposure to drugs and alcohol through friends.
- Voice your strong disapproval of the use of alcohol and other drugs.
- Set clear limits and enforce them.
- Monitor your children's social activities; make sure adult supervision is available at all activities outside the home.
- Establish and enforce a curfew.
- Give your children chores and other responsibilities.
- Convey that you value success at school and expect your children to do well.
- Promote involvement in extracurricular activities.
- Teach your children never to let anyone force them to drink alcohol or use other drugs, and never to take part in drinking games or contests, which can be fatal.
- Set a good example by never using recreational drugs yourself. Drink alcohol only in moderation.

Preventing teen tobacco use

Many teenagers experiment with cigarettes, and most think that they can stop smoking easily. Only 3 out of 100 high school smokers think they'll be smoking in five years. But in reality, 60 of those 100 will still be smoking seven to nine years later—and will be hooked. It usually takes 16 to 20 years of addicted smoking and more than one effort to quit before the average person who starts smoking as a teen will be able to quit successfully.

Kids whose parents smoke are more likely to see smoking as a normal part of being an adult. If you smoke, quit now, not only for your health, but for the health of your children. If you have tried quitting and couldn't, talk to your teen about how addictive nicotine is and how, when you were younger, you thought you could quit any time you wanted. Never smoke in the house or car.

Cigarettes

Teens start smoking cigarettes because they think it makes them look sophisticated and grown-up. Many teenage girls start smoking to lose weight or to keep from gaining weight. Cigarette advertising is especially alluring to young people, many of whom will become addicted to nicotine and die prematurely from the effects of smoking (see page 126). Nearly all adults who currently smoke became addicted to nicotine by age 17. If smoking rates stay the same, more than 6 million children living today will die of a smoking-related disease. After declining steadily for more than a decade, the rates of daily smoking among early and middle teens stopped declining in 2006.

For many teens, knowledge about the harmful health effects of smoking keeps them from starting. Many kids have known people—including relatives and family friends—who have suffered these devastating effects and died from smoking. Also, many kids now consider smoking a sign of poor judgment.

Light and menthol cigarettes

Kids sometimes think that "light" cigarettes are not as bad for them as regular cigarettes. But they are wrong. Light cigarettes put smokers at the same risk for smoking-related health problems as regular cigarettes. Some cigarette packs say that light cigarettes have lower levels of tar and nicotine than regular cigarettes. But these claims are misleading. Tobacco companies use smoking machines to determine the amount of tar and nicotine in cigarettes. These machines "smoke" every brand of cigarette in the same way, but people don't smoke cigarettes the same way machines do. People who smoke light cigarettes usually inhale more deeply, take more puffs, or smoke extra cigarettes to get the same "hit" of nicotine. As a result, they end up inhaling just as much tar, nicotine, and other chemicals as people who smoke regular cigarettes.

Menthol cigarettes have a minty taste that makes some smokers think they're healthier than regular cigarettes, but they are not. In fact, menthol cigarettes contain even more chemicals than regular cigarettes. Also, the soothing menthol can make it easier for a smoker to inhale deeply, allowing more chemicals to enter the lungs. As a result, menthol cigarettes may be even more harmful than regular cigarettes.

Smokeless tobacco: Snuff and chewing tobacco

Smokeless tobacco is not a safe alternative to cigarettes. It's addictive and can cause cancer, even in young people. Smokeless tobacco comes in two forms—snuff and chewing tobacco. In both forms, nicotine enters the bloodstream through the skin lining the mouth.

- **Snuff**   Snuff is a finely ground tobacco that is the most popular type of smokeless tobacco in the United States. Users put a pinch of snuff (also called a "dip" or a "rub") between their cheek and gum or lower lip and gum and hold it there.

- **Chewing tobacco**   Chewing tobacco, also called spit tobacco, is bulkier than snuff and is chewed. It comes in leaf and plug forms.

Like all forms of tobacco, smokeless tobacco contains nicotine, the addictive substance that gets you hooked. Holding one pinch of smokeless tobacco in your mouth for 30 minutes delivers as much nicotine as three or four cigarettes. Smokeless tobacco contains at least 3,000 other chemicals. As many as 28 of these chemicals can cause cancer. Using smokeless tobacco can cause serious health problems, including cancers of the mouth, throat, and esophagus, and shrinking of the gums around the teeth, which can lead to tooth loss.

Alternative or "natural" cigarettes

Alternative or so-called natural cigarettes include clove cigarettes (known as "kreteks") and flavored cigarettes (called "bidis" or "beedies"). Both types are imported, mainly from Southeast Asia. In addition to tobacco, they contain a variety of flavorings. Kreteks contain ground cloves and clove oil. Bidis contain candy-like flavors such as chocolate, vanilla, and cherry, which appeal to kids.

Some young people believe that kreteks and bidis are safer than regular cigarettes because of the "natural" flavorings, and because the packs often don't have warning labels. They'd be surprised to learn that both kreteks and bidis deliver more nicotine, tar, and carbon monoxide than regular cigarettes. And, like smoking regular cigarettes, smoking kreteks and bidis can eventually cause lung cancer and other serious diseases.

Another type of "natural" cigarette is the herbal cigarette. This product is made from a blend of herbs, such as passionflower, jasmine, and ginseng,

---

IF YOU'RE A TEEN WHO WANTS TO QUIT SMOKING

If you are like most teens who smoke, you want to quit but you're not able to or don't know how. The first step is to ask for help. Talk to your parents or another trusted adult (maybe someone who has successfully quit smoking) or your doctor; they may be able to recommend a smoking-cessation program designed especially for teens. You can also look for programs in your school. For example, the American Lung Association has developed a program that schools can use to help teens avoid tobacco or stop using it. Called N-O-T for Not On Tobacco, the program provides a 10-week session and booster sessions to help kids stay off tobacco over the long term.

N-O-T divides teen groups by gender, with a group leader of the same gender, to allow teens to discuss issues that might relate to them specifically as males or females. This grouping tends to make teens more open to expressing their feelings and experiences. The program teaches life-management skills to help teens deal with stress, decision-making, and peer and family relationships. To promote healthy lifestyle behaviors, the program helps teens learn how to avoid alcohol or illegal drugs, eat a healthy diet, and be physically active. To find out about programs in your area, contact the American Lung Association by calling 1-800-LUNG-USA or visiting its Web site (www.lungusa.org).

and contains no tobacco. Herbal cigarettes are easy to find and easy to buy, and it's legal to sell them to kids who are not old enough to buy tobacco. They look exotic and come in tempting flavors such as chocolate, cherry, or mango. Although herbal cigarettes contain no tobacco or nicotine, their smoke contains tar, carbon monoxide, and other toxins, so they can still be harmful to health.

Hookah pipes

Middle Eastern men have smoked hookah pipes for hundreds of years. A hookah is a water pipe that holds tobacco. This exotic form of smoking has become popular in the United States, especially among young people. The tobacco in a hookah may be mixed with honey, molasses, or dried fruit to give flavor to the smoke. When a person inhales from a hose attached to the hookah, the smoke is filtered through water in the base. Passing the smoke through the water partially filters tar and small particles from the smoke.

Because the pipe filters the tobacco smoke, hookahs are advertised as being safer than cigarettes. But in fact, hookah smoke contains levels of nicotine, carbon monoxide, and tar that are as high as or higher than those found in the smoke from many filtered cigarettes. Also, users typically inhale massive amounts of smoke and smoke longer at one session. Smoking from a hookah for one hour delivers 100 to 200 times the amount of smoke inhaled from one cigarette. Several types of cancer, as well as gum disease, have been linked to hookah smoking.

Teenagers and unsafe sex

The hormonal changes of puberty can trigger intense sexual urges and emotions. Many teenagers respond to these urges by becoming sexually active. But even though teenagers are physically able to act on their strong sexual desires, many lack the emotional and intellectual maturity needed to deal with a sexual relationship responsibly. And many may not understand the potentially harmful consequences of early sexual relationships.

Communicating your values about sexuality in ongoing conversations, beginning when your children are young, will help them make responsible choices. Don't be afraid to express your hope that your teen will wait until he or she is older and more mature before having sex. Teens who have a close relationship with their parents, set high goals for the future, and are informed about safe sex and reproduction are more likely than other teens to postpone having sex and to be responsible when they become sexually active.

Oral sex

Among teens ages 15 to 19 who have not had sexual intercourse, almost one in four reports having had oral sex with a partner of the opposite sex. As parents, it's important to broaden the discussions you have with your adolescents about sex to include oral sex. In surveys, teenagers rate oral sex as being much less risky than vaginal sex. Many teens also believe that oral sex is more acceptable than vaginal sex for adolescents their age, and that oral sex is less of a compromise to their values and beliefs.

Many teens think that having oral sex is not having sex. But oral sex is having sex. Oral sex is linked to a number of sexually transmitted diseases (STDs; see page 166), including gonorrhea, syphilis, and herpes. Many of these STDs can be transmitted from the mouth of one person to the genitals of another, or from the genitals to the mouth, where they can cause infections in the mouth, on the vocal cords, or in the respiratory system. For example, cold sores are caused by the herpes simplex virus, which also causes genital herpes, which has no cure. Oral sex can also transmit HIV (the virus that causes AIDS), whether the infected person is performing or receiving oral sex. Human papillomavirus (HPV), which can cause cervical cancer in women, can also raise the risk for oral cancer when contracted during oral sex; in fact, HPV now causes as many cases of oral cancer in men as smoking and drinking alcohol do.

Using condoms and other barriers such as dental dams or even plastic food wrap can lower the risks involved with oral sex, but few adolescents engaged in these activities use them. (A dental dam is a square piece of rubber that dentists use during oral surgery and other procedures. Dental dams can be purchased at most stores that sell condoms.)

A condom can be used on the penis for oral sex. A dental dam, a natural rubber latex sheet, a cut-open condom that forms a square, or a sheet of plastic food wrap can be placed over the vagina for oral sex. These barriers can also be used for protection during oral-anal contact.

Avoiding sexually transmitted diseases

Teenagers are at high risk for infection with STDs. By the twelfth grade, 65 percent of high school students have had sexual intercourse, and one in five has had four or more sexual partners. Teens account for a high proportion of the estimated 19 million new STD infections in the United States each year. For example, 40 percent of new chlamydia cases occur among young people ages 15 to 19. Girls in this age group have the highest rates of gonorrhea of any other group. Many STDs, such as chlamydia, can cause serious health problems if they are not detected and treated. And having some STDs, such as chlamydia and gonorrhea, make people more likely to become infected with HIV if they are exposed to the virus. (For more detailed discussions of specific STDs, see pages 166 to 178.)

Make sure your teenager knows these facts about STDs:

- Sexually transmitted diseases affect more than 19 million Americans each year, many of whom are teenagers or young adults.

- Using drugs and alcohol increases the chances of getting STDs because they interfere with judgment and the ability to use a condom properly.

- The more partners you have, the higher your risk of being exposed to HIV or other STDs.

- You cannot tell by looking at someone if he or she is infected with HIV or another STD.

- You can never know (unless someone tells you) whether a person has had sex with someone who is infected with an STD or who is an intravenous drug user. (IV drug users are at increased risk for HIV and hepatitis B.)

- Your risk for STDs increases dramatically if you have sex with strangers or in unfamiliar or public places.

- Most STDs do not cause symptoms in the early stage, so infections can be spread without either partner knowing it.

The latex male condom provides the best protection against STDs, including HIV. Many adolescents are embarrassed to talk about condoms, especially with their parents, but they need the information to be able to protect their health and their future. If you are embarrassed to discuss the topic with your child, give him or her a book (this book, perhaps), direct him or her to a reliable Web site (such as www.plannedparenthood.org), or arrange for your child to talk to his or her doctor. Even before your child becomes sexually active, make sure he or she knows how to use a condom; you might buy one and show him or her how to use it. (See page 177 for a complete explanation of how to use a condom.) To provide adequate protection against most STDs, it is very important to use a condom correctly every time a person has sex. Incorrect use is the major reason that condoms fail.

Teach your daughter that if a boy refuses to use a condom she should refuse to have sex with him. No discussion. If the boy insists, threatens her, or says he'd rather break up than wear a condom, she needs to end the relationship right then. She does not need to have a relationship with a person who does not respect her or himself enough to use protection against STDs.

Health issues for gay and lesbian teens

The same diseases that can be transmitted during heterosexual sexual activities can also be spread during gay or lesbian sex. If your child is gay or lesbian, make sure he or she knows the risks and how to protect himself or herself. Many lesbian girls also have male sex partners or have had male sex partners in the past, and many homosexual boys have or have had female partners. Teach your adolescent to protect against STDs by taking the following measures:

- Always use latex condoms to protect against STDs; sexually transmitted diseases can be spread during vaginal, oral, or anal sex.
- Lesbians and bisexual girls should always protect themselves from STDs and pregnancy by using latex condoms or dental dams.
- Don't use alcohol or other drugs before or during sex; these substances can impair your judgment.
- Don't have sex with strangers.
- Never have sex in unfamiliar or public places.
- Get regular health exams. Don't be afraid or embarrassed to ask your doctor about any health concerns you have.

Make sure all of your immunizations are up to date. Ask for the hepatitis B vaccination, given in three doses. Hepatitis B is a bloodborne virus that can be transmitted through sexual contact or sharing intravenous needles.

23

WOMEN'S REPRODUCTIVE HEALTH AND WELLNESS

THIS CHAPTER PROVIDES a full discussion of the importance of prenatal care to help you avoid potential complications of pregnancy and some common birth defects, and help ensure that your baby is born healthy. If you are planning a pregnancy, take measures before you get pregnant by adopting healthy lifestyle habits such as eating a nutritious diet and quitting smoking if you smoke.

A healthy pregnancy

You should start taking care of yourself long before you start trying to get pregnant. At least three months before starting to try to conceive, make an appointment for a prepregnancy checkup. Your doctor can help you build a strong foundation for a healthy pregnancy. If you have a family history of genetic disorders or birth defects, or if you're adopted and don't know your family history, your doctor can refer you to a genetic counselor (see page 212), who can help you evaluate your chances of having a child with an abnormality.

Get your body ready for pregnancy by establishing healthy habits and stopping any unhealthy habits that could harm your pregnancy or your baby. Here are some ways to take care of yourself even before you get pregnant:

- Eat a healthy diet (see chapter 1), including plenty of vegetables, fruits, whole grains, and lean sources of protein. Stay away from junk food and foods that are high in saturated and trans fats or that have excessive amounts of sugar and salt.

- Exercise regularly (see chapter 2)—at least 30 minutes a day most days of the week. Aim for an hour a day, every day, if you can.

- Get sufficient rest and sleep.

- Consume 400 micrograms (mcg) of folic acid (one of the B vitamins) every day to help prevent birth defects such as spina bifida. Many breakfast cereals and breads are now enriched with folic acid; check food labels. The best way to get enough folic acid is to take a daily multivitamin or a prenatal vitamin that contains 400 micrograms of folic acid.

- Make sure you have had all your shots, especially for rubella (German measles), which can cause serious birth defects. Chickenpox can also be dangerous during pregnancy. If you have had chickenpox and rubella in the past, you should be immune to them. If not, talk to your doctor about having blood tests to check your immunity. If you need to be vaccinated, then you must wait three months before you start trying to get pregnant.

- Tell your doctor about any prescription or over-the-counter medications (including herbal remedies) you are taking. Some medications and supplements are not safe to take during pregnancy.

- Stop smoking if you smoke. Quitting now, before you become pregnant, can give you time to completely withdraw from the nicotine. Smoking during pregnancy can cause premature birth, low birth weight, and an increased risk for frequent respiratory problems and attention deficit disorder in children.

- Stop drinking alcohol. There's no safe amount of alcohol during pregnancy. Drinking during pregnancy can cause fetal alcohol syndrome (see page 494), the most common preventable cause of mental retardation in children.

- Do not take illegal drugs. Taking illegal drugs during pregnancy can cause miscarriage, low birth weight, and premature birth, and can be fatal for both the pregnant woman and her fetus.

Regular prenatal care

Prenatal care refers to the regular medical checkups that a woman has throughout the nine months of pregnancy. With proper prenatal care, you can reduce your baby's risk for potentially serious health problems. It's important to start getting prenatal care early in your pregnancy. If you know you are pregnant, or think you might be, call your doctor to schedule a visit. Your doctor will schedule many appointments over the course of the pregnancy. Don't miss any, because they are all important. And follow your doctor's advice. As your pregnancy progresses, you will see the doctor according to the following schedule:

- A first visit during your second or third month of pregnancy (eight to twelve weeks)
- About once a month for the first six months of pregnancy
- Every two weeks during the seventh and eighth months of pregnancy
- Every week in the last month, until the baby is born

If you are over 35 or your pregnancy is considered high risk because of a chronic health problem (such as diabetes or high blood pressure), you will probably need to see the doctor more often.

SCREENING TESTS

Screening tests evaluate the risk of having a baby with certain birth defects. Birth defects are caused by mutations, or changes, in a baby's genes, which can be inherited or can occur randomly for the first time in a baby with no family history of a disorder. Genetic mutations can also occur when a pregnant woman is exposed to a toxin in the environment, such as radiation. Women over age 35 have a higher risk than younger women of having a baby with a birth defect.

The benefit of screening tests during pregnancy is that they don't pose any risk to a pregnant woman or her fetus. But screening tests can't tell for sure if a fetus has or does not have a birth defect. Instead, they give the odds of a woman's having a baby with a birth defect based on her age. Women under age 35 can find out if their risk is as high as that of a 35-year-old woman. For women over age 35, screening tests can show whether the risk for their age is higher or lower than average. Common screening tests used during pregnancy include ultrasound, maternal serum marker screening test, and nuchal translucency screening.

Ultrasound screening

Ultrasound uses sound waves to show a picture of the fetus on a computer screen. The best time to have the ultrasound screening test is between the 18th and 20th weeks of pregnancy, when most abnormalities can be detected.

Using ultrasound, a doctor can determine if a fetus has a neural tube defect (abnormal development of the brain and spinal cord). Neural tube defects, such as spina bifida (an opening in the spinal column), are common birth defects that can cause infant death or severe disability. However, ultrasound is not the most accurate test for determining if a fetus has Down's syndrome. Only one in three babies with Down's syndrome has an abnormal second trimester ultrasound. Ultrasound can miss some other problems too, such as clubbed feet and heart defects. One

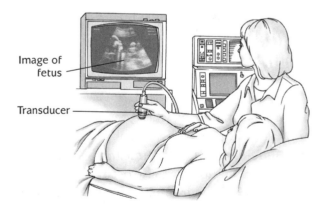

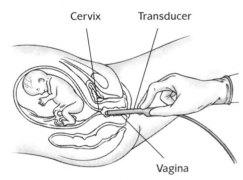

Abdominal ultrasound

During a prenatal abdominal ultrasound, the doctor or a technician passes a handheld device called a transducer across the pregnant woman's abdomen to view the fetus. The woman might feel some pressure as the doctor moves the transducer over her abdomen, but will probably not feel any pain.

Vaginal ultrasound

To perform a vaginal ultrasound, the doctor inserts a thin transducer into the vagina to produce images on a computer monitor. Doctors use vaginal ultrasounds during the first trimester of pregnancy to confirm or rule out a pregnancy, or to look for any abnormalities in the fetus.

advantage of ultrasound is that your doctor will probably be able to determine the sex of your baby using the technique—and will tell you, if you want to know it.

Maternal serum marker screening test

Doctors refer to the maternal serum marker screening test by many different names, including multiple marker screening test, triple test, and quad screen. This test is usually given between the 15th and 20th weeks of pregnancy. It helps doctors detect some genetic disorders called chromosome abnormalities (such as Down's syndrome) or open neural tube defects (such as spina bifida, in which the spinal cord has not closed). The doctor takes a sample of blood from the woman and has it tested for three chemicals: alpha-fetoprotein (AFP, a protein made by the liver of the fetus) and two pregnancy hormones, estriol and human chorionic gonadotropin (hCG). Sometimes doctors test for a fourth substance in the blood called inhibin-A. Testing for inhibin-A may improve a doctor's ability to determine if a fetus has a high risk for Down's syndrome. High levels of AFP may signal the presence of an open neural tube defect. Estriol levels show the general health of the fetus. Abnormal levels of hCG can indicate a defect caused by a chromosome abnormality such as Down's syndrome.

Nuchal translucency screening

The nuchal translucency screening (NTS) test can be performed between the 11th and 14th weeks of pregnancy. It uses an ultrasound exam and a blood test to calculate the risk for certain birth defects. The doctor uses the ultrasound to evaluate the thickness of the back of the fetus's neck. The blood test detects levels of a protein called pregnancy-associated plasma protein and a hormone called human chorionic gonadotropin (hCG). Doctors use this information to determine if the fetus has a normal or greater-than-normal chance of having some birth defects.

As with all screening tests, the results can sometimes be misleading. In 5 percent of women who have NTS, results show that their fetus has a high risk of having a birth defect when in reality it does not. This is called a false positive. To find out for sure if the fetus has a birth defect, NTS must be followed by a more precise diagnostic test such as chorionic villus sampling (CVS) or amniocentesis. NTS is not yet widely used, so a woman should talk to her doctor if she is interested in having the test. She should also call her health-care plan to see if it covers the procedure.

If you are over 35

More and more women are waiting to have children until their 30s or even 40s. While many women this age have no problems getting pregnant, fertility does decline with age. Women over 40 who don't get pregnant after six months of trying should see their doctor for a fertility evaluation.

As you age, your chances of having a baby with a birth defect also rise, although most women in their late 30s and early 40s have healthy babies. See your doctor regularly before you start trying to get pregnant. He or she will tell you about how age can affect pregnancy. Women over age 35 have an increased risk for the following:

- Fertility problems
- High blood pressure
- Diabetes
- Miscarriage
- Placenta previa (a condition in which the placenta is in the wrong place and covers the cervix)
- Cesarean delivery
- Premature labor and delivery
- Stillbirth
- A baby with a genetic disorder such as Down's syndrome

Because of these increased risks for women over 35, prenatal care is especially important for them. The doctor will probably recommend some additional tests to evaluate the health of the fetus.

√ Getting help with prenatal care

Every state in the United States has a program to provide medical care, support, and advice to pregnant women to help them have a healthy pregnancy and a healthy baby. These programs also offer information about health insurance and other services that a pregnant woman needs. To find out about prenatal services in your community, call 1-800-311-BABY (1-800-311-2229). For Spanish, call 1-800-504-7081. These toll-free telephone numbers will connect you to the health department in your area code. Or contact your state or local health department directly.

Healthy eating for a healthy pregnancy

While you are pregnant, you will need additional nutrients to keep you and your baby healthy. But this does not mean you need to eat twice as much. You should eat only about an extra 300 calories per day. Considering that 1 cup of cooked pasta has nearly 200 calories and an 8-ounce glass of fat-free milk has 80 calories, getting those extra 300 calories does not take a lot of food.

Don't restrict your diet during pregnancy, because your fetus might not get enough of the essential nutrients such as protein, vitamins, and minerals. Low-calorie diets can break down a pregnant woman's stored fat, leading to the production of substances called ketones. Ketones can be found in a pregnant woman's blood and urine and are a sign of starvation. The constant production of ketones can cause mental retardation in the fetus.

If you have been eating a healthy diet before you become pregnant, you may need to make only a few changes to meet the special nutritional needs of pregnancy. A pregnant woman needs a total of 2,500 to 2,700 calories every day. These calories should come from a variety of healthy foods. But what pregnant women eat is more important than how much. When you're pregnant, you need more of many important vitamins, minerals, and other nutrients than you did before pregnancy. To help ensure that you are getting enough nutrients, you should take a multivitamin or prenatal vitamin and eat a wide variety of healthy foods every day.

FRUITS AND VEGETABLES

Pregnant women should try to eat 7 or more servings of fruits and vegetables combined (3 servings of fruit and 4 servings of vegetables, for example) daily. Fruits and vegetables are rich sources of fiber, vitamins, and minerals. One serving of fruit equals one medium apple, one medium banana, ½ cup of chopped fruit, or ¾ cup of fruit juice. A serving of vegetables equals 1 cup of raw leafy vegetables, ½ cup of other vegetables (raw or cooked), or ¾ cup of vegetable juice.

WHOLE GRAINS

Pregnant women should eat 6 to 9 servings of whole-grain or enriched breads and cereals every day. Whole-grain products and enriched products such as bread, rice, pasta, and breakfast cereals contain iron, B vitamins, minerals, and fiber. Some breakfast cereals are enriched with 100 percent of the folic acid (see page 487) your body needs every day. (Folic acid has been shown to help prevent some serious birth defects such as spina bifida.) One serving of grains equals 1 slice of bread; ½ cup of cooked cereal, rice, or pasta; or 1 cup of dry breakfast cereal.

DAIRY PRODUCTS

Pregnant women should try to eat 4 or more servings of low-fat or nonfat milk, yogurt, cheese, or other dairy products each day. Dairy products provide the calcium they and their fetus need for strong bones and teeth. Dairy products are also good sources of vitamin A and D, protein, and B vitamins. One serving of a dairy product equals 1 cup of milk or yogurt, 1½ ounces of natural cheese, or 2 ounces of processed cheese. If you are lactose intolerant, you can get sufficient calcium by consuming lactose-free or reduced-lactose products. In some cases, doctors recommend that pregnant women take calcium supplements.

PROTEIN

Pregnant women should eat 60 grams of protein every day—10 more grams than normal. Protein builds muscle, tissue, enzymes, hormones, and antibodies that you and your fetus need to be healthy. Protein-rich foods also have B vitamins and iron, which are important for healthy blood. Two or more 2- to 3-ounce servings of cooked lean meat, fish, or poultry without skin, or 2 or more 1-ounce servings of cooked meat contain about 60 grams of protein. Eggs, nuts, and dried beans and peas also are good sources of protein. Most women in the United States regularly eat more protein than they need. So you probably won't have to make an extra effort to get 60 grams of protein a day.

One serving of protein equals 2 to 3 ounces of cooked lean meat, poultry, or fish; 1 cup of cooked dried beans or peas; 2 eggs; 1 cup of tofu; ⅔ cup of nuts; or 4 tablespoons of peanut butter.

ESSENTIAL NUTRIENTS FOR A HEALTHY PREGNANCY

Even women who plan carefully to eat healthy every day sometimes fail to get important nutrients. That's why most doctors recommend that pregnant women or women who are trying to get pregnant take a multivitamin or prenatal vitamin every day. Taking a daily multivitamin or prenatal vitamin will guarantee you a daily dose of needed nutrients, such as folic acid. But don't overdo it. Taking more than one multivitamin daily can be harmful. Here is a list of the most important nutrients for a healthy pregnancy:

HOW TO PREVENT MORNING SICKNESS

Morning sickness and nausea are common during pregnancy. Most nausea occurs during the early part of pregnancy and usually improves during the second trimester. For some women, however, morning sickness and nausea last longer, sometimes for the entire pregnancy.

The changes in your body can cause nausea and vomiting when you smell certain things, when you eat certain foods, when you're tired, when you're stressed, or even for no obvious reason. You may be able to reduce nausea by changing when and what you eat. Try these tips:

- Eat smaller meals, such as six to eight small meals instead of three larger ones each day.
- Don't go for long periods without eating.
- Drink fluids between, but not with, meals.
- Avoid foods that are greasy, fried, or highly spiced.
- Avoid strong and unpleasant odors.
- Rest when you're tired.

Severe nausea and vomiting in pregnancy are rare, but constant vomiting can cause excess water loss and lead to dehydration. If you think that your nausea or vomiting is keeping you from eating properly or from gaining enough weight, talk to your doctor.

- **Folic acid**   Pregnant women need 400 micrograms (mcg) of folic acid every day to help prevent birth defects such as spina bifida, cleft lip, and congenital heart disease. Folic acid is important for women to get even before they become pregnant. These birth defects often occur before most women know they are pregnant. So even before you start trying to get pregnant, make sure you are getting enough folic acid. Women who are already pregnant need to get enough folic acid every day.

    An easy way to get your daily dose of folic acid is to take a multivitamin containing it. Another way is to eat a serving of breakfast cereal that contains 100 percent of the daily value for folic acid, but you have to do this every day. Check the nutrition label on the cereal box to be sure. It should say "100 percent" next to folic acid. Orange juice, spinach, and legumes are also good sources of folic acid.

- **Iron** Pregnant women need twice as much iron (30 milligrams per day) as other women because of the greater volume of blood in their body. In addition, the fetus needs to store iron in his or her body to last through the first few months of life. Too little iron can cause a condition called anemia. If you have anemia, you might look pale and feel very tired. Doctors check for signs of anemia with routine blood tests taken at different stages of pregnancy. If a blood test shows that you have anemia, your doctor will probably recommend iron supplements. You should also eat lots of iron-rich foods such as lean red meat, fish, poultry, dried fruits, whole-grain breads, and iron-fortified cereals. And make sure to take your prenatal vitamin every day.

- **Calcium** Pregnant women between ages 19 and 50 should get 1,000 milligrams of calcium a day. Younger pregnant women need even more—1,300 milligrams a day. Most women in the United States don't get enough calcium. Low-fat or fat-free milk, yogurt, cheese, and other dairy products are good sources of calcium. Eating green leafy vegeta-

---

EATING FISH DURING PREGNANCY

Fish and shellfish can be part of a healthy diet during pregnancy. They're a great source of protein and heart-healthy omega-3 fatty acids. But almost all fish and shellfish contain some mercury, a heavy metal that can have extremely harmful effects on the brain of a developing fetus. Mercury occurs naturally in the environment. It can also be released into the air through industrial pollution and fall into surface water, accumulating in streams and oceans. Fish absorb mercury from the water as they feed.

Mercury gets into your body mainly from the fish you eat. The amount of mercury you might ingest from fish and shellfish depends on the amount and type of fish you eat. Use the following guidelines to get the healthy protein and omega-3 fatty acids in fish while avoiding high mercury levels:

- Never eat shark, swordfish, king mackerel, or tilefish (also called golden or white snapper) because these fish have the highest levels of mercury.

- Never eat raw, uncooked fish or shellfish—such as sushi or oysters—while you are pregnant. They could contain harmful bacteria that could make you very sick.

- Don't eat more than 2 servings (12 ounces total) of fish each week.

- Don't eat more than 1 serving (6 ounces) of white (or albacore) tuna, tuna steak, halibut, or snapper a week.

- Choose shrimp, salmon, pollock, catfish, or chunk light tuna because they contain the least amount of mercury.

- In general, the smaller and younger the fish, the less mercury it has absorbed.

bles and calcium-fortified foods such as orange juice and breakfast cereal can also provide calcium. If your diet is not providing 1,000 milligrams of calcium a day, talk to your doctor about taking a calcium supplement.

- **Water**   Pregnant women should drink at least six 8-ounce glasses of water each day, plus another glass of water for each hour of activity. Water plays a key role in a woman's diet during pregnancy: it carries the nutrients from the food she eats to her fetus. It also helps prevent constipation, hemorrhoids, excessive swelling, and urinary tract or bladder infections. Drinking enough water, especially during the last trimester, prevents dehydration. Getting too little water can lead to premature or early labor. Fruit juices also contain water, but they have a lot of calories that can promote extra weight gain. Caffeine-containing beverages such as coffee, soft drinks, and teas promote water loss from the body, so you can't count them toward the total amount of water you need every day.

How much weight should you gain during pregnancy?

Most doctors recommend an average weight gain of 25 to 30 pounds during pregnancy. But the amount of weight you should gain depends on your weight before you became pregnant and your height. Here is a rough guide for assessing weight gain during pregnancy, but check with your doctor to find out how much weight gain is healthy for you:

- If you were underweight before becoming pregnant, you should gain between 28 and 40 pounds.
- If you were overweight before becoming pregnant, you should gain between 15 and 25 pounds.

You should gain weight gradually during your pregnancy, with most of the weight gain during the last trimester. Doctors recommend that women gain weight at the following rate:

- 2 to 5 pounds during the first three-month period (the first trimester)
- 3 to 4 pounds each month for the next six months (the second and third trimesters)

Women who gain more than the recommended amount of weight during pregnancy and who don't lose the extra weight within six months after giving birth are at much higher risk of being obese 10 years later. Your total weight gain during pregnancy includes the weight of the baby, fluid, larger breasts, a larger uterus, and the placenta (the tissue that nourishes the fetus). Make sure that you visit your doctor throughout your pregnancy so he or she can check on your weight gain. If you gain too much weight during pregnancy, it can be hard to lose the excess weight after you have your baby. During pregnancy, fat deposits can increase by more than 33 percent. Most women who gain the recommended amount of weight lose the extra weight in the birth process and in the weeks and months after delivery. Breast-feeding also can help you lose extra weight by burning extra calories—at least 500 calories a day.

Exercise and pregnancy

When you are pregnant, exercise is one of the best things you can do for your physical and emotional health and the health of your pregnancy. Doctors recommend that pregnant women without health problems or pregnancy complications exercise moderately for 30 minutes or more on most—or, even better, all—days of the week. Here are some good reasons to get regular exercise during your pregnancy:

- Exercise can help ease and prevent the aches and pains of pregnancy including varicose veins, backaches, and exhaustion. It also helps reverse constipation.
- Active women seem to be better prepared for labor and delivery and to recover more quickly.
- Exercise may lower the risk for high blood pressure and diabetes during pregnancy.
- Fit women have an easier time getting back to a healthy weight after delivery.
- Regular exercise may improve sleep during pregnancy.
- Staying active can improve a woman's emotional health. Pregnant women who exercise seem to have better self-esteem and a lower risk for depression and anxiety.

Women with the following problems may not be able to exercise during pregnancy: heart disease, lung disease, obesity, severe diabetes, thyroid disease, or seizure disorder. Also, pregnant women may need to avoid

DO YOUR KEGELS

Some exercises that strengthen the muscles in the pelvis can help prepare a woman's body for delivery. The pelvic-floor muscles support the rectum, vagina, and urethra in the pelvis. Pelvic-floor exercises, also called Kegel exercises (see page 498), strengthen these muscles and can help make delivery easier. Doing these exercises regularly can also prevent urine leaking during pregnancy and, later in life, can help women avoid urinary incontinence.

exercise if they have persistent bleeding in the second or third trimester, complications with past pregnancies, premature labor, or pregnancy-related high blood pressure.

Low-impact exercise that produces moderate exertion is the best type of physical activity while you're pregnant. Many different types of exercise can be safe for most pregnant women, including walking, swimming, dancing, and biking. Follow these precautions when developing your pregnancy exercise plan:

- Avoid activities in which you could get hit in the abdomen, such as kickboxing, soccer, basketball, or ice hockey.

- Avoid activities that could cause you to fall, including horseback riding, downhill skiing, and gymnastics.

- Do not scuba dive during pregnancy. Scuba diving can create gas bubbles in the fetus's blood that could cause serious health problems.

Here are some tips for having safe and healthy workouts:

- When you exercise, start slowly, progress gradually, and cool down slowly.

- You should be able to carry on a conversation while exercising. If you can't, you may be exercising too intensely.

- Take frequent breaks.

- Do not exercise on your back after the first trimester. It can put excessive pressure on an important vein and limit blood flow to the fetus.

- Avoid jerky, bouncing, and high-impact movements. Connective tissues stretch much more easily during pregnancy, so these types of movements put you at risk for joint injury.

- Do not exercise at high altitudes (more than 6,000 feet above sea level). It can prevent the fetus from getting enough oxygen.

- Make sure you drink fluids before, during, and after exercising.

- Don't work out in extreme heat or humidity.
- If you feel uncomfortable, short of breath, or tired, take a break, and take it easier when you resume exercising. Your body will tell you when you're overdoing it.

How to prevent some common health problems during pregnancy

There's no denying it: pregnancy can be uncomfortable. But you can prevent or minimize your discomfort by following the advice below:

- **Nausea** In the morning, sit on the edge of the bed for a few minutes before standing up. Nibble on crackers or dry toast whenever you feel nauseous. Try to keep something in your stomach throughout the day. Drink plenty of fluids to prevent dehydration. If you can't keep anything down, chew crushed ice.
- **Heartburn** Don't eat too much at once, and avoid spicy, greasy, or acidic foods. Eat small, frequent meals; take small bites; and chew your food thoroughly. Avoid bending over. Sleep with your head at a 30-degree angle. Don't smoke; it promotes stomach-acid production.
- **Leg cramps** Be sure to get 1,500 milligrams of calcium every day. Stretch and massage your calf muscles before going to bed and when you wake up in the morning.
- **Swollen ankles and hands** Reduce your intake of sodium (salt). Elevate your legs while resting. Try not to stand for long periods.
- **Tooth and gum problems** Brush and floss your teeth at least twice a day. See your dentist regularly for checkups.
- **Anemia** Eat foods that are rich in iron, such as beef, fortified whole grains, eggs, and dried fruit. Consume fruits and vegetables containing vitamin C, which helps the body absorb iron. Take your prenatal vitamins as directed by your doctor.
- **Constipation** Eat plenty of high-fiber foods, including beans, fruits, vegetables, and whole grains. Exercise regularly.
- **Varicose veins** Don't wear clothes that fit tightly around your waist or upper legs. Avoid standing for long periods, but take a walk every

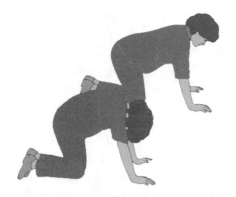

Preventing back pain

Get on your hands and knees and position your head in line with your spine without allowing your spine to sag. Curve your back up, tightening the muscles in your abdomen and buttocks and lowering your head. Gradually raise your head and lower your back to its original position. Repeat several times.

day. Rest with your feet up. Don't gain more weight than your doctor recommends.

- **Sleep problems**   Avoid napping after 3 p.m. Take a warm bath and drink a glass of milk before bedtime (the milk will also boost your calcium intake). Cut back on or eliminate caffeine-containing drinks, or avoid having any after noon. Get plenty of exercise during the day, but not too close to bedtime.

- **Back pain**   Try not to gain too much weight. Wear low-heeled shoes. Don't slouch when sitting, and use a small cushion to support your back. Sleep on a firm mattress and put a pillow under your knees to relieve pressure on your lower back.

What to avoid during pregnancy

A wide variety of substances can harm a growing fetus during pregnancy. If you have any questions about what to avoid during pregnancy, ask your doctor at your next prenatal visit.

ALCOHOL

There is no safe amount of alcohol for a woman to drink during pregnancy. That's why doctors recommend that women not drink any alcohol at all during pregnancy. Heavy drinking can cause a serious birth defect called fetal alcohol syndrome (see the box on the next page). But even small amounts of alcohol during pregnancy can affect a child's learning and memory—even as late as adolescence.

Women who are sexually active and don't use effective birth control should also refrain from drinking because they could become pregnant and not know for several weeks. When you drink alcohol, the alcohol that gets absorbed by your blood gets into your fetus's body through the umbilical cord. A pregnant woman's alcohol intake can slow the fetus's growth, damage his or her brain, and cause serious birth defects. In severe cases, excessive drinking during pregnancy can result in death of the fetus.

Not all pregnant women who drink alcohol have babies with fetal alcohol syndrome. But the only sure way to prevent problems is to not drink any

FETAL ALCOHOL SYNDROME

Fetal alcohol syndrome is a term that describes a range of abnormalities that can occur in a child whose mother drank alcohol during pregnancy. It is the most common preventable cause of mental retardation in American children. The effects of fetal alcohol syndrome are permanent and cannot be cured—but the condition is 100 percent preventable by not drinking alcohol during pregnancy.

Prenatal exposure to alcohol can cause severe brain damage in the fetus. A fetus's brain can be harmed at any time during pregnancy, because the brain develops throughout pregnancy. Children with fetal alcohol syndrome may have a smaller-than-normal brain and often have trouble with learning, attention, memory, and problem solving. They may have poor coordination, be impulsive, and have speech and hearing problems. Children with fetal alcohol syndrome can also have physical defects, including the following:

- Abnormal facial features, including a thin upper lip, a short nose, short eye openings, and flat cheeks
- Growth problems; they are often small and short for their age
- Heart defects
- Cleft palate
- Dislocation of the hip

alcohol during pregnancy. If you are pregnant and have been drinking, stop now. If you need help to stop (see page 151), talk with your doctor. He or she can refer you to a program that can help you safely stop drinking.

SMOKING

Smoking during pregnancy can have harmful effects on a developing fetus. Smokers take in substances—such as nicotine, carbon monoxide, and cancer-causing chemicals—that can enter the placenta (the tissue that nourishes the fetus) and reduce the amount of nutrients and oxygen to the fetus. Smoking during pregnancy can have long-term harmful effects on children as well. If you smoke, ask your doctor about a smoking-cessation program (see page 135) that would be safe and effective for you. Compared with nonsmokers, women who smoke during pregnancy are at greater risk for the following problems:

- Miscarriage or ectopic pregnancy (a pregnancy that develops in a fallopian tube, which is life-threatening)
- Serious pregnancy complications involving the placenta
- Baby with a low birth weight
- Preterm delivery

- Having a child with birth defects such as clubfoot, cleft lip, or cleft palate
- Having a child die of sudden infant death syndrome (SIDS)
- Having a child with attention deficit disorder or learning disabilities
- Having a child with more colds and other, potentially serious, lung problems such as asthma

The best time to quit smoking is as soon as you start planning a pregnancy or think you could get pregnant in the near future. If you quit, your baby will probably weigh the same as the baby of a woman who has never smoked. If you quit during the first three or four months of pregnancy, you can increase your baby's chance of being born at a normal weight and without health problems. After birth, breastfeeding is the best way to feed a baby. However, smoking while breastfeeding can cause problems in a nursing child. Nicotine and other harmful chemicals can be passed to a child in breast milk—another reason to quit if you have not done so yet.

CAFFEINE

Caffeine is a stimulant found in colas, coffee, tea, chocolate, cocoa, and some over-the-counter painkillers and prescription drugs. Consuming large quantities of caffeine during pregnancy can cause irritability, nervousness, and insomnia as well as babies with a low birth weight. Also, caffeine is a diuretic, which promotes water loss from the body. Most experts agree that small amounts of caffeine (equal to one to two 8-ounce cups of coffee a day) are safe during pregnancy. The safety of consuming larger amounts of caffeine is controversial. Until conclusive evidence is available, pregnant women should limit their caffeine intake. Talk to your doctor about your caffeine intake during pregnancy and follow his or her recommendation.

MEDICATIONS

While you are pregnant, do not take any type of medication without talking to your doctor first. Even over-the-counter medications—such as antihistamines or pain medications that contain aspirin or ibuprofen—can be harmful to a developing fetus. It's especially important not to use aspirin during the last three months of pregnancy, because it could cause problems in the fetus or cause excessive bleeding during delivery. Be careful with vitamins, too. Take the prenatal vitamins prescribed or recommended by your doctor, but don't take any additional supplements on your own. Although pregnant women need more of some nutrients, such as iron, calcium, and folic acid, too much of other nutrients can harm a fetus.

ILLEGAL DRUGS

Illegal drugs can severely damage a fetus. Yet, according to a national survey, more than 5 percent of all U.S. women who give birth used illegal drugs while they were pregnant. The survey also uncovered a strong link between cigarette smoking and the use of both alcohol and illicit drugs, primarily marijuana and cocaine. Some babies born to women who used marijuana during their pregnancy have an unusual quavering of their voice and a high-pitched cry, which experts think may indicate problems with brain and nervous-system development. During the preschool years, children who were exposed to marijuana during pregnancy seem to perform tasks needing sustained attention and memory more poorly than other children. In school, these children are more likely to have deficits in problem-solving skills, memory, and the ability to stay attentive.

Babies born to mothers who abused cocaine during pregnancy are often premature, have a low birth weight and smaller head circumference, and are often shorter in length. Exposure to cocaine during fetal development may also lead to later problems in some children, including deficiencies in some aspects of intellectual ability such as information processing and attention to tasks—abilities that are important for success in school.

FOODS TO AVOID

Some foods that might cause only a brief illness or not affect you at all during your pregnancy can severely harm a developing fetus. Avoid eating the following foods during pregnancy:

- **Raw meat**   Microorganisms such as salmonella can contaminate raw meats such as steak tartare or a rare hamburger.
- **Raw fish**   Many ocean and freshwater fish are contaminated with microorganisms and chemical pollutants.
- **Unwashed fruits and vegetables**   Residual amounts of pesticides can be present on the surfaces of fruits and vegetables. Also, other people have handled the produce and may not have washed their hands after using the toilet, spreading germs to the produce. Always wash fresh produce well under running tap water before eating.

- **Unpasteurized soft cheeses**   Soft cheeses such as Brie and Camembert can contain harmful bacteria.

OTHER THINGS TO AVOID DURING PREGNANCY

It may seem as if there is no end to the list of things you can't do during pregnancy, but taking precautions while you are pregnant is the best way to help ensure that you have a healthy pregnancy and a healthy baby. Here are a few more things you should avoid during your pregnancy:

- **Hot tubs and saunas**   The high temperatures of the water in hot tubs and saunas could be unsafe for a developing fetus.

- **X-rays**   Diagnostic X-rays can give your doctor valuable information about your health, but X-rays pose small risks. For this reason, X-rays are generally not performed on pregnant women unless they are absolutely necessary. Make sure you tell any doctor who orders a diagnostic X-ray if you are, or think you might be, pregnant. If you are pregnant, the doctor may choose to cancel the X-ray, postpone it, or change it to lower the amount of radiation you'll be exposed to.

- **Cat litter boxes**   If you have a cat, ask your doctor about toxoplasmosis, an infection caused by a parasite sometimes found in cat feces. When left untreated, toxoplasmosis can cause birth defects. Your doctor may suggest that, while you are pregnant, you avoid handling cat litter and working in garden areas used by cats.

- **Chemicals**   Stay away from chemicals such as insecticides, solvents (including some cleaners and paint thinners), lead, and mercury. Not all potentially harmful products have pregnancy warnings on their label. If you are unsure if a product is safe, ask your doctor about it before using it.

Pelvic support problems

The pelvic organs—the uterus, bladder, urethra, rectum, and vagina—are held in place by strong muscles, ligaments, and connective tissues. These supporting tissues are attached to the sides of the pelvis, the pelvic organs, and the openings of the urethra, vagina, and anus. If the supporting tissues become stretched, they can slacken, causing the organs they normally support to slip out of position or bulge into the vagina. Occasionally an organ such as the uterus or bladder drops down so much that it protrudes out of the vagina. These pelvic support problems can cause urinary incontinence or difficulty urinating or having complete bowel movements.

Vaginal childbirth and loss of muscle tone that can accompany aging are the major causes of pelvic support problems. Vaginal deliveries can stretch the supporting tissues and may weaken them. But pelvic support problems also occur in women who have not had vaginal deliveries. Declining levels of the female hormone estrogen at menopause may cause these tissues to become thinner and weaker. Other possible contributors to pelvic sup-

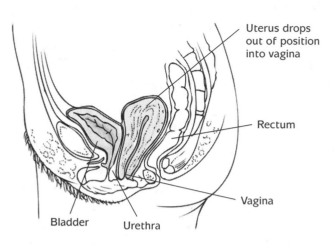

Uterus drops out of position into vagina

Rectum

Vagina

Bladder   Urethra

Prolapse of the uterus

Uterine prolapse occurs when the uterus sags from its normal position into the vagina. A prolapsed uterus may develop as a result of pregnancy, vaginal childbirth, or aging.

KEGEL EXERCISES

Kegel exercises are pelvic-floor exercises that can help reduce the risk for urinary incontinence (see page 365) and pelvic support problems such as prolapse of the uterus. Strengthening these muscles by doing Kegel exercises may help you avoid these problems.

First, you need to identify the muscles you need to exercise. The pelvic-floor muscles are the muscles you would use to stop the flow of urine. You can be sure you're exercising the right muscles if, when you squeeze them during urination, you stop urinating. You can do Kegel exercises standing, sitting, or lying down. Here's how:

- Tighten the pelvic-floor muscles for 5 to 10 seconds, then relax them for 5 seconds.
- Repeat 10 to 20 times.
- Do a set of 10 to 20 contractions at least 3 to 5 times a day (for a total of at least 50 contractions daily).

port problems include being overweight, having a chronic cough or chronic constipation, or repeated heavy lifting—all of which put extra strain on the supporting tissues.

PREVENTION

The most effective way to prevent pelvic support problems is to perform exercises that strengthen the supporting muscles in the pelvis. Doing these pelvic-floor exercises, or Kegel exercises as they're usually called, every day can significantly strengthen these muscles. The key, of course, is to do them every day. (For instructions on how to do Kegels, see the box on the previous page.) In addition to Kegels, here are some other ways to help you avoid putting extra stress on your pelvic organs and supporting tissues:

- Control your weight.
- Maintain a healthy lifestyle, including not smoking, which can cause a chronic cough.
- Avoid heavy lifting and lifting with your legs.
- Avoid becoming constipated by eating high-fiber foods (see page 4).

24

MEN'S REPRODUCTIVE HEALTH AND WELLNESS

THIS CHAPTER DESCRIBES PREVENTION strategies for the most common disorders of the male reproductive system, with the exception of cancers of the male reproductive system, which are covered in chapter 9 (starting on page 290). Most male reproductive health problems occur in the prostate gland or penis.

Male reproductive system

Unlike females, whose sex organs are located inside the body, males have reproductive organs that are both inside and outside the body. The most visible parts of the male reproductive system are the penis and the scrotum, which contains the testicles. The two testicles produce sperm and the primary male sex hormone testosterone. From the testicles, sperm pass through a duct called the vas deferens into a pair of sacs called the seminal vesicles. The seminal vesicles produce a fluid that is added to the sperm to form semen, the fluid that is ejaculated during orgasm.

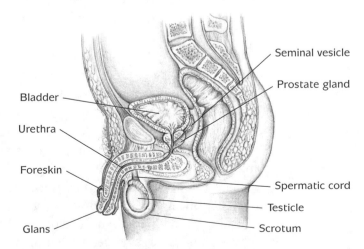

Bladder

Urethra

Foreskin

Glans

Seminal vesicle

Prostate gland

Spermatic cord

Testicle

Scrotum

Prostate problems

The prostate is a walnut-sized gland that forms part of the male reproductive system. The gland is made of two lobes enclosed by an outer layer of tissue. The prostate is located in front of the rectum and just below the bladder. The prostate also surrounds the urethra (the tube through which urine passes out of the body). It is common for the prostate gland to become enlarged as a man ages.

Benign prostatic hypertrophy

The prostate goes through two major periods of growth. The first occurs early in puberty, when the prostate doubles in size. At about age 25, the gland begins to grow again. This second growth phase often results, years later, in benign prostatic hypertrophy (BPH), noncancerous enlargement of the prostate gland.

Although the prostate continues to grow during most of a man's life, the enlargement does not usually cause problems until late in life. BPH rarely causes symptoms before age 40, but more than half of men in their 60s and up to 90 percent in their 70s and 80s have some symptoms of BPH.

As the prostate enlarges, the layer of tissue surrounding it stops it from expanding, causing the gland to press against the urethra like a clamp on a garden hose. The bladder wall becomes thicker and irritated. The bladder begins to contract even when it contains only small amounts of urine, causing more frequent urination. Eventually the bladder weakens and loses the ability to empty itself, causing some urine to remain in the bladder. The narrowing of the urethra and partial emptying of the bladder cause many of the symptoms of BPH.

The cause of BPH is not well understood and there is no definitive information on risk factors. Many symptoms of BPH are caused by obstruction of the urethra and gradual loss of bladder function, resulting in incomplete emptying of the bladder. The symptoms of BPH vary, but the most common ones involve changes or problems with urination, such as a hesitant, interrupted, weak urine stream; urgency and leaking or dribbling; or more frequent urination, especially at night.

The size of the prostate does not necessarily determine how severe the obstruction or the symptoms will be. Some men with a very enlarged prostate gland have little obstruction and few symptoms, while other men whose gland is less enlarged have more blockage and problems.

Sometimes a man may not know he has any obstruction until he suddenly finds himself unable to urinate at all. This condition, called acute urinary retention, may be triggered by taking over-the-counter cold or allergy medications. These medications contain a decongestant drug substance called sympathomimetic, which may prevent the bladder opening from relaxing and allowing urine to empty. With a partial obstruction, urinary retention also can be brought on by alcohol, cold temperatures, or a long period of immobility.

It is important to tell your doctor about any urinary problems you have. In 8 out of 10 cases, the symptoms suggest BPH, but they also can be a sign of other, more serious conditions that require prompt treatment. These conditions, including prostate cancer (see page 291), can be ruled out only by a doctor's examination.

PREVENTION

Doctors do not fully understand why the prostate gland tends to enlarge as men age. For this reason, effective prevention strategies remain speculation. Still, several studies have pointed to specific factors that may accelerate cell growth in the prostate and possibly lead to prostate enlargement. Many of these factors are related to lifestyle behaviors, including the following:

- **Zinc deficiency** Zinc is a mineral that is a powerful antioxidant that slows cell division and growth and protects against cell-damaging free radicals. A zinc deficiency could make cells vulnerable to damage, alter the balance of hormones in the body, and stimulate cell growth in the prostate. Foods rich in zinc include red meat, seafood, and pumpkin seeds.

- **Diet** Although results are not conclusive and the specific mechanisms are unknown, some studies have found a link between prostate enlargement and a diet high in starch and low in fruits and vegetables. For example, lycopene, an antioxidant present in cooked tomatoes, has been found to slow the growth of prostate cells in medical studies.

- **Obesity** Excess body fat can affect hormone levels, which has been linked to prostate enlargement.

- **Lack of exercise** Physical activity affects hormone levels and helps control weight, thereby affecting cell growth and prostate enlargement.

Prostatitis

Prostatitis (inflammation of the prostate gland) accounts for up to 25 percent of all office visits by young and middle-aged men for problems with the genital and urinary systems. The term "prostatitis" describes four disorders: chronic prostatitis, acute bacterial prostatitis, chronic bacterial prostatitis, and asymptomatic inflammatory prostatitis.

- **Chronic prostatitis** Also known as chronic pelvic pain syndrome, chronic prostatitis is the most common but least understood form of prostatitis. Found in men of any age, its symptoms go away and then return without warning. In one form, urine, semen, and other fluids from the prostate show no evidence of an invading microorganism but contain the kinds of cells (antibodies) the body usually produces to fight infection. In another form, no evidence of infection can be found.

- **Acute bacterial prostatitis** Acute bacterial prostatitis is the least common of the four types of prostatitis, but it is the easiest to diagnose and treat effectively. Men with acute bacterial prostatitis often have chills, fever, pain in the lower back and genital area, urinary frequency and urgency mainly at night, burning or painful urination, body aches, and a urinary tract infection. The disorder can be cured with antibiotics, but it may require a prolonged course of treatment.

- **Chronic bacterial prostatitis** Chronic bacterial prostatitis is relatively uncommon. In this condition, an underlying defect in the prostate becomes a focal point in which bacteria can colonize. Once the defect is found and removed, the infection can be treated with antibiotics.

- **Asymptomatic inflammatory prostatitis** This form of prostatitis is diagnosed when a man feels no pain or discomfort but laboratory tests detect infection-fighting cells in his semen. This form of prostatitis is usually detected during testing for infertility or prostate cancer.

WARNING

Severe pain in the scrotum or testicles: Don't ignore it.

Sudden, severe pain in the scrotum or in a testicle signals a medical emergency. If you feel intense pain in these areas, get immediate medical attention. You could have testicular torsion, a serious condition in which the spermatic cord that supplies blood to the testicles is twisted, blocking blood flow to the testicle. Immediate medical attention, possibly including emergency surgery, will be necessary to correct the problem and save the testicle.

Not all types of prostatitis are preventable, but the following steps can help reduce your risk:

- Always wash your hands well with soap and water after bowel movements and before handling your penis, to avoid transferring bacteria from the rectal area to the urinary tract.
- Avoid sexually transmitted infections (STDs, see page 166) by practicing safer sex (see page 175).

Erection problems

At some point in their lives, all men experience erection problems, but for more than 30 million men in the United States, erection problems are a chronic condition. The following types of erection problems can occur:

- Inability to have an erection
- Ability to have an erection only occasionally
- Inability to maintain an erection
- Ability to have an erection but cannot control ejaculation

Erections occur when blood flow to the penis is increased as a result of sexual arousal or stimulation, and outflow of blood from the penis is restricted by valves. The result is engorgement and enlargement of the penis. Many factors can interfere with the ability to have an erection, including hormonal imbalances, nerve problems, abnormal blood flow, smoking, some prescription medications, some illegal drugs, and emotional factors such as stress or anxiety. Although mental and emotional factors such as depression, guilt, anger, or anxiety can contribute to erection problems, the vast majority of erection problems have a physical cause. At the same time, erection problems from physical causes can lead to depression and stress, making erection problems worse.

Being able to have an erection depends on healthy nerves, blood vessels, muscles, and fibrous tissue, as well as adequate blood levels of the male hormone testosterone. Don't assume that erection problems are part of the normal aging process. There may be an underlying cause or contributing factors such as the following:

- Conditions that lead to heart disease—including high blood pressure and unfavorable cholesterol levels—can damage the arteries that supply blood to the penis. In other words, anything that is bad for your heart can be bad for your sexual health.

- Diabetes can damage blood vessels and the nerves that control erections.
- Alcohol and drug abuse can cause erection problems by damaging blood vessels and deadening the nerves that control erections.
- Some prescription drugs, such as some antidepressants and antihypertensive drugs, can cause erection problems. Your doctor may be able to change your medication, but do *not* stop taking a prescribed drug without talking to your doctor first.
- Lifestyle behaviors such as smoking, overeating, and being physically inactive can contribute to erection problems.
- Leaking valves in the veins of the penis resulting from injury or disease can cause erection problems.
- An injury to the spinal cord can cause erection problems by interfering with nerve signals.
- Treatments for prostate cancer, including radiation and surgical removal of the prostate, can damage the nerves that control erections.
- Diseases that affect the nerves, such as multiple sclerosis, can also lead to erection problems.
- In rare cases, reduced levels of the male hormone testosterone can lead to erection problems.

PREVENTION

Lifestyle factors can affect your ability to have an erection. Take the following measures to help prevent the problem:

- **Don't smoke.** Smoking can damage the blood vessels inside the penis, making it harder for blood to engorge the penis during arousal.
- **Drink alcohol only in moderation.** Alcohol depresses the central nervous system, including the nerves in the penis.
- **Don't use illegal drugs.** Some illegal drugs decrease sexual desire. Like smoking cigarettes, smoking marijuana can damage blood vessels to the penis.
- **Keep your weight within the normal range.** Being overweight is a risk factor for conditions that can damage nerves and blood vessels in the penis, including high blood pressure, heart disease, and diabetes.

- **Ask your doctor about your medications.** Some prescription drugs can contribute to erection problems.

- **Exercise regularly.** Being physically active is one of the best ways to keep your blood vessels healthy and improve your overall health.

- **Check your bicycle seat.** Long-distance bicycle riding on a hard, narrow bike seat can numb the nerves around the penis temporarily. Look for a bike seat with a cut-out center to help prevent this problem.

Practicing safer sex

The single best way (other than abstinence) to protect yourself from sexually transmitted diseases (STDs; see page 166) is to use a condom each and every time you engage in sexual activity, including sexual intercourse or oral or anal sex. Condoms are inexpensive and available over the counter in most drugstores, grocery stores, and convenience stores. Buy condoms made of latex or polyurethane; condoms made of natural materials such as lambskin are more porous and may allow entry of microorganisms such as HIV/AIDS. When buying condoms, check the expiration date on the package. Never use a condom past the expiration date; condoms can become damaged and spermicides can lose their effectiveness over time.

Condoms come lubricated (which can make vaginal or anal penetration more comfortable) or nonlubricated (which can be used for protection during oral sex). You can also buy a lubricant to use with condoms; use only water-based lubricants because oil-based lubricants such as massage oils, baby oil, lotions, or petroleum jelly can weaken a condom, possibly causing it to tear or break. Store condoms away from sunlight in a cool, dry place—not in a wallet or glove compartment. If you keep them in a hot place (such as a wallet or glove compartment), the latex can break down, which increases the likelihood that the condom will tear or break. A condom can be used only once.

How to use a condom correctly

Using a condom correctly every time you have sex not only greatly reduces your risk for STDs, but also helps prevent pregnancy. Follow the guidelines below to make sure you are using a condom correctly:

- Do not allow contact between your erect penis and your partner's genital or anal area or mouth until the condom is on. This protects against

STDs and also pregnancy (because drops of semen can leak from the penis before ejaculation).

- With the lubricated side out, put the rolled-up condom over the tip of your erect penis. (If you are not circumcised, pull your foreskin back before putting on the condom.)

- Leaving about ½ inch of space at the tip of the condom for ejaculated semen to collect, squeeze the tip of the condom with one hand and use your other hand to roll the condom down over the penis to the base. (Leaving space at the tip reduces the chances of an overly stretched condom ripping.)

- If you can't insert your penis easily into your partner because you don't have enough lubrication, add some. Too much friction can cause a condom to tear.

- Withdraw the penis immediately after sexual activity to keep the condom from slipping off as the erection subsides. As you withdraw your penis, hold the rim of the condom on the base of the penis to prevent semen from leaking into your partner.

- Remove the condom from the penis, check it for leaking, and discard it. Never reuse a condom.

√ Health risks of anal sex

The risk of acquiring and spreading HIV/AIDS and other STDs is increased during anal sex. HIV is present in the blood, semen, preseminal fluid, or vaginal fluid of an HIV-infected person. Generally, the person who is receiving anal sex is at greater risk because the lining of the anus and rectum is thin, allowing easier entrance of viruses and other microorganisms. However, a person who inserts his penis into an infected partner is also at risk because HIV can enter through the urethra (the opening at the tip of the penis) or through small cuts, scratches, or open sores on the penis. The risk of HIV infection during anal sex is increased even further if a person has other STDs, including chlamydia, gonorrhea, or syphilis.

Other than abstinence, using a condom is the most effective way to reduce your risk of acquiring STDs during anal sex. However, keep in mind that condoms are more likely to break during anal sex than during vaginal sex. For this reason, even with a condom, anal sex can be risky. If you engage in anal sex, you should use a generous amount of a water-based lubricant on the condom to reduce the chances of the condom breaking.

Foreskin problems

In uncircumcised men, the penis and foreskin can become inflamed for a number of reasons, but sometimes the cause remains unknown. The two most common foreskin problems are balanitis and phimosis. Many cases can be prevented with simple measures such as those described below.

Balanitis

"Balanitis" is a term that refers to inflammation of the head of the penis. The inflammation can be caused by infection, using harsh soaps, or failing to completely rinse off soap when bathing. It can also result from a urinary tract infection or an allergic reaction to clothing or detergents. The condition usually results from poor hygiene in uncircumcised men, which increases the risk for infection. In circumcised men, balanitis occurs primarily in those who have a weakened immune system such as from diabetes, cancer, or AIDS. Balanitis can make it difficult and painful to retract the foreskin to expose the tip of the penis, a condition called phimosis (see below). It can also make it hard to reposition the foreskin over the head of the penis, a condition called paraphimosis (see below).

Symptoms of balanitis include the following:

- Redness of the foreskin or penis
- A rash on the head of the penis
- Foul-smelling discharge
- Pain in the penis and foreskin
- Scarring and a narrowed opening of the penis

PREVENTION

In most cases, balanitis can be prevented or relieved by washing daily with warm water. In some cases, however, antibiotic or antifungal creams are needed.

Phimosis and paraphimosis

About 10 percent of uncircumcised men will, at some time, develop phimosis (shrinking or tightening of the foreskin of an uncircumcised penis). This tightening is normal in an infant, but the foreskin usually loosens by puberty. In older men, the disorder can result from prolonged irritation and can interfere with urination or sexual activity. Phimosis has been linked to cancer of the penis. The usual treatment for phimosis is circumcision (see box).

Phimosis sometimes gets so severe that it progresses to a condition called paraphimosis (squeezing of the head of the penis by an extremely tight, retracted foreskin). Swelling and pain develop if the foreskin cannot be returned to its normal position over the head of the penis. The squeezing may obstruct blood flow to the head of the penis—a medical emergency that doctors usually treat with emergency circumcision.

An alternative option is a procedure called a dorsal slit, in which a cut is made down the top of the foreskin, freeing it from the head of the penis. A dorsal slit is a simple and safe procedure, with few complications. However, some boys and men express dissatisfaction over the appearance of the foreskin after the procedure. A nonsurgical treatment for minor cases of phimosis is the application of a steroid cream to the foreskin.

CIRCUMCISION

Male circumcision is the surgical removal of some or all of the foreskin from around the head of the penis. Circumcision is very common in the United States, and is performed most often soon after birth. However, the trend is toward fewer circumcisions because of a growing concern among many parents that circumcision is not medically necessary. Complications from circumcision are uncommon, and those that occur are usually minor, such as infection or bleeding.

Some studies have indicated that circumcision may lower the risk for urinary tract infections in infants, some sexually transmitted diseases (STDs; see page 166), and cancer of the penis. Because the foreskin provides a favorable environment for viruses, some experts speculate that women whose partners are uncircumcised may face a higher risk of developing cervical cancer from human papillomavirus (HPV; see page 170) infection. However, research in this area is inconclusive. Circumcised men do seem to have a lower risk for the STDs syphilis and chancroid, both of which produce sores (ulcers) in the genital area.

25

PREVENTING PREMATURE AGING

MORE PEOPLE THAN EVER BEFORE are enjoying good health and productivity well into their 70s, 80s, and beyond. The average life expectancy for Americans, about 49 years in 1900, increased over the last century to about 77, thanks to improvements in health care, nutrition, and the overall standard of living for most people. Experts predict that life expectancy for men and women with the healthiest lifestyles will continue to increase. In fact, centenarians (people 100 years of age and older) are a fast-growing segment of the U.S. population.

Not only are Americans living longer on average, but many are also remaining healthier and more active well into older age. Although most people over age 65 have some form of chronic disease, these disorders are often less debilitating than in the past, thanks to new ways to treat and control them. Growing older does not necessarily mean growing weaker and sicker. This chapter will discuss how you may be able to avoid aging prematurely and to stay healthy and active well into older age.

How the body changes with age

As we age, our body undergoes changes. For example, muscle strength can diminish, bones can weaken, and movement may become limited, threatening independence. But our lifestyle choices—especially what we eat, how active we are, how much we weigh, and whether we smoke—can slow or speed these changes. Here are some of the ways your body may change as you get older:

- Bones lose calcium and may become more brittle, which can result in fractures.

- The gel-like disks between the vertebrae of the spine lose fluid and get thinner; the vertebrae themselves can collapse, causing the spine to curve and become compressed. Height decreases, and a person may look stooped.

- The proportion of fat to lean muscle in the body tends to get altered—more fat (up to 30 percent more) and less muscle.

- More fat gets deposited around the middle of the body, especially around the abdomen. (Fat in the abdominal area raises the risk for type 2 diabetes and heart disease.)

- Joints become less flexible. Cartilage starts to rub against bone inside the joints because of reduced fluid levels and tissue breakdown, potentially causing the inflammation, pain, and stiffness of osteoarthritis (see page 331).

- Muscles lose tone and cannot contract as well—even with regular exercise. Loss of lean muscle lowers overall strength.

- The skin becomes thinner and may take longer to heal.

- The immune system declines, increasing susceptibility to infection.

- The nervous system declines, making movements, intellect, and sensation less sharp. We learn more slowly and may need to have information repeated (which is normal and not a sign of Alzheimer's disease).

- Hair turns gray as the follicles make less pigment. The age at which a person's hair turns gray depends on inherited factors, and no amount of vitamins or other nutritional supplements can reverse the change.

- Hair gets thinner; many men and women may develop hair-thinning and baldness.

- Nails grow more slowly and may become brittle and sometimes turn yellow.

Some of these changes depend on race or gender. For example, bone loss is lower in black women than in white women. Both men and women can develop osteoporosis (see page 325), but women develop it more often because of the sharp drop in female hormone levels after menopause. Also, women tend to start out with lower bone mass than men, so they have less bone to lose before developing osteoporosis.

While some of these changes are genetically determined, people can often control the extent and the speed at which they occur by living a healthy lifestyle. Health-promoting lifestyle factors—including eating a healthy diet, getting regular exercise, maintaining a healthy weight, not smoking, and not drinking excessively—can overcome many genetic susceptibilities.

Maintaining a healthy lifestyle

Maintaining a healthy lifestyle as you get older is vital to helping you stay healthy and independent. Much of the illness and disability brought on by chronic disease is avoidable through known prevention measures. Healthy eating, regular physical activity, mental stimulation, not smoking, drinking alcohol only moderately, maintaining a safe environment, having social support, and getting regular recommended screening tests and health checkups are essential components of a healthy lifestyle. For complete discussions of the major lifestyle measures and prevention strategies—such as eating a healthy diet, exercising regularly, and maintaining a healthy weight—see chapters 1 through 6.

Eating a healthy diet

When it comes to a healthy diet (see chapter 1), the whole is much greater than the sum of its parts. It seems as though combinations of nutrients found in foods protect against adverse aging better than any given nutrient taken alone. That's why it's essential to consume a varied diet, with a heavy emphasis on vegetables, fruits, whole grains, fish, and legumes (cooked dried beans and peas)—foods that contain lots of beneficial substances, including vitamins, minerals, omega-3 fatty acids, and plant stanols and sterols.

Older people may be more susceptible to dehydration than younger people. In older people, the kidneys, which are responsible for maintaining water balance, function less well. Older people don't sense as well or as quickly when they are thirsty, and older people whose mobility is restricted may find it difficult to get sufficient fluids. As we age, our body tends to have a larger proportion of body fat, which contains less water than lean tissue, lowering the total amount of water in the body. As a result, older people can become dehydrated more quickly if, for example, they have a fever or diarrhea or the weather is extremely hot.

To avoid dehydration, older people should try to drink six to eight glasses of water a day. Some foods, such as fruit and some vegetables (broccoli and tomatoes), also provide fluid. Older people should limit their intake of alcohol and caffeine-containing drinks such as coffee and tea because they tend to promote water loss from the body.

ANTIOXIDANTS

Antioxidants are plentiful in fruits and vegetables, as well as in nuts, whole grains, and fish. The list below shows food sources of some of the most common antioxidants:

- **Vitamin A and beta carotene** These are essential for growth and development and for maintaining healthy vision and skin.

- **Lutein and zeaxanthin** Much of the pigment in the retina of the eye is made up of lutein. Getting sufficient lutein and zeaxanthin in the diet may lower the risk for the common vision-robbing eye disorders cataracts (see page 408) and age-related macular degeneration (see page 413).

- **Lycopene** Lycopene in the diet has been linked to a decreased risk for prostate cancer.

- **Selenium** Selenium may help reduce the risk for some cancers.

- **Vitamin C** Vitamin C is necessary for healthy bones, teeth, and skin, and helps in wound healing.

- **Vitamin E** Researchers are studying whether vitamin E might delay the onset of Alzheimer's disease symptoms or reduce the risk for blood clots.

STEROLS AND PLANT STANOLS

Plant sterols and stanols (see page 9) may reduce the risk for heart disease by significantly improving blood cholesterol levels—lowering total cholesterol and LDL (bad) cholesterol. Although you probably take in these substances every day in the foods you eat, the amounts are often too small to have any substantial cholesterol-lowering effects. You've probably seen—or maybe tried—the margarines that contain plant sterols and stanols. To get the most benefit, you need to consume 1.3 grams of plant sterols or 3.4 grams of plant stanols each day. If you take a cholesterol-lowering statin drug, you may be able to lower your cholesterol levels even more by consuming sterol-containing spreads and margarines.

CALCIUM AND VITAMIN D

Calcium and vitamin D are two nutrients that are essential for strong bones and teeth and for reducing the risk for osteoporosis (see page 325). Calcium is also essential for healthy functioning of the heart, muscles, and nerves, and it helps blood clot normally. Vitamin D helps the body absorb and use calcium. In addition to absorbing vitamin D from the diet and supplements, the body makes vitamin D in the skin after direct exposure to sunlight. The amount of vitamin D produced in the skin varies depending on the time of day, season, latitude, and a person's skin color. Vitamin D production falls

---

BREAKING NEWS   **Vitamin D: A wonder vitamin?**

Vitamin D has long been known to promote strong bones and teeth. Now researchers are saying that it may have beneficial effects on other parts of the body as well—and may even help you live longer. Some studies have linked a deficiency of vitamin D to an increased risk for cardiovascular disease, cancer, and type 2 diabetes—diseases that are responsible for 60 to 70 percent of all deaths in the United States. Without supplements, it is not easy for many people to get the daily 800 to 1,000 IUs (international units) of vitamin D3 (also called cholecalciferol) that are recommended for people age 50 and over. To get that amount, you would need to spend about 10 minutes a day in the sun in the middle of the day, when the sun is at its peak (except during winter months in northern latitudes), or drink about 2 quarts of fortified milk. Most calcium supplements also contain vitamin D.

in older people and in people who are housebound and therefore not exposed to enough sunlight. Some medications (such as anti-inflammatory steroids) also lower vitamin D levels. In these situations, people may need to take vitamin D3 (cholecalciferol) supplements to ensure a daily intake of 800 to 1,000 IUs (international units) of vitamin D, the amount recommended by the National Osteoporosis Foundation for helping to prevent osteoporosis and related fractures. Ask your doctor about taking calcium supplements; most calcium supplements also contain vitamin D.

OMEGA-3 FATTY ACIDS

Doctors and nutritionists have long recommended eating fish to help reduce the risk for heart disease. Now studies suggest that the omega-3 fatty acids (see page 8) found in the oil of certain fish may also benefit the brain by lowering the risk for Alzheimer's disease. The two most common types of omega-3 fatty acids—EPA and DHA—are contained in oily fish such as salmon, lake trout, tuna, and herring.

THE MEDITERRANEAN DIET

The typical American diet that is high in unhealthy fats (especially saturated fats, cholesterol, and trans fats; see page 11) is known to lead to unfavorable blood cholesterol levels and increase the risk for heart disease. The traditional Mediterranean diet, by contrast, is loaded with plant foods such as fruits, vegetables, whole-grain breads and cereals, legumes, and nuts. Olive oil and fish play starring roles. The Mediterranean diet is also packed with antioxidants, which may be at least partly responsible for its many notable health benefits.

Studies of people who eat a diet that is typical of the Mediterranean region have shown that this type of diet leads to reductions in heart disease. Several studies of people with either existing heart disease or risk factors for heart disease have shown a reduction in the number of heart attacks when people followed a Mediterranean diet. In addition to lowering your risk for heart disease, the Mediterranean diet may help you live longer and healthier by reducing your risk for type 2 diabetes and cancer and by lowering your blood pressure. Even among older adults ages 70 to 90 years, those who follow a Mediterranean-type diet (compared with people who don't) have much lower rates of death from all causes, and a longer life.

Exercise

If doctors were asked if they could produce a fountain of youth, they would probably say that it would have something to do with exercise. Indeed, if exercise could be packed into a pill, it would probably be the most frequently prescribed medication. Millions of older people have discovered the key to feeling better and living longer—staying physically active. Finding an exercise program that works for you and sticking with it can pay big health dividends. (If you are over 50 and have been inactive and are just starting out on an exercise program, check with your doctor first.)

Regular exercise is known to prevent or delay type 2 diabetes, heart disease, and some cancers; help relieve arthritis pain, anxiety, and depression; improve strength, balance, and energy; and help people reach and maintain a healthy weight. See chapter 2 for a complete discussion of the benefits of exercise.

You can exercise even if you have a chronic condition such as heart disease or diabetes. In fact, physical activity can help improve these conditions. For most older adults, walking, riding a bike, swimming, lifting weights, and gardening are safe, especially if they build the pace up gradually.

Adults over 50 can benefit from including strengthening exercises (see page 52) in their regular physical activity. (Strengthening exercises are also called resistance training, weight training, or strength training.) As people age, they tend to lose muscle. Strengthening exercises can build muscle and slow the rate of age-related loss. In addition to building muscles, strength training can promote mobility, improve health-related fitness, and strengthen bones.

Here are some things you can do to make sure you are exercising safely:

- Start slowly, especially if you have not been active for a long time. Gradually build up the duration of your activities and then their intensity.
- Don't hold your breath during strength-training exercises. It could cause harmful increases in blood pressure. It may seem strange at first, but the rule of thumb is to breathe out on exertion (such as when you lift something) and breathe in as you relax (or lower the weight).
- Use safety equipment. Wear a helmet for bike riding and the proper shoes for walking or jogging.
- Be sure to drink plenty of water when you're active. Many older people don't feel thirsty even if their body needs fluids.

- Always bend forward from your hips, not your waist. If you keep your back straight, you are probably bending the right way. If your back "humps," you are bending wrong.

- Warm up your muscles before you stretch. Try walking or marching and doing light arm-pumping first.

Staying mentally active

In the past, the loss of the ability to remember, learn, think, and reason—skills referred to collectively as cognition—was considered a normal part of aging. Doctors now know that most people can remain both alert and mentally able as they age, and that severe mental deterioration is the result of disease—not an inevitable part of aging. In older people who do become confused, mental decline usually precedes the loss of physical ability that can affect everyday activities, from driving to following instructions for taking a medication.

Certain mental exercises may offset some of the normal age-related decline in thinking skills and keep mental abilities sharp for everyday tasks such as shopping, making meals, and handling finances. Frequent participation in mentally stimulating activities—such as reading newspapers or magazines, reading books, playing cards and other games, doing crosswords or other puzzles, going to museums, taking a class or watching lectures on DVDs, or traveling—may lower your chances of developing Alzheimer's disease. Mental stimulation helps keep the brain alert and agile. Think of the brain as a muscle: if you don't use it, you'll lose it.

The following factors seem to influence a person's risk for mental decline with age. Some of these factors lower the risk, while others raise it:

- **Education**   Higher levels of education correlate with good mental and emotional health in later life. Researchers speculate that education may provide a kind of mental reserve from which you can draw in old age.

- **Income**   Affluent people seem to experience mental decline less often and less severely than those who are less well-off economically.

- **Social support**   Having close relationships with friends and family provides emotional and social support and seems to confer good mental and emotional health, as well as sharp mental skills in later life.

- **Physical activity**   Older adults who exercise at least three times a week have been found to be much less likely to develop dementia than those who are less active.

Volunteering is associated with better health

Several studies have shown that volunteers help themselves to better health while helping others. Volunteers live longer, function at a higher level, and have lower rates of depression and heart disease than nonvolunteers. In adults age 65 and older, the positive effect of volunteering on physical and mental health seems to stem from the personal sense of accomplishment they gain from volunteer activities. The volunteering threshold linked to health benefits is about 100 hours per year, or about 2 hours a week.

- **Depression and anxiety**   Some studies have found a link between depression or anxiety and poor mental and emotional health later in life. Researchers have recognized a possible connection between mood disorders and future mental decline.

- **Genetics**   The risk for Alzheimer's disease has an inherited component. The siblings of centenarians who are mentally fit have a better chance than the general population of living into their 90s and also being alert.

Staying at a healthy weight

Maintaining a healthy weight can reduce your risk for many common chronic diseases and may also help you move better and stay mentally sharp as you age. If you are underweight, overweight, or obese, you place yourself at risk for health problems. For example, obesity is strongly linked to heart disease, type 2 diabetes, and some cancers. These chronic conditions can ultimately shorten life and lower a person's quality of life.

Although people who maintain a stable weight in young adulthood and as they approach middle age tend to have fewer risk factors for health problems, it's never too late to reach and maintain a healthy weight. On average, men put on weight until about age 55, and then start to lose weight. This change may be related to a decline in levels of the male hormone testosterone, which can shift the balance to less muscle and more fat. (Muscle weighs more than fat.) Women gain weight until about age 65, and then start to lose weight. As in men, the weight loss is triggered in part by the loss of muscle.

Eating right and getting regular exercise can help you maintain a healthy weight as you get older and help compensate for the common middle-age weight gain.

Ask your doctor what is a healthy weight for you. If you start to gain or lose weight and don't know why, talk to your doctor to see if this change is healthy for you.

Preventing the symptoms of menopause

Menopause is the time in a woman's life when menstruation stops. It's a normal change in a woman's body. You have reached menopause when you have not had a period for 12 months in a row—and no other causes, such as pregnancy or illness, can account for this change. The years leading up to menopause are called perimenopause. During this time, a woman's body slowly makes less and less of the female hormones estrogen and progesterone. This process usually occurs between ages 45 and 55.

Menopause affects every woman differently. Your only symptom may be your periods stopping, but if you are like most women, you will probably have some other symptoms. Common symptoms of menopause include hot flashes, insomnia, excessive sweating, heart palpitations, anxiety, headaches, depression, and irritability. About 80 percent of women have at least hot flashes.

Hormone replacement therapy

Not too long ago, doctors encouraged most women to take hormone replacement therapy to relieve the symptoms of menopause, believing that it also lowered a woman's risk for heart disease, osteoporosis, and cancer, and improved her quality of life. But then, starting in 2002, research from clinical trials emerged that found that hormone replacement therapy poses some risks, including a slightly increased risk for heart attack, stroke, and possibly breast cancer.

These findings alarmed many women and their doctors, and the use of hormone replacement therapy dropped suddenly. But many women continue taking hormone replacement therapy because they believe that the relief it provides for their menopausal symptoms (such as hot flashes, insomnia, and night sweats) is worth the small increase in risks that the therapy poses. Hormone replacement therapy remains the most effective available treatment for relief of menopause symptoms.

The bottom line on hormone replacement therapy: carefully consider the benefits and risks of hormone replacement therapy for your menopausal symptoms and discuss these with your doctor. Evaluate your personal risk profile for heart disease, stroke, breast cancer, osteoporosis, colon cancer, and other conditions. Discuss quality-of-life issues with your doctor and alternatives to hormone replacement therapy (see below). If your major concern is vaginal dryness, you might consider using topical vaginal products (creams or gels that you apply to the vagina). If your symptoms (such as hot flashes and night sweats) are so severe that they are affecting your quality of life and your ability to function, you may want to consider hormone replacement therapy. If women choose to use hormone replacement therapy, most doctors recommend taking the lowest dose for the shortest amount of time (less than five years). Although estrogen has been found to help reduce bone loss and slightly reduce the risk for colon cancer, doctors do not prescribe estrogen solely for these purposes.

Alternative therapies

There are currently no treatments (including those discussed here) that are nearly as effective as hormone replacement therapy for relieving menopause symptoms. But many women who don't want to take estrogen and are having problems with menopause symptoms try alternative therapies such as the following to see if they have any effect on their symptoms. Some of these therapies may have small effects, some have no effect, and some are questionable or have not been adequately tested for safety. You should always tell your doctor if you are considering trying any "natural" remedies for treating your menopause symptoms. Herbal remedies can have unknown effects and adverse reactions with other medications you are taking.

- **Lifestyle changes** To help prevent hot flashes and night sweats, it's a good idea to take measures to avoid being too warm. For example, wear layered clothing so you can remove a layer when you have a hot flash. Sleep in a cool room. Avoid spicy foods, caffeine, and hot drinks. Reduce stress; try deep-breathing and stress-reduction techniques (see page 114), including meditation and other relaxation methods. Doctors recommend against eating a diet that is either too low or too high in protein. (See page 6 for the recommended allotment of protein in the diet.)

- **Vaginal lubricants**   The loss of estrogen at menopause can make the vagina less lubricated, which can make intercourse painful. Water-based and estrogen-containing lubricants can be very helpful; these products are available over the counter at most drugstores.

- **Medications**   Doctors sometimes prescribe medications used for treating other disorders, such as high blood pressure or depression, to relieve symptoms of menopause. Antidepressants such as venlafaxine, paroxetine, and fluoxetine have been proven in clinical trials to be moderately effective in relieving hot flashes.

- **Acupuncture or biofeedback**   Alternative therapies such as acupuncture or biofeedback can be effective in some women for helping to relieve hot flashes.

- **Phytoestrogens**   Phytoestrogens are estrogen-like compounds found in many plants. Soybeans and some soy-based foods—including tofu, tempeh, soy milk, and soy nuts—contain phytoestrogens. Other plant sources of phytoestrogens include black cohosh, ginseng, wild yam, dong quai, and valerian root. However, there is no solid evidence that the phytoestrogens in soybeans, soy-based foods, other plant sources, or dietary supplements relieve hot flashes. In addition, the risks of taking the more concentrated forms of soy phytoestrogens, such as in pills and powders, are not known. Dietary supplements with phytoestrogens do not have to meet the same quality standards as drugs, and little is known about the safety or effectiveness of these products. Dong quai, for example, contains psoralen, a known cancer-causing agent and blood thinner.

  - **Procainamide hydrochloride**   This over-the-counter supplement is made from red clover phytoestrogens. At 40 milligrams a day, it is the one phytoestrogen product approved by the FDA in the United States for short-term use in relieving symptoms of menopause.

- **Vitamins**   Some vitamins—vitamin E, vitamin B6, and vitamin C—may be helpful for hot flashes in some women. The recommended daily doses for menopause symptoms are 400 to 800 IUs of vitamin E, 400 to 500 milligrams of vitamin B6, and 500 milligrams of vitamin C.

- **Progesterone creams and oils**   Many women are trying these over-the-counter products to relieve menopause symptoms but there is no scientific evidence that they are effective. Also, their absorption by the body is questionable.

Preventing age-related medication mistakes

Many older people see several doctors and may use several different pharmacies for their prescriptions, or they order their medications by mail. They may not have one doctor or other health professional who knows all the medications they are taking and could help them avoid dangerous drug combinations.

Age-related changes in body systems can also increase medication risks, even if a person is taking only two or three drugs. Major organs function less efficiently in older people. For example, the heart doesn't pump as well, the liver is not as good at breaking down drugs, and the kidneys are less able to excrete the drugs. The increase in body fat and decrease in muscle that come with aging can affect how much of a drug reaches the bloodstream, how well it is distributed in the body, and how effectively it is cleared from the system.

Aging can also affect how the body responds to some drugs, especially blood pressure medications and drugs that affect the brain (such as sedatives and antidepressants). Antihistamines can also have different effects in older people. These medications can have adverse side effects such as sleepiness, depression, delirium, agitation, and worsening dementia in older people.

Be aware of the following factors when taking medications:

- Some medications cannot be taken with other medications, including over-the-counter drugs and herbal remedies; when combined, they could cause serious health problems.

- Weight gain or loss can affect the amount of medicine you need to take and how long it stays in your body.

- Circulation can slow with age, which can affect how quickly medications get to the liver and kidneys. The liver and kidneys may also work more slowly, affecting how a drug breaks down and gets eliminated from the body. This means that drugs can stay in the body longer, raising the risk for an adverse interaction with another medication.

If you are taking more than one medication, trying to remember what each drug is for and when to take it can be tricky. Ask your doctor and pharmacist to explain what your medications are for, and how and when to take them, to make sure you're using them correctly. Take the steps on the next page to make sure you don't unintentionally make dangerous mistakes with your medication:

- Read the labels of your medications carefully, and follow the instructions exactly.

- Look for warnings on your prescriptions and follow the advice. For example, a label might tell you to take the medication with food, or one hour before meals, or not to take it if you are taking specific other medications, or not to drink alcohol if you are taking it. For example, if you are taking medication for sleep, pain, anxiety, or depression, it is unsafe to drink alcohol.

- Ask your doctor and pharmacist if your medications interact adversely with other drugs, either over-the-counter or prescription drugs.

- Check the label on the container before you take a drug to make sure it's the right one and that it is prescribed for you.

- Never take medications in the dark.

- Never take an over-the-counter or herbal remedy without checking with your doctor. Or ask the pharmacist if the remedy is safe to take with the other medications you are taking.

- Make copies of a checklist of all the medications you take every day, including the name, amount, and times to take them. Check off each medication as you take it.

- Become familiar with how your medication makes you feel so you notice any changes that occur as you get older.

- Tell your doctor about all medications you take, including prescription and over-the-counter medications and dietary or herbal supplements. Bring a list of all the medications you take and their dosages to each doctor's appointment. If it's easier, put all your labeled medication containers in a bag and bring it to the doctor's office. To be extra cautious, show the list to your pharmacist when you have a new prescription and ask him or her to review it for possible drug interactions.

- Tell your doctor about any food or medication allergies you have.

- Ask your doctor what side effects you can expect from a particular medication and what potentially harmful side effects warrant an immediate call to the doctor. Keep track of any side effects and let your doctor know right away about any unexpected symptoms or changes in the way you feel.

- Go through your medicine cabinet at least once a year to get rid of old or expired medications. But don't flush them down the toilet (because of possible harm to the environment). Ask your pharmacist what is the safest way to dispose of old medications.

- Have all of your medications reviewed by your doctor at least once a year.
- Never stop taking a medication unless your doctor tells you it is okay to do so—even if you feel better.
- Never take a drug that has been prescribed for someone else.
- Keep all medications in a locked cabinet or drawer and out of the reach of children.
- Consider using a container that organizes all of your pills for the day or the week.

Sexuality and aging

Many factors determine whether an older person remains sexually active, including the normal physical changes of aging, disorders that could affect sexual function, desire, the availability of a suitable partner, and having enough privacy for sexual expression.

Physical changes in men

After age 40, the incidence of erection problems in men increases, and the intensity of sensation can fall, as can the quickness of attaining erections and the force of ejaculation. Unlike younger men, middle-aged men are more likely to experience orgasm in one stage, which includes a shorter orgasm and a more rapid loss of the erection after ejaculation. The amount of time needed before having another erection increases. Men over 50 sometimes have only partial orgasms. Changes in hormone levels account for some of the age-related changes in male sexuality. Testosterone levels, after rising in adolescence, fall steadily after that throughout a man's life.

Physical changes in women

The loss of the female hormone estrogen at menopause can affect a woman's sexuality. Some women may experience a decrease in sexual desire, some don't experience any change in sexual desire, and others find that their sex

STDs: An increasing risk for older people

Sexually transmitted diseases (see page 166) do not discriminate by age. Many older Americans who find themselves single because of divorce or the death of a partner do not think they are at risk for STDs, even when they have multiple sex partners. As a result, increasing numbers of older Americans are acquiring STDs, including HIV/AIDS, from unprotected sex.

But older people may be even more vulnerable than younger people to acquiring STDs. For example, aging can weaken the immune system. Older men who are taking one of the popular impotence drugs may be more likely to engage in risky sexual behaviors with more than one partner. In women who are past menopause, thinning of the vaginal walls and a decrease in vaginal lubrication may make them more likely to acquire an infection during sexual intercourse. Another problem is that STDs often go undiagnosed in older people because doctors may not think their older patients are sexually active. For this reason, HIV/AIDS and other STDs may go untreated for a longer time, worsening the course of the disease.

If you are a sexually active older person who is not involved in a mutually monogamous sexual relationship, you are at risk. Educate yourself about how STDs are spread (see page 175) and how you can protect yourself and your partner by practicing safer sex (see page 177), especially the use of condoms.

life becomes more satisfying because they no longer have to worry about pregnancy or birth control.

The drop in estrogen production at menopause can cause the lining of the vagina to thin, making the vagina more prone to irritation and infection. These changes, along with a lack of vaginal lubrication, can make intercourse painful. Using a water-based lubricating gel can help relieve pain and discomfort during sexual intercourse. Hormone replacement therapy (see page 520) can relieve vaginal dryness and other symptoms of menopause, and may help restore sexual desire; but hormone replacement therapy may raise a woman's risk for heart disease and breast cancer. Maintaining muscle tone in the pelvic area can help women continue a pleasurable sex life. Performing daily pelvic-floor (Kegel) exercises (see page 498) is especially important at this time.

INDEX

Page numbers in *italics* indicate illustrations.
A "t" inserted after a page number indicates a table.

condoms *(continued)*
   correct use, 177, 322, 478, 507–508
   oral sex, 476, 507
constipation, 5, 343, 344, 345
   pregnancy, 489, 490, 492, 499
convulsions, 390
COPD. *See* chronic obstructive pulmonary disease
corticosteroids, 327, 353, 375, 409, 411
cortisol, 102, 103, 119, 149
cosmetics, 447, 464, 465
coughing, 365–366, 367, 380, 445, 499
cough syrups, 298–299
crabs (STD), 169–170
crack cocaine, 156
cranberry juice, 362
Crohn's disease, 103, 130, 131, 265
cross-contamination, 39, 306, 318–319
Cryptosporidium, 319
cutting (self-injury), 463
cyanocobalamin, 17, 30–31, 420
cystitis, 360, 361
cysts, 281, 363–364, 396
cytomegalovirus, 276

dairy products, 4, 6, 11, 13, 15, 22, 25–30, 33
   adolescents, 465
   allergies, 372
   children, 450
   intolerance, 327, 337, 338, 371, 486
   pregnancy, 486
   unpasteurized, 27, 38, 39, 317, 321, 497
dander, 380, 384
DASH eating plan, 23, 26, 27–29, 37, 231, 237, 240
deer ticks, 309, *309,* 310

DEET, 309, 311, 312, 313
dehydration
   exercise, 7, 49, 459
   older adults, 514, 517
   pregnancy, 487, 489, 492
dementia, 46, 419–428, 518
   alcohol-related, 140, 147, 419, 422
   identification, 423
   See also Alzheimer's disease
dental care
   brushing/flossing, 26, 429–434, *433,* 492
   exams, 210–212, 235, 277, 432, 434
   pregnancy, 492
   tooth structure, *429*
   vitamin D, 14, 515–516
dentures, 336, 337
depression
   adolescents, 462, 463
   dementia, 419, 420, 428
   eating disorders, 95, 98
   erection problems, 505
   exercise, 43, 52, 53, 157
   family history, 186
   headaches, 390, 393
   insomnia, 108, 109
   meditation for, 124
   menopause, 520
   older people, 420, 519
   optimism vs., 119
   pregnancy, 490
   sleep deprivation, 108
   stress, 101, 103, 120
   yo-yo dieting, 94
DES, 288, 290
DEXA (dual-energy X-ray absorptiometry), 208
diabetes. *See* gestational diabetes; type 2 diabetes
diabetic retinopathy, 416–417
diaphragm (contraceptive), 361
diarrhea, 9, 14, 38, 298, 319

food safety, 40, 320
   hemorrhoids, 344
   irritable bowel syndrome, 345, 346
diet. *See* nutrition
Dietary Guidelines for Americans, 23–27, 438
dietary supplements
   colds, 297–298
   interactions, 21, 144, 523, 524
   megadoses, 14, 18, 21
   sources of, 447
   vegetarians, 30, 31
   when to use, 21
   See also specific types
dieting, 92, 93–94, 95
diet pills, 89, 365
digestive system, 9, 250, 335–357
   fiber-rich foods, 4–5
   lactose intolerance, 327, 337, 338, 371, 486
   smoking and, 126, 130–131
   stress and, 103
   See also gastroesophageal reflux disease; peptic ulcer
digital rectal exams, 197, 198, 199
dilated eye exam, 210, 253, 412, 416, 417
dilation and curettage, 286
diphtheria, 301
diuretics, 95, 97, 98, 495
diverticular disease, 5, 335, 342–344, *343*
dopamine, 134, 155, 156, 157–158
douching, 175, 176, 317, 362
Down's syndrome, 482, 483, 484
driving
   adolescents, 458, 460, 467
   drinking and, 27, 143, 144, 454, 467
   older adults, 163
   sleep problems and, 108, 403

weight, 84, 88
See also type 2 diabetes
gonorrhea, 166, 167–168, 173, 174, 321, 476, 477, 508
gout, 6
Graves' disease, 133
gum cancer, 129, 274
gum disease, 429, 430–434, *432*
   dental exams, 211, 212, 432, 434
   pregnancy, 432, 492
   prevention, 210–211
   tobacco use, 128, 432, 434, 473, 475

Haemophilus influenzae type b vaccine, 304, 444
hallucinogens, 154, 159–162
hand sanitizers, 297, 303, 305, 445
hand washing, 303, 306, 350, 505
   colds, 297, 445, *445*
   food handling, 27, 39, 40, 295, 306, 318, 320, 496
   pet handling, 305, 320, 371
hashish, 153, 154, 155
hay fever, 370, 404
headaches, 63, 389–394, 395, 411, 412, 520
hearing loss, 395–401
   decibel levels, 397
heart attack, 7, 224–230, *227*
   anabolic steroids, 470
   angina vs., 222, 226
   arrhythmias, 224, 242
   aspirin for, 223, 224, 227, 229, 266
   atherosclerosis, 218, 219, 221
   chest pain, 223, 226
   emergency action, 225, 227
   hormone replacement therapy, 520
   napping benefits, 107
   NSAIDs, 266
   plaque rupture, 75–76, 128, 218, 224, *224*

sleep apnea, 110, 403
smoking, 126, 128, 226, 228
warning signs, 76, 226
women, 128, 227–228, 329
heartburn, 104, 130, 335, 338–340, 492
heart disease, 84, 217–224, 240, 242, 244
   abdominal fat, 43, 87, 94, 512
   alcohol use, 140, 147
   antioxidants, 18
   bacterial endocarditis, 235
   cardiomyopathy, 147, 231, 243
   children, 448, 449
   congenital defects, 76, 231, 232, 235, 242, 243, 482, 487
   DASH eating plan, 28, 231
   dental work cautions, 235
   erection problems, 505–506
   exercise, 25, 42, 43–44, 49, 51, 53, 63, 73, 75–76, 187, 218, 228–229, 250, 517
   family history, 179, 186, 187, 200, 220, 221, 223, 228, 234
   gum disease, 128, 431
   heroin addiction, 159
   hormone replacement therapy, 112, 229, 266, 520, 526
   Mediterranean diet, 516
   metabolic syndrome, 82
   mitral valve prolapse, 235
   nutrition benefits, 3, 4, 6, 7, 9–13, 14, 27, 28, 30, 187, 218, 226, 515
   palpitations, 520
   screening, 199
   secondhand smoke, 126, 134, 135
   sleep deprivation, 106, 442
   smoking, 43, 126, 128, 135, 187, 218, 220, 222, 223, 226, 228
   stress, 44, 101, 103, 104, 218
   sudden sniffing death, 455

type 2 diabetes, 43, 45, 87, 246, 251, 253
waist size, 82, 87, 88, 94
weight, 43, 81–84, 187, 218, 220, 223, 226, 228
See also angina; arrhythmias; cholesterol level
heart failure, 44, 230–232, 428
   alcohol use, 140, 147
   arrhythmias, 231, 242, 243
   atherosclerosis, 219, 231
   heart attack, 224, 231
heart rate, 50, 459
   target, 49, 64–66
heart valves, 231, 235, 243
Heimlich maneuver, 405, *405*
Helicobacter pylori, 104, 130–131, 272, 341, 342
hemorrhagic stroke, 229, 238
hemorrhoids, 194, 344–345, *344*, 489
hepatitis, 165, 269–270, 347–351
   alcoholic, 143, 144–145, 146, 353, 354, 355
hepatitis A, 319, 347, 348, 350
   vaccine, 304, 349, 350, 351, 444
hepatitis B, 166, 173, 269–270, 321–322, 347–350, 477
   vaccine, 173, 270, 304, 349–350, 351, 444, 478
hepatitis C, 153, 269–270, 271, 348, 349, 350–351
hepatitis D and E, 348
herbal cigarettes, 474–475
herbal supplements, 297, 480
   interaction risks, 21, 144, 523, 524
   menopausal symptoms, 521, 522
hernias, 55, 339
heroin, 153, 158–159
herpes simplex virus, 171, 276, 476. *See also* genital herpes
herpes zoster vaccine, 304

improvement tips, 40

meal planning, 31–36, 40, 249

meal skipping, 90, 92

Mediterranean diet, 516

older people, 513–516

portions and servings, 33–36, 40

pregnancy, 480, 485–489, 492, 496–497

sleep improvement, 113

smoking cessation, 138

stress reduction, 114–115

weight loss, 88–90

See also dietary supplements

Nutrition Facts. *See* food labels

nuts, 8, 9, 26, 29

  allergies, 371–373

  choking hazards, 406

oils, 8, 11–14, 26, 29, 32

older adults. *See* aging

olive oil, 8, 13, 32, 40, 516

omega-3 fatty acids, 5, 8–9, 10, 40, 229, 384, 415, 516

omega-6 fatty acids, 8–9

opiates, 154, 158

opioids, 144, 162

optic neuropathy, 133

optimism, 118–119

oral cancer, 128–129, 149, 211, 274–277, 473

oral contraceptives, 96, 128, 282, 283, 286

oral glucose tolerance test, 201

oral leukoplakia, 128

oral sex

  adolescents, 476

  condom use, 176, 476, 507

  STD transmission, 165–166, 167, 170, 171, 321

orange juice, 15, 338, 487, 489

organ transplants, 235, 306, 311, 349

orgasm, 525

osteoarthritis, 325, 331–333, *331*, 391, 512

  exercise, 42, 43, 52, 73, 118, 517

  stress, 104

  weight, 82, 83, 84

osteoporosis, 325–330, 466, 513

  alcohol use, 148–149, 327

  bone density, 52, 129, 207–209, 326, 329, 465

  calcium, 46, 327, 515–516

  DEXA test, 207–209

  exercise, 46, 52, 328

  female athlete triad, 96

  hormone replacement therapy, 329, 521

  risk reduction, 465–466, 468

  smoking, 126, 129–130, 327

ovarian cancer, 83, 265, 281–284

ovaries, 281, *281*, 283–284, 285

overweight. *See* weight

oxycodone, 153, 162, 163, 469

oxygen, 50, 217, 230, 336, 379, 384, 403

oysters, 38

Pacific Islanders

  sleep apnea, 403

  type 2 diabetes, 246

pain

  abdominal, 342, 345

  angina, 218, 221–224, *222*, 226

  back, 490, 493, *493*

  coronary artery spasms, 225

  exercise, 58, 63, 78–79

  in eyes, 407, 411, 412

  gallbladder attacks, 357

  headaches, 389–394, 411, 412, 520

  infections, 295

  meditation and, 124

  relaxation and, 122, 391

  scrotum/testicle, 504

pain relievers, 229, 341, 342, 364–365, 427, 469

abuse of, 153, 162

paint thinners, 497

pancreas, 14, 131, 140, 245, 247

pancreatic cancer, 83, 129, 276, 341

pancreatitis, 143, 145

  gallstone, 356

Pap test, 170, 171, 188–190, 277, 287–290, 443

paraphimosis, 509–510

parasites, 273, 304, 305–307, 497

Parkinson's disease, 51, 109

peanut allergy, 371, 372, 373

peanut butter, 6, 406

pelvic exam, 188, *188*, 277

pelvic inflammatory disease, 167, 168, 174

pelvic support problems, 497–499

penicillin, 374, 375

penis, 177, 507–510

  cancer of, 290, 293, 510

  circumcision, 293, 510

  correct condom use, 177, 507–508

  See also erection problems

peptic ulcer, 104, 130–131, 229, 327, 341–342

perforated eardrum, 396

periodontal disease. *See* gum disease

peripheral artery disease, 218, 219, 232–234, 252, 367

permethrin, 309, 312

personal trainers, 61, 71

pertussis, 300, 301, 304

pessimism, 119

pesticides, 496

pets. *See* animals

phimosis, 293, 509–510

physical activity. *See* exercise

phytochemicals, 18

phytoestrogens, 112, 522

picaridin, 312

Pilates, 55, 58, 61